Herbalist

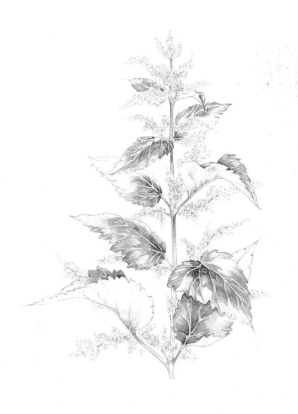

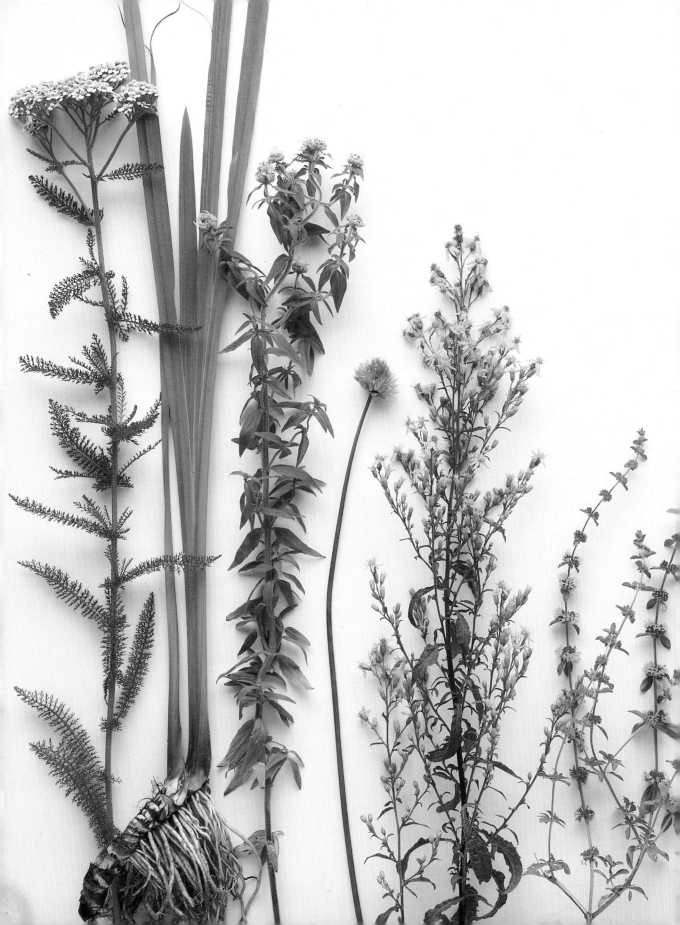

THE NEW AGE

Herbalist

*How to use herbs for healing, nutrition,
body care, and relaxation*

Consultant Editor

Richard Mabey

with

Michael McIntyre · Pamela Michael

Gail Duff · John Stevens

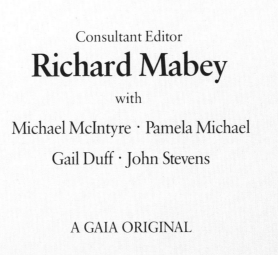

A GAIA ORIGINAL

A FIRESIDE BOOK
Published by SIMON & SCHUSTER INC
New York London Toronto Sydney

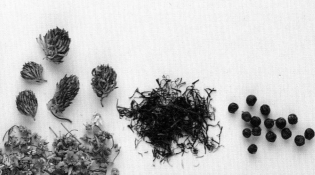

A GAIA ORIGINAL

Written by Richard Mabey with Michael McIntyre (Chapters 1 and 5), Pamela Michael (Chapter 3), Gail Duff (Chapter 4) and John Stevens (Chapter 6).

Project Editor	Phil Wilkinson
Editorial and research	Anna Kruger
	Rosanne Hooper
Project Designer	Kate Poole
Design	Bridget Morley
Illustrations	Jane Reynolds
	Nigel Hawtin (Glossary)
Photography	Philip Dowell
Production	Susan Walby
Direction	Joss Pearson, Patrick Nugent,
	Lucy Lidell

A Fireside Book
Published by Simon & Schuster
New York

Previously published by Collier Books

Library of Congress Cataloging-in-Publication data

Mabey, Richard, 1941–
  The new age herbalist.

  1. Herbs—Therapeutic use.   2. Herbs—Utilization.
I. McIntyre, Michael, 1946–   . II. Title.
RM666.H33M32   1988b   615'.321   87–38210
ISBN-13:   978-0-684-81577-0
ISBN-10:   0-684-81577-X

20 19 18 17 16 15 14

Typeset by Fakenham Photosetting Ltd., Fakenham, Norfolk
Printed in China

Plants for photography provided by Suffolk Herbs, Sawyers Farm, Little Cornard, Sudbury, Suffolk

Dried herbs for photography supplied by G. Baldwin & Co., 171–3 Walworth Road, London SE17 1RW.

How to use this book

This is a new herbal for the modern age. You can use it both as a general information source and as a practical guide to herb applications in everyday life. The information and practical applications are presented in different sections of the book, and you will need to cross refer between them.

The information sections

The wider perspectives of the history of herbalism and the human uses of plants are presented in the main Introduction, in feature spreads (with tinted borders) throughout the book, and in the general introductory texts to chapters. Chapter 1, Glossary of Herbs, is an extensive reference section listing and illustrating the herbs used elsewhere in the book and explaining their properties according to herbalists' knowledge and modern scientific evidence. You should **not** use this section for self-prescription or other practical applications. However, you should **always** refer to it, before using any herbs or following any instructions in the practical chapters, since it also features any cautions or contra-indications for particular herbs, alerting you to possible restrictions on use. Chapter 2, Practical Herbalism, is a short introductory section, which also gives basic herb preparation methods common to all subsequent sections. Again, you should **not** use it alone (or with the Glossary only). You should refer back to it as necessary when you are using the practical sections.

The practical sections

Chapters 3, 4, and 5, contain specific practical information on using herbs in body care, relaxation, home care, nutrition, and healing. Here you will find recipes for preparations as diverse as cold remedies and herb shampoos, household soaps and herbal relaxants. Use these chapters, especially the Healing chapter, in conjunction with the Glossary and chapter 2. The final practical section, Chapter 6, provides a complete programme for organic herb gardening, from soil analysis to harvesting, and includes sections on symbiotic planting and organic fertilizers.

While we have taken great care to detail the negative evidence associated with particular herbs, herbalism is a kinder technique than conventional medicine. In orthodox medicine many damaging drugs are freely available with inadequate cautions to the user. Herbalism is a gentle art, fun to practice, and kinder to our minds and bodies than modern synthetic living. But herbs can be powerful, and should be treated with as much respect and sense as any other medicine, food, or item used for home or body care. Used wisely, we hope this book will bring you great pleasure.

Note: Neither the publisher nor the authors accept responsibility for identifications made by persons who use this guide. In addition, they do not accept responsibility for any effects that may arise from ingesting any wild herb. Although many species are known to be edible for many people, it is not possible to predict an individual person's reactions to particular species. Therefore, neither the publisher nor the authors can accept responsibility for any personal experimentation.

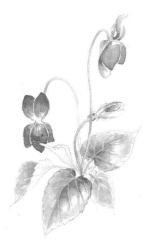

The Lord hath created medicines out of the earth; and he that is wise will not abhor them.

Apocrypha, Ecclesiasticus 34:4

Why should a man die, who has sage in his garden?

Anon, Regimen Sanitatis Salernitanum, Medieval herbal

The Great Spirit is our father, but the earth is our mother. She nourishes us; that which we put into the ground she returns to us, and healing plants she gives us likewise.

Big Thunder, North American Indian, 1900

There is life on earth – one life, which embraces every animal and plant on the planet. Time has divided it up into several million parts, but each is an integral part of the whole. A rose is a rose, but it is also a robin and a rabbit. We are all of one flesh, drawn from the same crucible.

Lyall Watson, Supernature, 1973

In the last decade interest in traditional medicine has been renewed, and much is now being done worldwide to give it the respect it deserves – green medicine is being born again.

Anthony Huxley, Green Inheritance, 1984

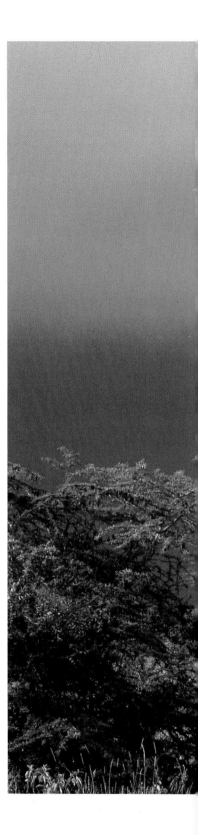

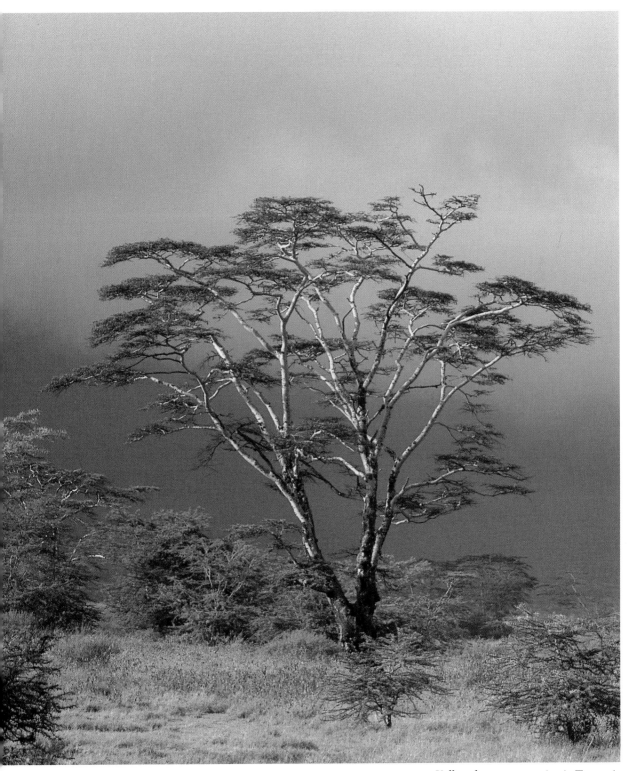

Yellow fever tree growing in Tanzania

Contents

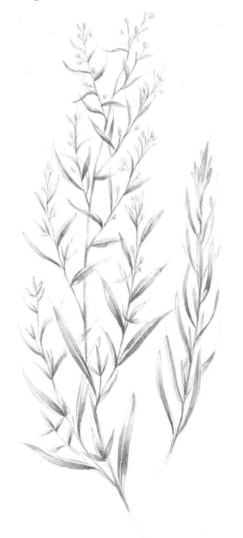

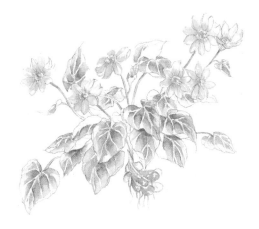

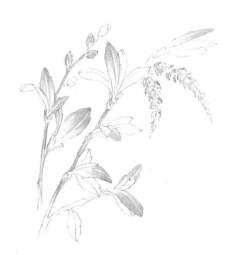

Introduction

Plants have become one of the totems of our times. In a world where the damaging effects of food processing, over-medication, and agribusiness are daily more evident they have come to stand as symbols of a more natural and healthy way of life.

Useful plants have already gone beyond being the concern of small minorities to become commercial successes in both Europe and America. There are new meat substitutes, organic fertilizers, insecticides, and fuels – all based on plant products. Herbs are being embraced on a scale unmatched for two centuries – not only in cosmetics, foods and teas, but in domestic products, alternative medicines, even veterinary remedies. Just what proportion of the original plant ingredients find their way into some of these products may be open to question. The advertising world in particular has not been slow to play on worries about the increasing quantities of man-made chemicals in the environment and the images and virtues associated with herbs have often been merged into a vague green wholesomeness that may have little to do with a specific plant or product. But collectively their message is clear and the western world has seen an unprecedented resurgence of interest in herbalism and useful plants in the last two decades. Even their images are ubiquitous – on fabrics, furniture, and street decorations. So as fossil fuels and the chemicals that depend on them run out, it may not be fanciful to see the Chemical Age replaced by the Age of Plants.

A global balancing act

The growing interest in herbs and economically useful plants is part of the movement towards "greener" economics and lifestyles. It is, for example, clearly linked with the concern for renewable energy, conservation of resources, holistic medicine and organic farming. All these movements share a belief in the vast potential of plants and a new respect for their role on the earth.

Plants, to begin with, trap the sun's energy and make it available to the rest of the planet's inhabitants. En masse, they not only produce the bulk of the world's oxygen but actively regulate the amount of carbon, water and hydrogen in the atmosphere, and even seem to control the basic temperature range of the earth. (For more information about the ways in which the global environment is regulated, see James Lovelock, *Gaia: A New Look at Life on Earth* 1979). Their role as a collective chemical factory is equally indispensable. Out of nothing more than sunlight, air and water, they produce proteins, sugars,

American mandrake
This herb, which should not be confused with the European mandrake of myth and legend (see p. 19), is common in damp places in the eastern USA and Canada. It has a long history of medicinal use. Like many other herbs, it was highly valued by the North American Indians before being adopted by herbalists in the USA and Europe. It is a powerful herb, used to stimulate the liver and bowel, but is poisonous in large doses. In common with a number of the more potent remedies, American mandrake should only be used as prescribed by a qualified herbalist.

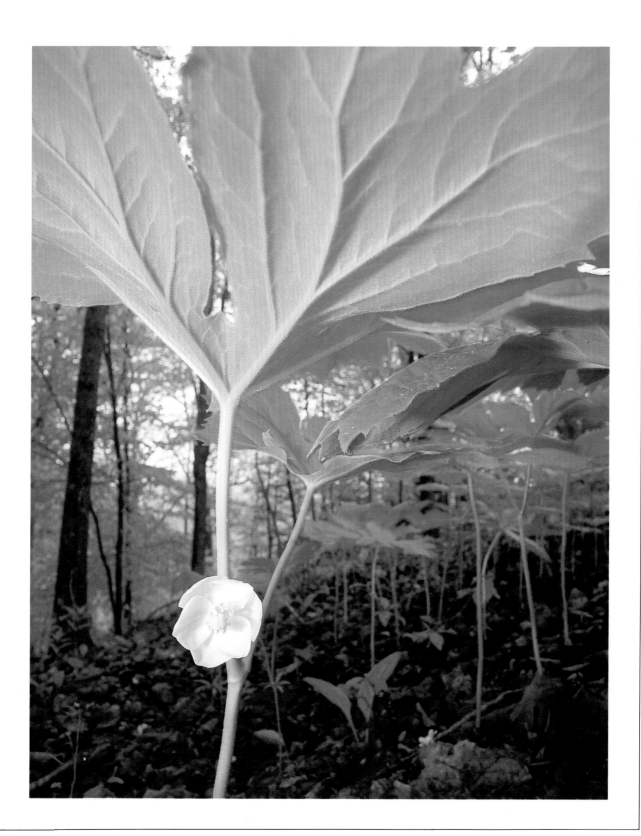

enzymes and hormones to control their growth, oils to regulate their temperature, and pesticides to protect themselves against attack.

On a smaller scale, plants are inextricably linked in symbiotic relationships with the rest of the living world. The only food source for higher organisms, and the major provider of shelter, plants have, until recently, provided almost all basic human raw materials, such as timber, cloth, paper, dyes, and oils. In turn, plants rely on animals for pollination, and on scavenging organisms to break down their dead remains and return their elements to the nutrient cycle in the air and soil. In short, the world's vegetation is not only a crucial source of energy and chemicals, but a model of sheer ingenuity, of the frugal use of resources and of energy conservation.

What is a herb?

You could argue that all useful plants are herbs. This, more or less, is how the Oxford English Dictionary defines the term, specifying that it is "applied to plants of which the leaves, or stems and leaves, are used for food or medicine, or in some way for their scent or flavour". Looking at the immense range of modern herbs and their current uses, one would be tempted not so much to narrow this definition as to make it even broader. It would now, for instance, include flowers and roots as well as stems and leaves, plants used as detergents and dyes as well as for food and medicine, and part of the raw materials of people as far removed as cocktail drinkers, historic gardeners, and holistic healers. To expand on the Oxford definition, therefore, a herb can be any plant used for medicine, as an ingredient in food or drink for its preservative flavouring, or health-giving properties, or for its perfuming, cosmetic, or cleansing actions in any other product. This embraces a large variety of plants used in many ways – the herbal revival is, thankfully, a long way from being a movement with a single set of beliefs and aims. One of its strengths is its diversity and a range of ideas that can be worn as lightly or as seriously as you please.

Yet, intriguingly, the common understanding of "herb" has more limited and specific connotations in everyday usage. We tend, for example, to exclude plants when they are being used purely as food. Watercress as a salad is a vegetable, pure and simple. But in the 18th century recipe in which it was simmered with scurvy grass and oranges to make a "spring cleansing" drink, it was unquestionably a herb. We also exclude plants used purely for decorative or utilitarian purposes. No one would seriously regard willow twigs woven into a basket as a herb, yet originally they were used in an infusion for colds and headaches, and their active constituents led to the production of aspirin. Two common meanings, however, remain attached to herbs. One is the idea that they are small-scale, domestic, "traditional"

Pollination
The process of pollination is crucial to a plant's survival. Plants have many different mechanisms to enable pollen to be transferred from flower to flower. The most common involves insects such as bees, which travel from one flower to another in search of nectar, transferring pollen as they go.

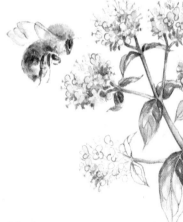

Marjoram
Herbs, while they account for a relatively small percentage of the total plant coverage of the earth, have their part to play in helping to balance the earth's energy, water, and temperature levels. But they are also useful to humans in other ways. What is remarkable about many herbs, such as marjoram, right, is the number of uses people have found for them – in cooking, healing and such processes as dyeing.

Plant and planet

From tall trees through herbaceous species to tiny sea algae, plants play a crucial part in supporting human and animal life on earth. By photosynthesis they convert sunlight into chemical energy and give out oxygen; they take in carbon, in the form of carbon dioxide, much of which passes into the food chain or into the soil. In doing this, they influence air temperature, since the carbon dioxide in the atmosphere acts as an insulator that stops heat from escaping into space. Another important role of plants is in the water cycle, the circulation of water between the oceans, the atmosphere, plants and animals. And they affect the soil, taking in elements such as nitrogen, phosphorus, and potassium, and passing these to the food chain, from where they are recycled once more to the soil in the form of animal waste.

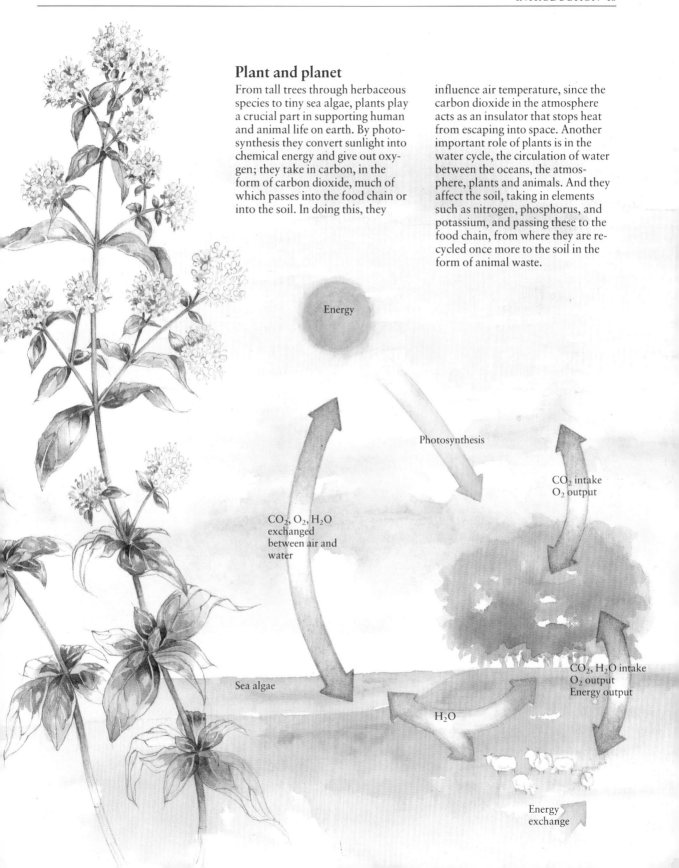

Energy

Photosynthesis

CO_2 intake
O_2 output

CO_2, O_2, H_2O exchanged between air and water

Sea algae

H_2O

CO_2, H_2O intake
O_2 output
Energy output

Energy exchange

plants; the other that they must do you good in some way – improving your health, appearance or sense of well-being. A less sympathetic, parallel image is one of crankiness, amateurism and superstition. The history of herbalism is rich with mythology, and if it is still not taken seriously in some quarters, it is partly because much of the literature has failed to discriminate between good and bogus evidence from the past.

Herbal success stories

Recently, more respectful and inquisitive scrutiny of the way plants work has yielded a growing range of useful new substances and materials. The seed oil of the evening primrose has been shown to help a wide range of minor metabolic disorders, and is now in such demand that it has become a small-scale crop in arable regions. Another oil – from the jojoba, a small Central American desert shrub – has virtually replaced sperm-whale oil in the leather industry – and in the process has spawned a whole new future for itself as a cosmetic moisturizer. Potentially even more significant are a petrol substitute that has been obtained from a *Euphorbia* (a cactus-like plant) and insecticides that have been extracted from the roots of certain daisies.

What is striking about these newly exploited plants is that they often share similar paths to commercial success. Their use was either grounded in local tradition, or some kind of grass-roots practice; they were "discovered", tested and advanced into commercial production, frequently after a period of small-scale organic farming and local business. The resulting large-scale enterprises have shown that ecological principles can be compatible with economic practicalities.

The sunflower shows this process very clearly. When the first sunflowers were brought from Central America to Europe in the 16th century, almost nothing was known about their properties. Indian peoples in both South and Central America extracted oil from the seeds, and used the foliage as cattle feed, but, unusually, appeared to have no medicinal uses for the plant. Even John Gerard, compiler of the first widely popular herbal to be published in Britain in 1597, was unable to report any therapeutic virtues. But as the sunflower was dispersed around the world as a crop, it began to acquire a folk reputation as a treatment for bronchial troubles. In Russia, where vast quantities are cultivated today, the flowers and leaves were used in the treatment of coughs, bronchitis, and even malaria. A recent investigation of this practice proved that inulin, one of the constituents of sunflower oil, is very effective in the treatment of asthma. As a bonus – for health and commerce – the oil is very low in saturated fats and so regarded as kinder to the arteries than animal fats.

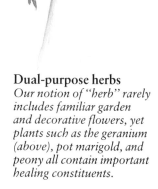

Dual-purpose herbs
Our notion of "herb" rarely includes familiar garden and decorative flowers, yet plants such as the geranium (above), pot marigold, and peony all contain important healing constituents.

Sunflower
One of the most useful plants – for both its seed and oil – the sunflower is now cultivated widely.

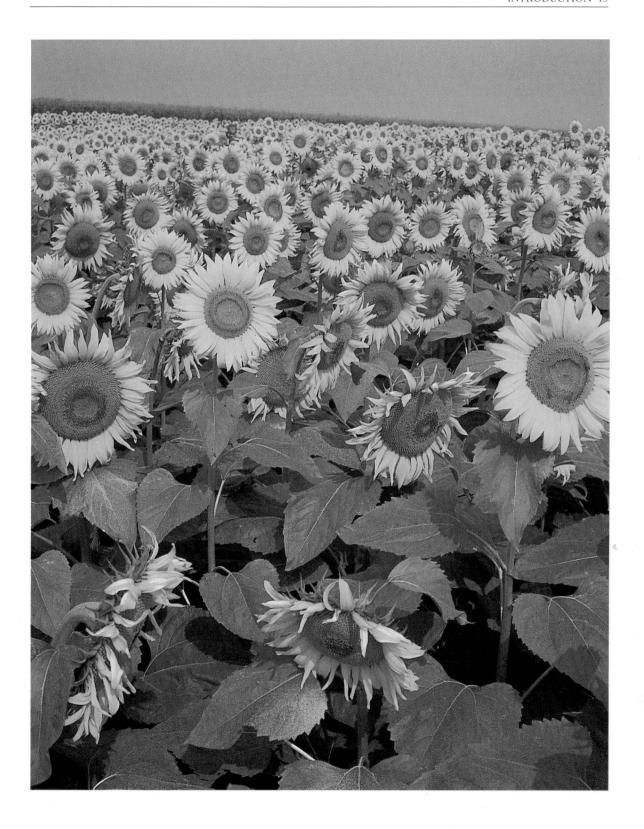

Herbs, healing and instinct

For most peoples and for much of history, there has been no clear division between the use of plants for food and for medicine. Wild vegetables for example, a necessary part of all subsistence diets, have always provided important vitamins and trace elements. The earliest physical evidence of a European prehistoric diet, from excavations in Neolithic lake-villages in western England and Switzerland, shows that our ancestors had a remarkably varied diet. In the pots and waste pits were the remains of mustard, bramble, wild rose, strawberry, crab apple, wild service tree (*Sorbus torminalis*), and orache (a spinach-like weed) amongst others – all nutritious foods, as well as remedies which have since been recommended by medical herbalists.

One of the important objectives of herbal medicine has always been a long-term nutritional one, an attempt to remedy deficiencies of minerals and trace elements. Medical herbalists prefer wild plants since they are usually richer in nutrients than cultivated varieties, which are often bred for appearance or size. But herbs have also been used to treat disease in the same way as conventional drugs. In some cases this may have happened accidentally. Strong-flavoured herbs like hyssop and rosemary, originally used to make none-too-fresh animal products palatable, may have offset the dangers of bacterial food poisoning because they contain small quantities of antiseptic chemicals.

Dosing with herbs even occurs in the animal world. Zoologists have observed some species of African chimpanzee taking regular doses of a member of the chrysanthemum family that contains a potent antibiotic – though whether as a preventative or as a cure, it is impossible to say. Domestic animals will also purposely seek out certain plants when they are sick – dogs are well known for eating grass.

All ancient human cultures had an understanding of "green medicine" that was part and parcel of a life lived close to the natural world, one which still survives, even in parts of the developed world. In North America, Indian herbal remedies have been recorded by researchers (one documented more than 150 separate herbs used by the Ojibwa alone) and some have been taken into the modern American herbal *materia medica*.

Sympathetic magic

The most basic herbal remedies must have been first discovered by trial and error. Species with fast and drastic effects – purgatives like buckthorn, and narcotic painkillers like henbane, for example – would have made their mark early. However, it is probably true that many other herbs with more subtle influences on human physiology

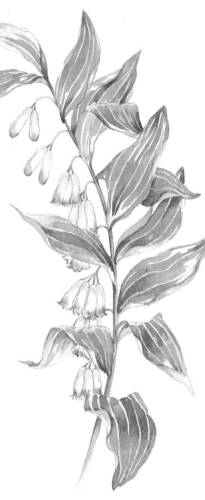

Herbalism in the wild
The North American Ojibwa people, also known as the Chippewa, successfully treat a vast range of ailments with wild plants. Treatments range from a decoction of Solomon's seal root (Polygonatum spp.) for coughs, and an eyewash of red maple bark (Acer rubrum), to infusions of sweet fern leaves (Comptonia peregrina) for diarrhoea, and of horsetail for kidney complaints.

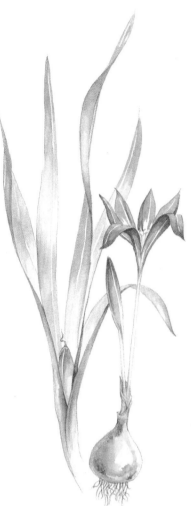

Meadow saffron
*The Doctrine of Signatures
was sometimes applied
rather fancifully. The root
of meadow saffron, consi-
dered to be shaped like a de-
formed, gouty foot, was
thought to be an effective
cure for gout. This was one
of several superstitions
founded on a degree of
truth. The root is in fact a
rich source of colchicine, an
alkaline painkiller that
helps to quell the pain of
gout, arthritis and rheumatism, when taken in small
quantities.*

(or perhaps none at all) were also believed to be effective from earliest times. It is hard for us to imagine the awe with which plants must have been held in a pre-scientific age. They could appear out of the ground, apparently by spontaneous generation. Barely distinguishable species could kill you, feed you, or drive you mad. The secrets of their growth and properties were beyond ordinary understanding. It is no real wonder that plants with suggestive appearances were credited with special powers, and that theories were developed to try to explain and predict their effect upon humans.

Most of these were variations on the principles of sympathetic magic. This was based on a search for similarity, contrast and pattern. Beliefs about the medicinal properties of plants were based on how they performed in other situations. Toadstools gathered from a dead tree, for example, would put life back in a corpse; ivy berries would cure drunkeness because ivy strangles vines; parasitic plants might in their turn overcome human "parasites", such as warts. Not all pre-scriptions were so solemn. Many classical authors believed that notor-iously windy foods like lentils would protect a garden from gale-damage if planted round the edge. This was our ancestors' science. We disparage it as magic and gullible superstition, but in an age when humans felt themselves to be part of nature, not its master, it was surely not unreasonable to believe that the way plants grew in some way mirrored their actions in the body.

Superstition to science

In the West, sadly, herbal medicine lost both the ecological instincts and the basis in observation that characterized sympathetic magic. For much of the Middle Ages, European scholars did little more than copy or attempt to decode the classical herbals, and in the process perpetu-ated a tangle of errors, misinterpretations and superstitions. Later, in the expansive, post-Renaissance mood of the 17th and 18th centuries, a new breed of commercial herbalists began to vulgarize sympathetic magic into the Doctrine of Signatures. This decreed that all plants were stamped with some physical manifestation of their medical qualities. So, eyebright, whose flowers had a mottled and bloodshot look, had been "signed" for sore eyes; parsley piert, rooting in stone walls, would break through kidney stones just as effectively.

Much of this was little more than a mystifying brand of sales talk aimed at the gullible – similar to the ritual brandishing of "ingredient X" in modern advertising. But sometimes, it appeared to be a way of rationalizing the properties of plants whose effectiveness was already known by trial and error. The lungwort lichens (*Lobaria* spp) for example, were recommended against chest disorders notionally on the grounds of their pouched, lung-like appearance. Yet they had a long

Plant myths

Myths and folklore develop for different reasons: Arab traders spun exotic fables about their spice sources to frighten off the competition; accounts of trees walking explained the movement of, say, a fruitful olive from a neighbour's land; the widespread belief in the Middle Ages that the barnacle goose was the fruit of the barnacle tree argued that it was thus plant matter, not meat, and therefore acceptable food during times of fast. And plants have, since pre-history and world-wide, been worshipped as deities or venerated as symbols of fertility.

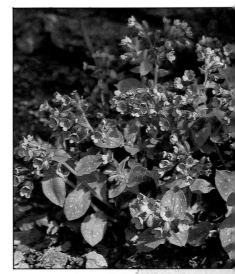

But is the folk-history of herbs of any value beyond being a source of colourful stories? It can certainly be a valuable source of clues to the usefulness of plants, and to the kinds of relationships that human communities have had with them. Traditional and vernacular names, for example, indicate their one-time uses even if the plants are no longer most appropriate for these purposes. Soapwort and pewterwort (horse-tail) are both herbs once used in domestic cleaning. Sauce alone (jack-by-the-hedge) and poor man's cabbage (bistort) were staple wild vegetables. Feverfew, whitlow grass (*Erophilia verna*), and boneset (comfrey) were named from the ailments they were employed against.

The seemingly convoluted rituals that were involved in the picking and preparation of herbs also begin to make some kind of sense if they are looked at without prejudgement. Picking herbs at dawn, for instance, ensured that they would be harvested before their essential oils had been evaporated by the sun (see p. 270).

Rewarding clues lie hidden, too, in the wilder fringes of herbal mythology. What was it about houseleek that nurtured the belief that it was an effective lightning deflector? Or about cyclamen that gave it so powerful a reputation as an abortifacient that pregnant women should not even touch or walk over it? Both beliefs seem patently absurd, yet they proved remarkably persistent. Were they just obscure cases of sympathetic magic (see p. 16), or corruptions of some more fundamental observations or experiences?

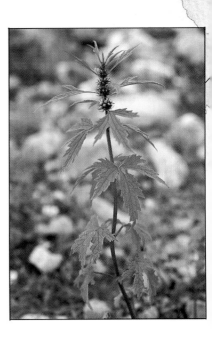

One of the most extraordinary botanical myths is that of the "vegetable lamb". It survived well into the 17th century and is figured on the frontispiece of John Parkinson's celebrated gardening-manual-cum-herbal, *Paradisi in sole*. The vegetable lamb supposedly grew in Tartary and developed from seed into a large melon-like fruit, carried on a stalk about two feet above the ground. When ripe the melon split open, revealing a woolly-coated lamb-like creature which then rotated slowly around its stalk, grazing the grass within its reach. When this was exhausted the creature died.

It is hard to think of any plant which, even viewed through the most imaginative eyes, could have given rise to this myth. Yet it remains a powerfully evocative and touching image, and the accounts of it in early herbals may well have been intended as parables rather than literal descriptions.

Lungwort

The medieval idea that a plant resembles the disease it can cure formed the superstitious basis for The Doctrine of Signatures. *This concept decreed that the small white speckles on the lungwort leaf (*Pulmonaria officinalis) *pointed to its effectiveness against lung diseases. It is a mild expectorant, but its healing power was over-estimated.*

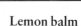

Lemon balm

Observation supports the old myth that lemon balm draws bees more than other plants, and science now confirms the medical value of this herb. Gerard's assertion in the 16th century that it "glueth together greene wounds" is supported by the discovery that hydrocarbons in balsamic oils starve germs of oxygen.

Motherwort

*The name motherwort (*Leonurus cardiaca) *derives from the ancient belief that it reduces anxiety in pregnant women. It has displayed sedative properties in scientific experiments. As well as pacifying the nervous system, motherwort also appears to act as a tonic without inducing feverishness.*

Mandrake

*The mandrake (*Mandragora officinarum) *root's bizarre "human" shape has earned it a worldwide reputation for magical powers. In its native Palestine and neighbouring Arab countries it was long thought to be an aphrodisiac and also had a reputation for increasing fertility. Later it was used as a narcotic and an anaesthetic for crucified criminals. Here too, it was named "Satan's apple" and thought to cause madness.*

history of use in folk-medicine and have recently been found to contain antibiotic chemicals, effective against the kind of bacteria that cause tuberculosis and many other chest infections.

Most plant remedies in popular use probably earned their place through this kind of mixture of personal experience, local custom and an added dash of faith. In the more urbanized areas of Europe this knowledge began to be lost from the 17th century, and the alternative cures peddled by the city apothecaries and herbalists became progressively more unscrupulous and dangerous. In Britain this led to a backlash by more responsible physicians, and a campaign against the unrestricted use of more toxic herbs, like deadly nightshade, by unqualified practitioners, especially apothecaries whose role in both diagnosing diseases and dispensing treatments was easily abused.

The crucial split between herbalism and orthodox medicine came with the unravelling of the effects of the foxglove in 1785, by the English physician William Withering. Withering had learned from herbalists that foxglove leaves could be a dramatic remedy for dropsy. But the effects were unpredictable and the dosage often proved fatal. He discovered that the principal effect was in fact on the heart, which in turn stimulated the kidneys to clear the body of the fluids that caused dropsy. From this he found that in small and accurately measured doses, the leaf – as digitalis – was an invaluable treatment for heart failure. This eventually led to the discovery and purification of the active principles digitoxin and digoxin, now used in orthodox medicine as standard heart stimulants.

In the years that followed, conventional medicine argued, with species like foxglove very much in mind, that plants would remain one of the major sources of effective new drugs, but that for safety's sake, the active ingredients need to be extracted, purified and given in accurate, monitored doses. Most of the industrial world's major drugs were originally discovered in plants which had a history of use in traditional medicine or ritual. The opium poppy produced hypnotics such as codeine and morphine; the root of *rauwolfia*, an Indian remedy for insomnia and certain types of insanity, led to the development of synthetic tranquillizers and anti-hypertensives; the South American paralysing dart-poison, curare, has become a vital muscle relaxant in surgery; the Peruvian "fever tree", cinchona, gave quinine; and most antibiotics were originally extracted from moulds – which may have been the reason why some ancient fungus-based remedies, such as mouldy hyssop, were effective.

The process of examining plants for drugs continues, although it can hardly keep pace with the speed at which plant species are being extinguished, especially in the tropical rain forests. A typical rain forest may hold more than 1,000 species potentially active against

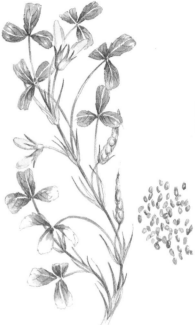

A birth control agent?
Fenugreek seed – thought to increase the flow of milk in cows – may well be a good source of diosgenin, the essential ingredient in the birth-control pill and anabolic steroids. Diosgenin was first discovered in the American yam (Dioscorea spp.) but when prices soared, drug companies began to explore other sources. If fenugreek passes clinical trials it will have some ecological advantages over the yam. In particular, its leaves and stems make good animal fodder, and the plant restores nitrogen to the soil.

cancer, although only a fraction of them have so far been subjected to a thorough programme of scientific testing.

What is medical herbalism?

Medical herbalism to some extent overlaps with conventional medicine and the more relaxed home-based herbal remedies – such as dandelion leaves as a diuretic and laxative, fennel and dill for indigestion and witch hazel for bruises. It differs from both, however, in important ways. First, it is committed to the use of whole, unextracted herbs, believing that the active principles are safer if they are not taken in isolation from other naturally occurring organic substances. Second, many of the herbs are individually prescribed to redress deep-seated nutritional or biochemical deficiencies in particular patients, and so can take a considerable time to work.

For these reasons, it is difficult to test and evaluate medical herbs in the same way as orthodox drugs. Yet it would be invaluable to have objective evidence about their effectiveness to back up empirical experience, so that their continued use does not have to rely purely on tradition and anecdote. Already, several governments, mindful of the increase in public use of herbal medicines, are beginning to impose stricter conditions on the ingredients of commercially available remedies, and on how their usefulness is described and justified. A thorough testing programme would be difficult and prohibitively expensive for most herb companies. But the results could be surprising and even attractive to pharmaceutical companies – as the case of feverfew bears out. When scientifically evaluated over a sufficient period of time, it was found to relieve migraine but with the possible side-effect of mouth ulcers after prolonged usage. Feverfew appears to act as a spasmolytic, preventing the spasms in small blood vessels that are known to be the immediate cause of migraine. The chief active ingredients, called sesquiterpene lactones, have been isolated, raising the possibility of preparing purified extracts. Orthodox physicians argue that extracts of the active constituents will make dosing more precise and allow side-effects to be eliminated. Medical herbalists, on the other hand, believe that a whole new range of side-effects may appear if active chemicals are given in a concentrated, isolated way.

Plants as pharmacists

The reason why plant chemicals have such a dramatic effect on human physiology is partly, of course, because all living things are composed of families of related organic compounds. Proteins, enzymes, sugars, vitamins and poisons from plants are bound to have some effect, however random, on similar substances in our own physiology. It is fascinating how frequently a plant chemical, when applied to humans,

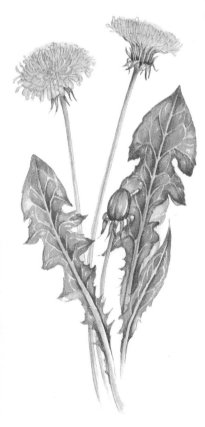

Home herbal remedies
The "household names" of medical herbalism, such as the dandelion, are fast-acting enough to be recognized by mainstream medicine, but safe enough to use at home. Dandelion, known to the French as "pissenlit", has a long history as an effective diuretic and mild laxative. Its leaves are served as salads and tea and its root roasted to make a good coffee substitute.

mimics its normal reaction inside the parent plant. Antibiotics are the classic example. In plants they are specifically evolved to ward off attacks by bacteria and fungi, and they do exactly the same in animals. It looks as if there may well be other similarly transferable processes. Chemicals that inhibit parasites and tumours in plants have been found to have the same effect on humans, and some promising anti-viral compounds have also been discovered.

Beyond this direct relationship, there are more subtle similarities between plant and animal biochemistry which may help to explain some apparently arbitrary reactions. Human sex hormones, for example, have been found in yeast and certain fungi. Many plants also contain compounds very similar to the endorphins and exorphins that control the human pain response. No doubt their role in plants is to help transmit information about damage and to stimulate repair.

Plant substances may have a comparable effect on humans because we have evolved from a common biological ancestry, and because some of the most basic elements in human cells share many properties with those in plants. Research in this whole field is still at a very early stage, but it does raise the exciting possibility of predicting the action a plant chemical will have on humans, once its role in the plant has been worked out. Attitudes towards scientific research, however, vary across the world. In China, more than 2,000 traditional plant re-medies are still in use today. When the United States Department of Health sponsored an investigation into Chinese herbal medicine in 1974, it found a much more sympathetic attitude in the medical establishment than exists in the West. China is anxious to improve its medical practice and to integrate it with western scientific medicine; but it seeks to modernize and validate herbalism instead of replace it.

The World Health Organization is making similar efforts else-where, in an attempt to safeguard the kind of medicine on which the bulk of the world still depends. Their fieldwork among aboriginal peoples is urgent. Much traditional knowledge is being lost with the disappearance of the forest habitats and the disposal of their human inhabitants.

In the West, mainstream sciences just as much as herbalism have suffered through lack of integration. The loss, however, extends beyond the passing over of many potentially effective remedies. More serious is the gradual fading of the kind of respect for and intimacy with the natural world that characterizes plant-based medicine.

An integrated approach

One of the aims of this book is to form a bridge both between orthodox medicine and herbalism and between the many principles in whose name herbs are prescribed – from the pragmatic to the mystical.

Chemical properties

Among the many constituents of herbs are certain chemicals that have useful actions for the plant and are also beneficial to human users. For example, many leaves contain tannins and other bitter chemicals. These deter insect predators and in herbal medicines act to promote the healing of wounds. As research into the actions of plant chemicals progresses, it may lend respec-tability to one of the bases of sympathetic magic – that a plant's physiology gives clues about its effect on the body.

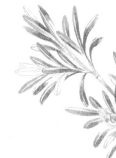

Cranberry
Many fruits have their own natural preservatives. Cran-berries contain benzoic acid and other bactericidal sub-stances which perform this role.

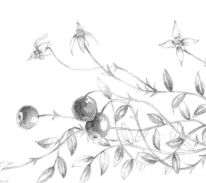

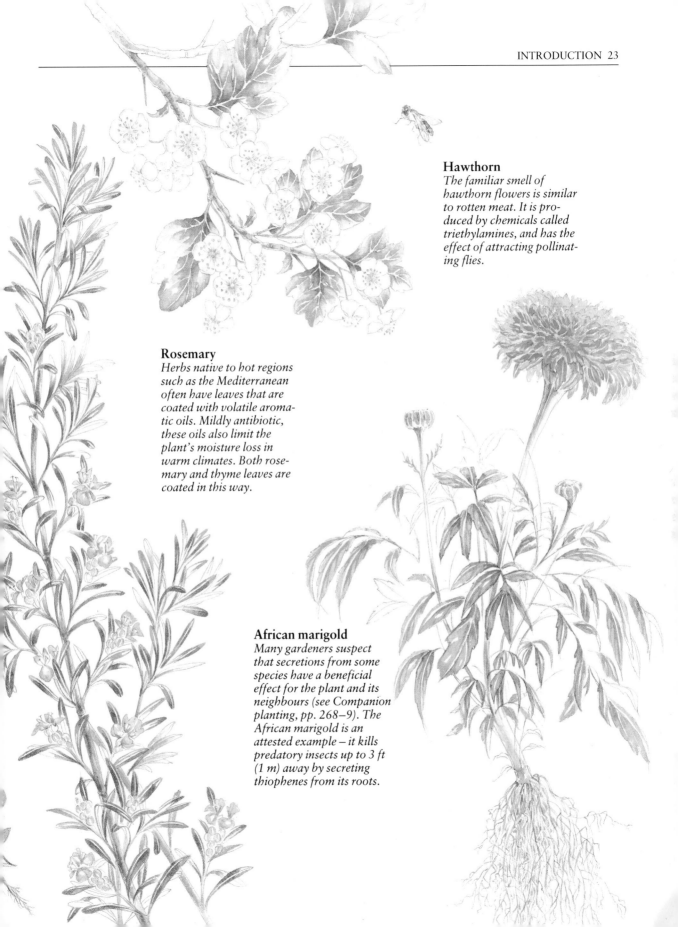

Hawthorn
The familiar smell of hawthorn flowers is similar to rotten meat. It is produced by chemicals called triethylamines, and has the effect of attracting pollinating flies.

Rosemary
Herbs native to hot regions such as the Mediterranean often have leaves that are coated with volatile aromatic oils. Mildly antibiotic, these oils also limit the plant's moisture loss in warm climates. Both rosemary and thyme leaves are coated in this way.

African marigold
Many gardeners suspect that secretions from some species have a beneficial effect for the plant and its neighbours (see Companion planting, pp. 268–9). The African marigold is an attested example – it kills predatory insects up to 3 ft (1 m) away by secreting thiophenes from its roots.

In general, we believe that no herbalists should regard their treatment as beyond scientific explanation and analysis, but should be prepared wherever possible to provide reliable objective evidence about how their herbs work.

At the same time we recognize that in some cases herbs work through more than direct biochemical channels. They also act psychosomatically, helped, for instance by the symbolic significance of their appearance, their associations, their history and the way they have been cultivated. This is one of the most powerful and intriguing healing pathways, yet conventional medicine dismisses it as part of the "placebo" effect, since it cannot be easily tested by existing techniques. In such cases, we have given the benefit of the doubt to "customary practice" and we have presented the case for unconventional herbal practice, such as Bach flower remedies, as fairly as possible, though this does not imply that we endorse them. Over 400 years ago, the herbalist John Gerard was wise to the more subtle curative properties of herbs when he wrote this appreciation of the sweet violet.

> "They have great prerogative above others, not onely because the minde conceiveth a certaine pleasure and recreation by smelling and handling of those most odoriferous flours, but also for that very many by these Violets receive ornament and comely grace: for there be made of them Garlands for the head, Nose-gaies, and poesies, which are delightful to look on, and pleasant to smell to, speaking nothing of their appropriate vertues; yea Gardens themselves receive by these the greatest ornament of all, chiefest beautie and most gallant grace; and the recreation of the minde which is taken thereby, cannot be but very good and honest: for they admonish and stir up a man to that which is comely and honest."

This brings us back full-circle to the idea that at no level – chemical, ecological, psychological – can plants be considered in isolation. The whole context in which they grow effects not just their chemical content, but their symbolic power – what John Gerard called their "grace". New respect for the significance and value of herbs will inevitably determine styles of cultivation in future. This, in turn, will influence our attitudes toward the soil, the conservation of species, even the purity of our water sources – a cycle of beneficial effects that can only rebound positively upon us.

Such a shift raises the possibility of a way back to the ancient idea of "herb" as a comprehensive term for useful plants. Perhaps all plants grown with their own complex nutritional, chemical and ecological relationships preserved, in a system that pays due respect to the harmony and integrity of the natural world – perhaps all such plants become herbs.

A symbolic plant
The oak – once common in Europe, North and South America and China – retains some of its symbolic power in spite of its decline. Sacred to the Greeks and the Druids it is still a symbol of strength and health. This may be linked to the healing properties of oak bark. Our future physical and psychological health may well rest on a renewed respect for the value of such plants.

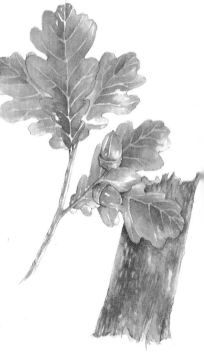

PART ONE

Understanding Herbs

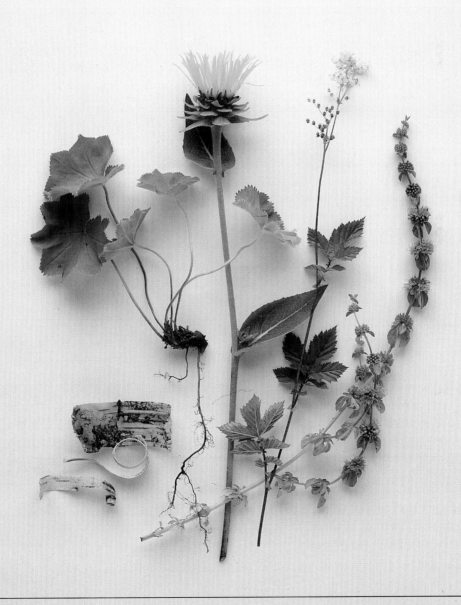

CHAPTER ONE

Glossary of Herbs

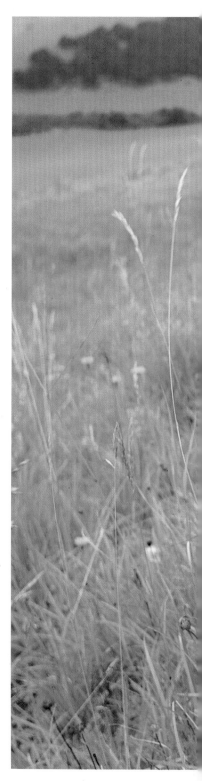

For a newcomer to the world of herbalism, the most extraordinary feature of herbs is their incredible versatility. You may think of a particular herb as useful for flavouring food or as a source of perfume, for example, then discover it has a wide range of other applications. A herb that is prized in cooking may also be of value against pests in the garden, one used in beauty care may also be a healing herb. A plant such as the elder can provide the raw material for wines, conserves, medicines, and dye. This chapter shows how the magical biochemistry of herbs makes possible these diverse properties.

The herbs in this glossary are listed under their botanical families, emphasizing the similarities between related plants. Many of the mint family (Labiatae), for example, are rich in essential oils, and important as culinary herbs, while a number of herbs in the daisy family (Compositae) are good for healing wounds and stopping bleeding. Within each family the herbs are listed alphabetically under their Latin names, with their common names also given in bold type. As well as the plants that have traditionally been used by herbalists, the glossary also contains a few plants that have been extensively used in orthodox medicine, such as the foxglove, and other more recently researched plants whose dramatic healing properties have lately been publicized. Superior numbers refer to notes on research on pages 281–2.

Each entry indicates the size of the herb (either its height or both its height and approximate spread on the ground) and gives a page reference to a photograph of the plant. Details of the parts of the plant used are followed by a list of its chemical constituents. (For more information about these, see the Chemical Glossary, p. 280). There follows a summary of the main uses of the herb and a detailed description of its history, its specific applications, how its chemistry affects the body, and where possible, research findings on its effects. It must be stressed, however, that for self-prescription you should use the Herbs for Healing chapter (see pp. 186–240) and not the glossary. Finally, if there are any circumstances under which the plant should not be used, or if part of the plant is poisonous, there is a caution. The word "Restricted" indicates a plant whose use is limited to registered medical herbalists, pharmacists, and doctors.

Caution Do not use the Glossary for self-prescription. See Chapter 5 for dosages for particular ailments.

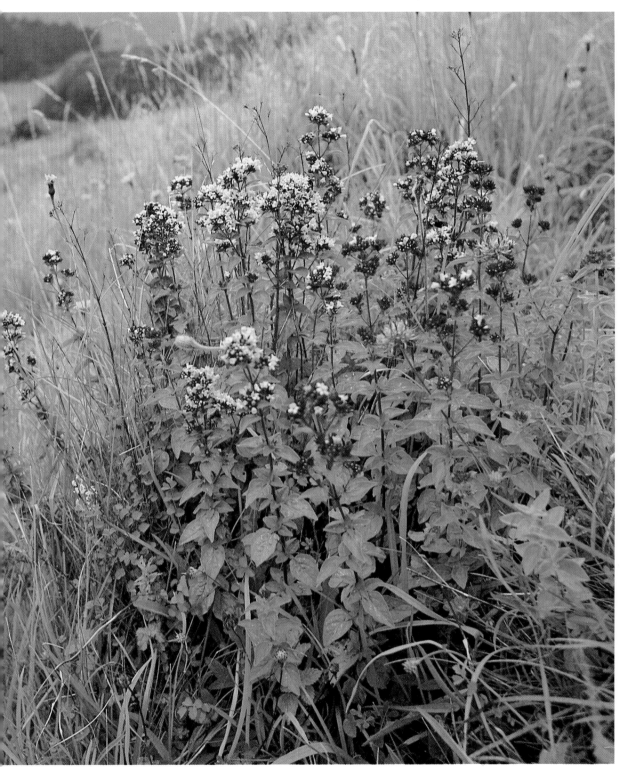

Wild marjoram growing on the South Downs in England

ARACEAE

Acorus calamus
Sweet flag

Sweet sedge, sweet grass, sweet rush, myrtle flag

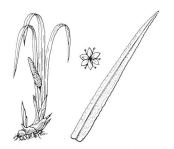

h 3 ft (1m). See p. 30.

Parts used Rhizome.

Constituents Volatile oil up to 3.5% (comprising aserone, cis-methyl isoeugenol, calamene, linalool, eugenol, azulene, pinene, cineole, camphor, etc), sesquiterpenes, acoric acid, tannin, resin, mucilage.

Main uses *Medical* Stomach and bowel complaints.

Mentioned in the book of Exodus and brought to Europe by the Tartars in the thirteenth century, sweet flag has a long reputation as a healing herb. In Europe, it is used for the stomach and bowel because it stimulates the salivary glands and production of stomach juices, helping to counter acidity and ease heartburn and dyspepsia. It also eases flatulence and relaxes the bowel, reducing catarrhal states of the mucous membranes. In traditional Chinese medicine sweet flag is used to treat deafness, dizziness and epilepsy. Sweet flag is sometimes chewed for toothache and to break tobacco addiction because it has a mild sedative effect.

NOTE The Food and Drugs Administration in the USA has prohibited the use of this as a remedy due to the presence of aserone in the essential oil. But rhizomes from Europe have low concentrations of aserone compared with those from India and no cases of malignancy have been reported in mill and mine workers who chew the rhizome.

Symplocarpus foetidus
Skunk cabbage

Meadow cabbage, polecat weed, skunkweed

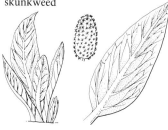

16×12 ins (40×30 cm)

Parts used Root.

Constituents Volatile oil, resin, acrid principle, silica, iron, manganese.

Main uses *Medical* Asthma, whooping cough, and bronchitis.

Skunk cabbage has an unpleasant smell when bruised but it is a highly useful herb nonetheless. It is antispasmodic and expectorant with somewhat sedative properties and is prescribed for tightness of the chest, irritable tight coughs and other spasmodic respiratory disorders. In addition, it is sometimes used to calm the nervous system. It also has a diuretic action. Skunk cabbage was introduced into Europe during the last century.

CAUTION The fresh plant can cause blistering.

ARALIACEAE

Panax ginseng
Oriental ginseng

Chinese ginseng, Korean ginseng, Japanese ginseng

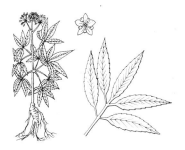

h 24–31 ins (60–80 cm). See p. 82.

Parts used Dried root.

Constituents About eleven hormone-like saponins (called ginsenosides by the Japanese and panaxosides by the Russians), volatile oil, sterols, starch, sugars, pectin, vitamins B1, B2 and B12, choline, fats, minerals (including zinc, copper, magnesium, calcium, iron, manganese, vanadium).

Main uses *Medical* As tonic, particularly for people weakened by disease, old age, or stress.

Ginseng (in Chinese, "Renshen", meaning "man root") is the king of tonics. For centuries in the East, top-grade roots have been valued more than gold. There are many different grades of ginseng. Wild ginseng, particularly that from Manchuria, is considered the best but is phenomenally expensive. Cultivated ginseng comes in two varieties, white and red. The red is cured by steaming which gives it its colour and reputedly a warmer nature than the white. Most Korean ginseng is of the red variety and is stronger or more yang in nature than that from China.

Unfortunately, the fame of ginseng has led to misconceptions about its use and to low grade or adulterated products being sold as ginseng in the West. Despite its Latin name Panax, meaning panacea, it is not universally applicable in every illness. It should not be taken during acute inflammatory disease or bronchitis since it can drive the disease deeper and make it worse. Moreover, in China, ginseng is rarely used on its own, but is usually combined with other herbs, such as licorice or Chinese dates, which temper its powerful nature. Ginseng is best taken by someone made weak by disease or old age. Modern research reinforces traditional views about ginseng.[1] The several hormone-like substances in the plant are thought to account for its simultaneously sedative and stimulating (adaptogenic) effect on the central nervous system.[2] Experiments in Russia carried out since 1948 indicated that ginseng improved concentration and endurance.[3] The effect of ginseng on nurses in a London hospital in another experiment was similar.[4] An often quoted work by the American scientist Siegal, entitled Ginseng Abuse Syndrome (GAS),[5] apparently compromising the safety of ginseng has recently been demonstrated to have little or no foundation.[6]

American ginseng (*Panax quinquifolium*) is considered by the Chinese to be less stimulating and warming than their own indigenous variety. It contains some but not all of the same ginsenosides. San Qi ginseng (*Panax pseudoginseng*) is probably the most important wound-healing herb in the Chinese pharmacopeia. It has been used successfully to treat angina pectoris.[7] Siberian ginseng (*Eleutherococcus sentiocosus*) is reputed to have similar properties to oriental ginseng.

ASCLEPIADACAE

Asclepias tuberosa
Pleurisy root

Canada root, flux root, orange swallow-wort, tuber root, white root, windroot, milkweed, butterfly weed

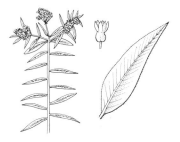

h 24 ins (60 cm). See p. 83.

Parts used Root.

Constituents Glycosides including asclepiadin, and possibly cardiac glycosides; volatile oil, resins.

Main uses *Medical* Wide range of respiratory complaints, specifically pleurisy. Formerly official to the United States Pharmacopeia.

This plant was revered as a healer by the North American Indians and called after the Greek god of medicine, Asclepias, by American doctors because of its power to save lives. Its powerful sweat-inducing and expectorant properties have ensured that it continues to be used for colds, flu, and respiratory problems.

CAUTION The fresh root may cause nausea and vomiting.

Piscidia erythrina
Jamaican dogwood

Fish-poison tree, fish fuddle

See p. 83

Parts used Bark.

Constituents Alkaloid, glycosides (piscidin, jamaicin, icthyone); flavonoids; plant acids; a saponin; glycoside; tannin.

Main uses *Medical* Insomnia, neuralgia, toothache, spasmodic dysmenorrhoea.

In South America, the pounded leaves and young branches of this tree are used to stupefy fish so they can easily be caught. But the chemicals in the plant are only poisonous to cold-blooded creatures. Its toxicity has been reported low in most animals and an extract of the plant has been shown to be sedative in cats. It also has an antispasmodic effect on smooth muscle. The main herbal use is as a sedative and painkiller. It is useful to treat insomnia, neuralgia and menstrual cramping. Scientific reports also indicate that Jamaican dogwood can calm the cough reflex and reduce fevers, which provides two further therapeutic possibilities.

BERBERIDACEAE

Berberis vulgaris
Barberry

Jaundice berry, pepperidge bush

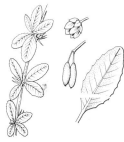

h 7 ft (2 m)

Parts used Bark, fruit.

Constituents Alkaloids (including berberine, berbamine, oxyacanthine, jatrorrhizine, columbamine, palmatine, isotetrandine, bervulcine and magnoflorine), tannin, resin, fat, starch.

Main uses *Medical* Stimulate the liver and gall bladder, and as a digestive tonic.

Barberry bark contains many active alkaloids, useful to the medical herbalist. The alkaloids berberine, oxyacanthine, and columbamine are all strongly antibacterial.[1,2,3] Berberine may also have antiviral properties[4] and research shows that it dilates the arteries so lowering blood pressure as well as being anticonvulsant.[5,6] It has been successfully used to treat Leishmaniasis (infections transmitted by sandfly). It is also effective in treating cholera.[7,8]

CAUTION This herb should not be used during pregnancy as the alkaloid berberine stimulates the uterus.

Caulophyllum thalictroides
Blue cohosh

Squaw root, papoose root, blue ginseng, yellow ginseng

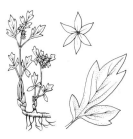

h 3 ft (1 m)

Parts used Root and rhizome.

Constituents Alkaloids, cystine (caulophylline), baptifoline, anagyrine, laburnine. Also caulosaponin, resins.

Main uses *Medical* For suppressed periods with cramping pain; labour pains; arthritis; stomach cramps.

It is sometimes said that blue cohosh should not be used during pregnancy, but this was not the experience of North American Indian women who drank the tea a few weeks before childbirth to make the birth process swift and easy, nor of experienced North American doctors in the Eclectic or Physiomedical herbal tradition who used it to counter restlessness and pain during pregnancy and to reduce labour pains. Blue cohosh eases the cramping

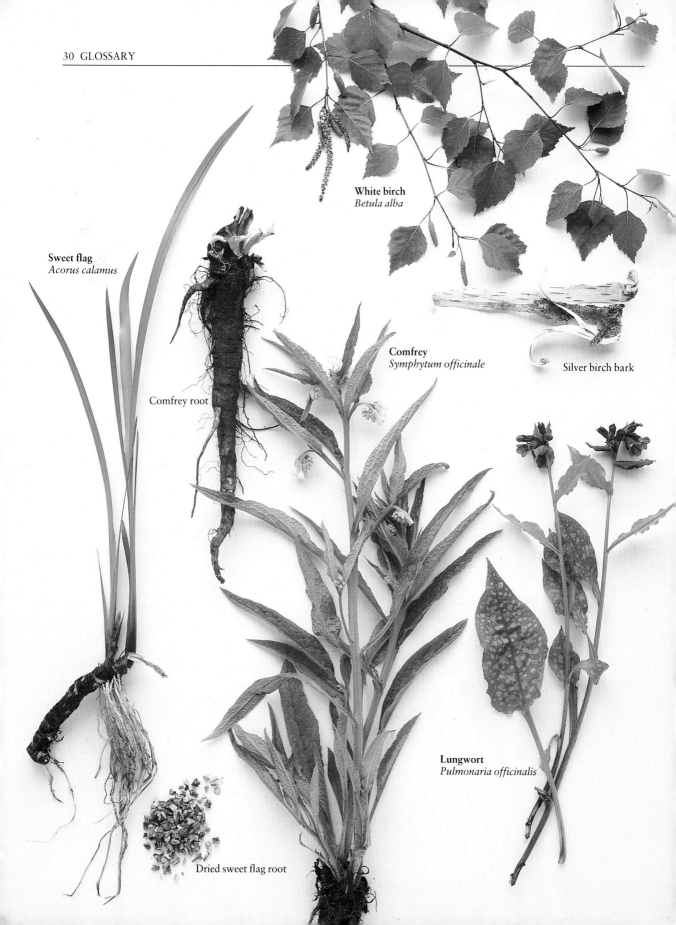

White birch
Betula alba

Sweet flag
Acorus calamus

Comfrey root

Comfrey
Symphytum officinale

Silver birch bark

Dried sweet flag root

Lungwort
Pulmonaria officinalis

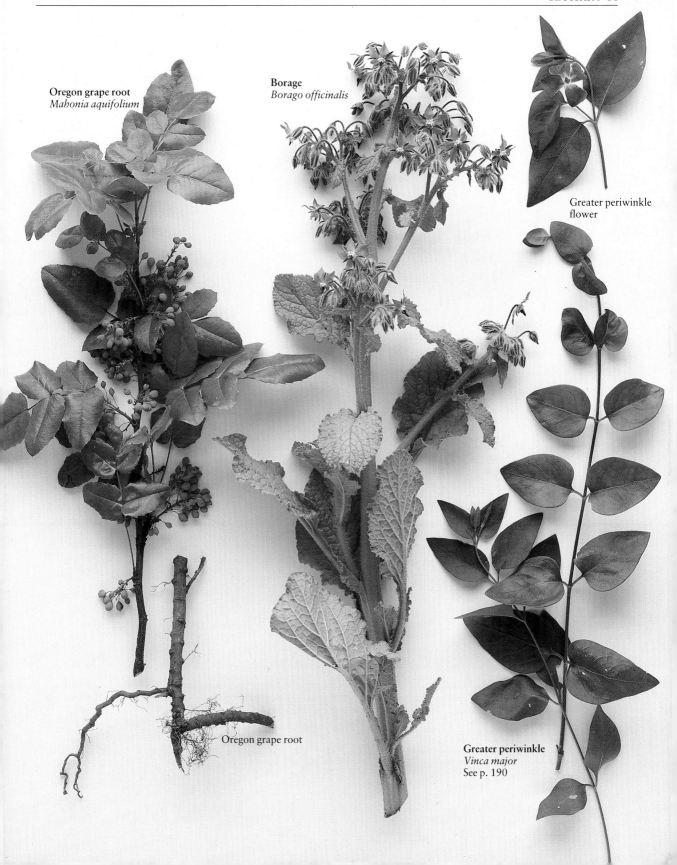

Oregon grape root
Mahonia aquifolium

Borage
Borago officinalis

Greater periwinkle
flower

Oregon grape root

Greater periwinkle
Vinca major
See p. 190

pain of dysmenorrhoea. It has also been used to treat arthritis and ease stomach cramps.

CAUTION The herb should not be used during pregnancy, or where there is high blood pressure or heart disease. The seeds are poisonous.

Mahonia aquifolium (also known as *Berberis aquifolium*)
Oregon grape root
Mountain grape, Rocky Mountain grape, holly leaved barberry

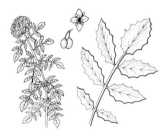

h to 6 ft (2 m). See p. 30.

Parts used Root and rhizome.

Constituents Alkaloids (berberine, berbamine, oxyacanthine, and herbamine).

Main uses *Medical* Liver and gallbladder complaints and chronic skin disease.

Oregon grape root has a considerable reputation as a blood purifier, cleansing the tissues and blood of toxins and waste products. Its bitter components stimulate the liver and gallbladder and are tonic to the digestion and mildly laxative. It is used for skin diseases such as psoriasis, eczema, acne, and cold sores.

CAUTION Like barberry bark and golden seal which also contain the alkaloid berberine, this herb should not be used during pregnancy.

BETULACEAE

Betula alba (plus *B. pendula*, *B. verrucosa*)
White birch
Silver birch, paper birch

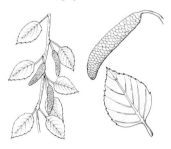

h to 65 ft (20 m). See p. 30.

Parts used Leaves, bark, oil, sap.

Constituents Buds: volatile oil which includes the camphor-like betulin. Young leaves: rich in saponins; also a flavonoid derivative, hyperoside resin, tannins, sesquiterpenes, betuloventic acid, vitamin C. Bark: betulinol and a glycoside.

Main uses *Culinary* Sap in wine or vinegar; used as a sweetening agent. *Medical* Fluid retention, arthritis, gout, urinary stones or infections.

The graceful birch has been immensely useful to northern peoples. They have made wheels, hoops for casks, brooms and switches from its wood.

The sap, preserved with cloves and cinnamon, was once taken to treat skin diseases like acne as well as rheumatism and gout.

Birch-leaf tea is a powerful diuretic capable of dissolving kidney and bladder stones.[1,2,3] It also kills off harmful bacteria in the kidneys and urinary tract. To obtain the full diuretic effect herbalists add a pinch of sodium bicarbonate (baking soda) to the infusion which promotes the extraction of the diuretic hyperoside. The leaves also have a substantial reputation for treating rheumatism, arthritis, and gout.

Birch leaves can be used to treat fluid retention due to heart or kidney malfunction. In addition the tea lowers blood cholesterol levels and stimulates the flow of bile.[4] A decoction of the bark has been used to allay intermittent fevers. Oil extracted from the buds or bark has been used externally in lotions to treat psoriasis and eczema. This oil should not be confused with sweet birch oil which is extracted from black birch (*Betula lenta*) native to North America.

BORAGINACEAE

Borago officinalis
Borage
Bugloss, burage

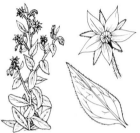

24×20 ins (60×50 cm). See p. 31.

Parts used Leaves, flowers, seed; cultivation see pp. 274–5.

Constituents Mucilage, tannin, essential oil, potassium, calcium, pyrrolizioline alkaloids.

Main uses *Culinary* Flowers to flavour summer wine cups (see p. 183); young leaves pickled. *Medical* Coughs, depression.

Borage is a plant which deserves more medical research. Folk use suggests a variety of medicinal properties, a potential which has lately been endorsed by the discovery of high levels of gamma linoleic acid in the seeds. This is useful in many disorders (see evening primrose p. 89).

The ancients extolled the virtues of borage, pointing out its ability to counter melancholic states. Pliny repeats an ancient verse "I, Borage always bring courage". The seventeenth-century diarist, John Evelyn, wrote that borage was "of known virtue to revive the hypochondriac and cheer the hard student". This use suggests a supportive effect on the adrenal glands which may well be the case since comfrey, a close relative, has been shown to affect the sex hormones which stimulate the ovaries and testes. Such a hormonal effect is also indicated by the traditional belief that the leaves and seeds of borage could increase the milk supply of nursing mothers.

Borage is also sweat-inducing in hot infusion, making it a good remedy for colds and flu, especially when these affect the lungs because it is also a good cough remedy.

This plant is also a useful culinary herb. The leaves have a taste reminiscent of cucumber.

CAUTION Avoid excessive consumption.

Pulmonaria officinalis
Lungwort

Beggar's basket, Jerusalem cowslip, Jerusalem sage, maple lungwort

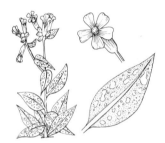

12×14 ins (30×35 cm). See p. 30.

Parts used Dried flowering plant; cultivation, see pp. 278–9.

Constituents Mucilage, saponin, allantoin, tannin, silica, potassium, iron, and other mineral salts.

Main uses *Medical* Bronchitis and other lung complaints.

The names of this plant reflect its use in the treatment of respiratory disorders. The speckled appearance of the leaf, thought to resemble a lung, convinced adherents of the Doctrine of Signatures (see p.17) that the plant was a specific for the lungs. In fact they were on the right track, since the plant is a soothing expectorant. The silica it contains restores the elasticity of the lungs. It reduces bronchial mucus. The tannin it contains makes it suitable for treating haemorrhoids, and the tannin and alantoin content explains its extensive folk use for wounds.

Symphytum officinale
Comfrey

Knitbone, boneset, bruisewort, consormol, knitback

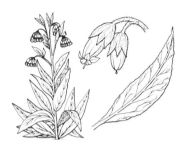

40×30 ins (100×80 cm). See p. 30.

Parts used Fresh or dried roots or leaves; cultivation see pp. 278–9.

Constituents Mucilage, allantoin (up to 0.8%), tannins, resin, essential oil, pyrrolizioline alkaloids, gum, carotene, glycosides, sugars, beta-sitosterol and steroidal saponins, triterpenoids, vitamin B12, protein (up to 35%), zinc.

Main uses *Culinary* Fresh leaves and shoots as vegetable or salad (see p. 170). *Medical* Fractures, bruises and burns (external); respiratory and digestive disorders.

Comfrey is one of the most famed healing plants. Its remarkable power to heal tissue and bone is due to allantoin, a cell-proliferant that promotes the growth of connective tissue, bone, and cartilage, and is easily absorbed through the skin. Recent American research has also shown that comfrey breaks down red blood cells, a finding that supports its use for bruises, hence its country name, bruisewort.[1] Comfrey is also useful externally as a poultice for varicose ulcers and as a compress for varicose veins. It also alleviates and heals minor burns.

Comfrey has always been a traditional remedy for gastric ulcers, and work at a London teaching hospital has shown that it inhibits a prostaglandin that causes inflammation of the stomach lining.[2] Comfrey is also traditionally used to treat colitis. It is a useful remedy for bronchitis and other respiratory disorders.

In 1968, Japanese scientists first reported the presence of pyrrolizidine alkaloids in comfrey.[3] Subsequent Australian research found these alkaloids

in several plants of the Borage family and reported that rats fed with up to 33% of comfrey leaf in their diet suffered liver cancer.[4] But one of the few investigations using the whole plant has shown that it is not carcinogenic but the very opposite.[5] Moreover, Japanese doctors recommend a vinegar extract of the herb for cirrhosis of the liver.[6]

Several studies have found that comfrey can influence the sex hormones (note its steroidal saponin content) which stimulates the ovaries and testes.[7] Gerard, prescribing comfrey for back pain, noted that it caused "involuntary flowing of the seed in men".

CAUTION In view of the controversy about the plant, avoid excessive consumption of comfrey.

BURSERACEAE

Commiphora molmol
Myrrh

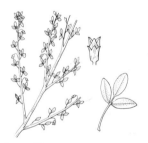

See p. 83.

Parts used Gum-resin.

Constituents Volatile oil, about 8%, (containing heerabolene, limonene, dipentene, pinene, eugenol, cinamaldehyde, cuminaldehyde, etc), resins, up to 40% (including commiphoric acids), gum (about 50%).

Main uses *Medical* Sore throats and infected gums; thrush (*Candida albicans*); athlete's foot.

Since ancient times myrrh has been the herbalist's cleansing agent, countering putrefaction and poisons throughout the body. Its antifungal, antiseptic and astringent action makes it a major ingredient of gargles and mouthwashes[1,2,3], and a useful agent for treating thrush (*Candida albicans*) and athlete's foot. It also stimulates the circulation and is expectorant.

Spices

Traditionally defined as the dried seeds of certain plants, and widely known for their culinary properties, spices are most familiar in the West in their dried form. This is because most are native to tropical regions or to the far east, although some will grow in North America and northern Europe. Because of the strong association of spices with certain types of flavours, a few non-seed parts of some plants, such as ginger roots and coriander leaves, are also included in the photograph. You will also find prepared spices such as ground and powdered seeds and roots and cinnamon sticks. Most of these plants are valued for important medical applications as well as for their culinary uses.

Key to photograph

1 Black mustard seeds 2 White mustard seeds 3 White mustard powder
4 Saffron 5 Green peppers 6 Black peppers 7 Szechuan peppers 8 Fresh peppers and leaves 9 Anise 10 Star anise 11 Birds-eye chillies and leaves
12 Selection of chillies 13 Dried green and red chillies 14 Fennel leaves 15 Fennel seeds 16 Lovage seed head 17 Caraway seed 18 Dill seed 19 Cumin 20 Black cumin
21 Fenugreek 22 Nutmeg 23 Mace
24 Cardamom leaves 25 Black cardamoms 26 Green cardamoms
27 Fresh cardamom stem 28 Turmeric powder 29 Fresh ginger root and leaves 30 Dried ginger root
31 Fresh ginger 32 Ginger powder
33 Juniper leaves 34 Juniper berries
35 Dried poppy seed heads 36 White poppy seeds 37 Blue poppy seeds
38 Cinnamon sticks 39 Cinnamon bark 40 Coriander leaves
41 Coriander seed 42 Cloves
43 Allspice 44 Allspice powder

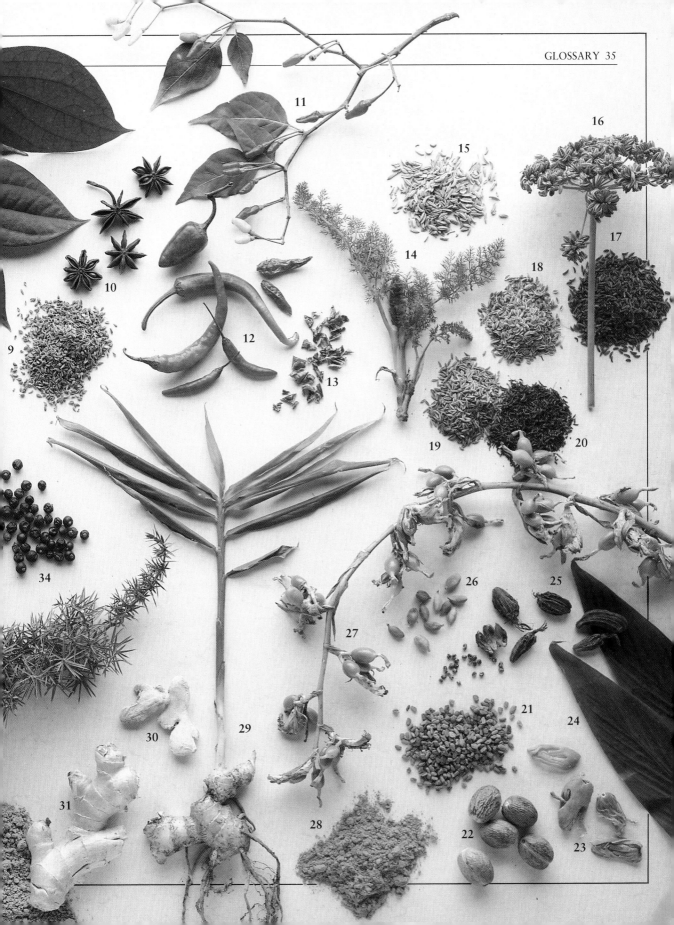

Commiphora opobalsamum
Balm of Gilead

Long prized for its sweet smell, the resin of this tree was the Queen of Sheba's gift to Solomon. Today, buds of *Populus candicans*, below, are used in its place.

Populus candicans (Salicaceae)
Balm of Gilead

Part used Leaf buds. See p. 83.

Constituents Volatile oil, up to 2% (including cineole, bisabolene, bisabolol and humulene), resins, palicin and populin, phenolic acids.

Main uses *Medical* Chest infections, sore throats.

Modern Balm of Gilead, *Populus candicans*, is used for its antibacterial and expectorant actions. It is excellent for chest infections and for sore throats (as a gargle). Salicin, a major constituent of this plant, is a painkiller, while bisabolol in the oil (see chamomile, p. 49) reduces inflammation and is antimicrobial. Balm of Gilead ointment eases rheumatic pain. Not to be confused with false Balm of Gilead, a garden plant, see p. 39.

CAMPANULACEAE

Lobelia inflata
Lobelia
Indian tobacco, asthma weed, pukeweed

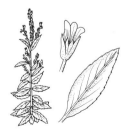

28×12 ins (70×30 cm). See p. 38.

Parts used Aerial parts.

Constituents Alkaloids (lobeline, isolobinine, lobelanidine, lobinaline), a bitter glycoside (lobelacrin), a pungent volatile oil (labelianin), resin, gum, fats, chelidonic acid.

Main uses *Medical* Asthma, whooping cough. Muscle spasm, sprains.

Lobelia, once a famous North American Indian remedy, was adopted by the Physiomedical school of herbalists as its major relaxant remedy. They used it to treat pain caused by spasm, which it does by relaxing the tissues rather than producing a narcotic effect like opium. It is most useful in asthma and bronchitis because it is also expectorant.

One of the plant's main alkaloids, lobeline, stimulates the respiratory system, whilst isolobinine is a respiratory relaxant. Lobeline is reported to have many of the pharmacological properties of nicotine, first stimulating the central nervous system and then subsequently strongly depressing it.[1] The North American Indians smoked it instead of tobacco, but today it is sometimes used to help tobacco withdrawal symptoms. Lobelia plasters and liniments are used to treat sprains, muscle spasms and bruises because of the plant's relaxing and stimulating effect. It is also good for insect bites, poison-ivy irritation, and ringworm.

Blue lobelia (*L. siphilitica*) is used in homeopathy for diarrhoea.

RESTRICTED

CANNABIDACAE

Humulus lupulus
Hops

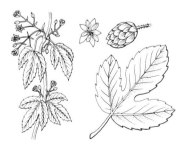

h up to 20 ft (6 m). See p. 38.

Parts used Dried female strobiles.

Constituents Volatile oil, up to 1%, (comprising mostly humulene, myrcene, B-caryophyllene and farnescene), plus over 100 other compounds including geraniol, linalool, citral, linionene and serolidol; also a bitter resin complex (3–12%) which includes valeronic acid, lumulone, and lupulone. The oil and bitter resins together are known as lupulin. In addition, condensed tannins; flavonoid glycosides (astralagin, quercitrin, rutin); fats; amino acids and oestrogenic substances; asparagin.

Main uses *Medical* Insomnia, nervous tension, gastrointestinal spasm.

Observing the tendency of hops to intertwine around willows and other trees, Pliny called the plant "willow wolf" from which it gained its Latin name *lupulus*. Although the use of hops in brewing was known since Roman times, their widespread introduction was resisted, particularly in England, until the 17th century. During the reign of Henry VIII, parliament was petitioned against the hop as "a wicked weed that would spoil the taste of the drink and endanger the people". After the introduction of hops into brewing, the drink flavoured in the old way with plants such as costmary and ground ivy was known as ale, while that brewed with hops was given the German name "bier".

Hops have been used as a medicine for at least as long as for brewing. The flowers are famous for their sleep-inducing sedative effect, whether drunk as a tea or slept on as a hop pillow (probably due to the valeronic acid, resin and oil).[1] The volatile oils released while sleeping on a hop pillow probably affect the brain directly through its olfactory centre.

Modern research shows that hop extracts relax smooth muscle, especially that of the digestive tract.[2] Hops are therefore used in combination with other herbs to treat such disorders as irritable bowel syndrome, Crohn's disease and nervous stomach. The ability of hops to relax and soothe is complemented by the antibacterial activity of components lupulone and humulone,[3] which reduce inflammation, and the plant's overall bitter-tonic effect.[4] Thus hops can allay infection of the upper digestive tract which may play a significant role in provoking gastric and duodenal ulcers.

Female hop pickers can suffer disruption or complete absence of menstruation due to the absorption of the oil through their hands. This is due to the oestrogenic principles in hops, and accounts for its traditional anaphrodisiac effect in men.[5] The hormonal properties of hops probably account for its use in skin creams and lotions, marketed for their alleged skin-softening properties. The asparagin in the plant gives it some diuretic effect.

CAUTION The pollen from the strobiles may cause contact dermatitis. Because of their sedative effect, hops are not recommended in the treatment of depressive illness.

CAPRIFOLIACEAE

Lonicera periclymenum
Honeysuckle

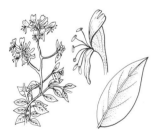

h variable. See p. 39

Parts used Aerial parts.

Constituents Mucilage, glucoside, salicylic acid, invertin.

Main uses *General* For its scent. *Medical* For skin infections.

This sweet-smelling shrub was once used extensively in medicine but is now valued mainly for its perfume. There are many different species, most of which are prized by gardeners for their fragrance. They include *L. caprifolium*, the Italian honeysuckle, *L. tartarica*, from Siberia, and *L. xylosteum* from Asia and eastern Europe.

Sambucus nigra
Elder

European elder, black elder, common elder, bore tree

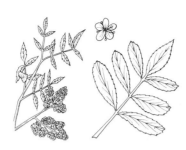

h 10 ft (3.5 m). See p. 39.

Parts used Flowers, berries.

Constituents Flowers: small quantity of essential oil (containing palmitic, linoleic, and linolenic acids), triterpenes, flavonoids (including rutin), also pectin, mucilage, sugar. Berries: sugar, fruit acids, vitamin C, bioflavonoids. Leaves: cyanogenic glycosides, vitamins, tannins, resins, fats, sugars, fatty acids.

Main uses *General* In eye and skin lotions (see p. 144). *Culinary* Flowers and berries used in wines, cordials, desserts, and jams. *Medical* Colds, flu, catarrh.

The elder is one of our most widely useful plants. The flowers are sweat-inducing in hot infusion (bioflavonoids in the plant encourage the circulation) and combined with yarrow and mint are specific for the treatment of colds and flu. Elderflowers also reduce bronchial and upper-respiratory catarrh and are used to treat hayfever. Externally a cold infusion of the flowers may be used as an eyewash for conjunctivitis and as a compress for chilblains. Elderflower ointment can be used for irritation of the skin and chilblains. A gargle made from elderflower infusion or elderflower vinegar alleviates tonsillitis and sore throats. Elderflowers have a mild laxative action and in Europe have a reputation for treating rheumatism and gout. The berries are mildly laxative and sweat-inducing, and simmered with sugar, make a winter cordial for coughs and colds.

CAUTION Elder leaves, roots, and bark should not be used internally.

Viburnum opulus
Crampbark

Guelder rose, highbush cranberry, snowball tree

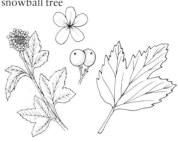

h 13 ft (4 m)

Parts used Stem bark.

Constituents Bitter resin (viburnin), valeric acid, salicosides, tannin.

Main uses *Medical* Cramps.

Crampbark is an excellent muscle and nervous relaxant good for cramping pains. It is particularly useful for easing painful periods and the cramping pains of pregnancy (it is used to prevent miscarriage for which it is often combined with black haw). Like black haw, crampbark is also used by herbalists to prevent excessive menstrual flow at the menopause.

CAUTION The fresh berries are poisonous.

Viburnum prunifolium
Black haw

Stagbush, sweet viburnum

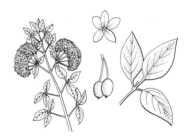

h 16 ft (5 ft)

Parts used Root bark.

Constituents Scopoletin, bitter principle (viburnin), triterpenoid saponins, salicosides, resin, plant acids (including valeric acid), tannin, arbutin.

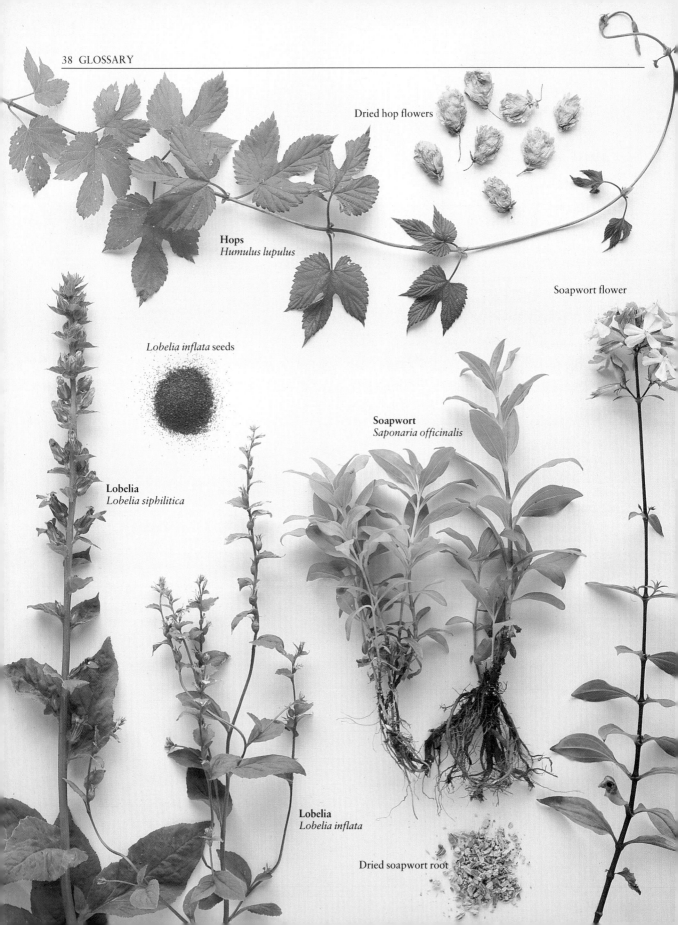

Dried hop flowers

Hops
Humulus lupulus

Soapwort flower

Lobelia inflata seeds

Soapwort
Saponaria officinalis

Lobelia
Lobelia siphilitica

Lobelia
Lobelia inflata

Dried soapwort root

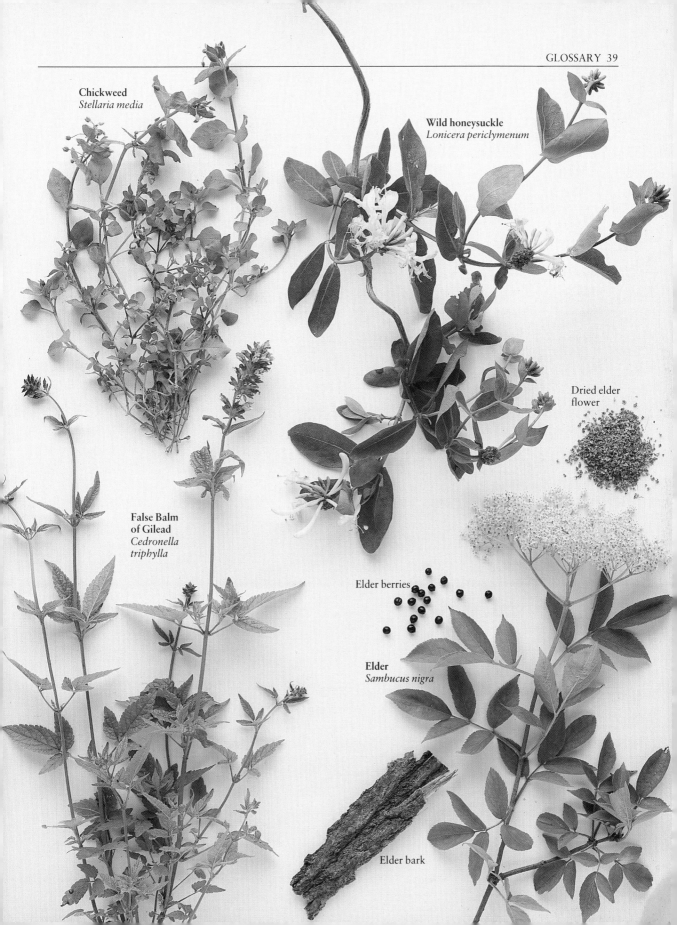

Chickweed
Stellaria media

Wild honeysuckle
Lonicera periclymenum

Dried elder
flower

**False Balm
of Gilead**
*Cedronella
triphylla*

Elder berries

Elder
Sambucus nigra

Elder bark

Main uses *Medical* Menstrual pains.

This is primarily a women's herb, often combined with crampbark: Scopoletin (a coumarin) in the plant has been identified as a uterine relaxant.[1] It is an excellent remedy for menstrual cramping, and is used by herbalists in helping to prevent miscarriage, and to prevent excessive flow at the menopause.

CARYOPHYLLACEAE

Saponaria officinalis
Soapwort

Bouncing Bet, fuller's herb

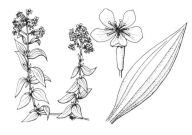

16×24 ins (40×60 cm). See p. 38

Parts used Rhizome; cultivation see pp. 278–9.

Constituents Saponins.

Main uses *General* Cleansing preparations. *Medical* Skin conditions.

Both the Latin and common names indicate a traditional use of this plant in washing. It was especially useful in the textile trades for cleaning cloth. This and the medicinal properties of soapwort are due to the hormone-like saponins it contains, which lower the surface tension of water and produce a lather. Within the body, these saponins are mildly irritant to the respiratory and digestive systems. Thus soapwort is expectorant and laxative in small doses (see Caution). It has an ancient reputation used both internally and externally for treating skin conditions such as psoriasis, eczema, boils, and acne. Its use for gout and rheumatism is probably effective because of the anti-inflammatory property of its saponins. Soapwort is also said to increase the flow of bile.

CAUTION In large doses soapwort is a strong purgative and even mildly poisonous, so it should only be used as prescribed by a qualified herbalist.

Stellaria media
Chickweed

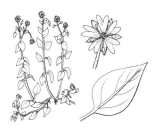

h 4–16 ins (10–40 cm). See p. 39.

Parts used Aerial parts.

Constituents Saponins, mucilage.

Main uses *Culinary* In salads and, lightly boiled, as a vegetable. *Medical* Skin diseases.

Chickweed has similar uses to soapwort but is safer to use internally. Its main use, however, is external as a poultice or ointment for skin irritation and inflammation as well as for skin ulcers. Boils, carbuncles, and abscesses respond well to a poultice. Internally chickweed has a reputation for treating rheumatism and bronchitis.

COMPOSITAE

Achillea millefolium
Yarrow

Nosebleed, millefoil, thousandleaf

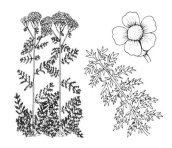

h 3–24 ins (8–60 cm). See p. 42.

Parts used Aerial parts, especially the flowering heads.

Constituents Up to 1.4% volatile oil (composed of up to 51% azulene; borneol, terpineol, camphor, cineole, isoartemesia ketone, and a trace of thujone), lactones, flavonoids, tannins, coumarins, saponins, sterols, a bitter glyco-alkaloid (achilleine), cyanidin, amino acids, acids (including salicylic acid), sugars (including glucose, sucrose and mannitol).

Main uses *General* In skin cleansers (see p. 142). *Medical* Colds and flu; digestive tonic; wound healing.

Yarrow is one of the best-known herbal remedies for fevers.[1] A hot infusion induces a therapeutic sweat which cools fevers and expels toxins. Like all sweat-inducing remedies, yarrow encourages blood flow to the skin and this helps to lower blood pressure, an action which is also due to the flavonoids in the plant which dilate the peripheral arteries.[2] The flavonoids also help to clear blood clots. The alkaloid in yarrow has been reported to lower blood pressure; the cyanidin influences the vagus nerve, slowing the heart beat.

Tannins in the plant are probably responsible for yarrow's reputation as a wound healer, hence its country name nosebleed.[3] Its Latin name is derived from a legend that Achilles used yarrow's wound-healing powers on his men. Yarrow is good for all kinds of bleeding, external and internal. It can be used internally for bleeding piles but conversely it can also be used to treat absent periods.

Yarrow also has anti-inflammatory properties,[4,5] a fact which has been confirmed by medical research which suggests that this is due to a mixture of protein carbohydrate complexes in the plant.[6] We know too that both cyanidin and azulene are anti-inflammatory, as is salicylic acid. This may account for the folk use of yarrow in treating rheumatism.

In China, yarrow is used fresh as a poultice for healing wounds. A decoction of the whole plant is prescribed for stomach ulcers, amenorrhoea, and abscesses.

CAUTION Taking yarrow orally may cause sensitivity to sunlight in some people.

Arctium lappa
Burdock

Great burdock, great bur, clotbur, cocklebur, beggars buttons, lappa, cockle buttons

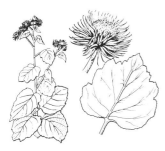

h 6 ft (2 m). See p. 42.

Parts used Fresh or dried roots, leaves, seeds.

Constituents Root: up to 50% inulin, polyacetylenes, volatile acids (acetic, proprionic, butyric, isovaleric), non-hydroxyl acids (lauric, myristic, stearic, palmitic), tannin, polyphenolic acids. Seeds: 15–30% fixed oils, a bitter glycoside (arctiin), chlorogenic acid. Leaves: arctiol, fukinone, taraxasterol.

Main uses *Culinary* Dandelion and burdock bitter (see p. 183); candied stalks; root as vegetable. *Medical* Skin disorders (eg boils and acne), arthritis.

Burdock purifies and cleanses the tissues and blood and for this reason should be used gently over a period of time. The whole plant has mild diuretic, sweat-inducing, and laxative properties. It is prescribed for skin diseases such as eczema and psoriasis. Burdock has an anti-microbial action which has been attributed to the polyacetylenes in the plant.[1] This explains its reputation for treating skin eruptions such as boils and acne. Its antimicrobial property, together with its diuretic action, also makes it useful for treating cystitis. Old-time North American herbalists particularly valued the seeds to treat skin problems, while in China the seeds are used to treat the eruptions of measles, sore throats, tonsillitis, colds, and flu. The roots and leaves can also be used to treat rheumatism and gout because they encourage the elimination of uric acid via the kidneys. The bitter taste of burdock is tonic to the digestive system; the leaves are said to stimulate the secretion of bile.

Research has shown that the seeds can lower blood sugar in rats.[2] In France, the fresh root is also used for lowering blood sugar, its inulin content making it particularly suitable for diabetes. Burdock leaves are useful externally as a poultice for bruises and skin problems. A lotion of the leaves or root massaged into the scalp is good for falling hair. Finally, all parts of the burdock plant have a reputation for curing cancers.[3]

Arnica montana
Arnica

Wolf's bane, mountain tobacco, mountain daisy

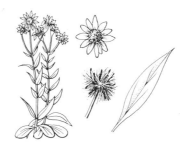

h 12–24 ins (30–60 cm). See p. 42.

Parts used Dried flowers or extract. Homeopathic ointments and other preparations available.

Constituents Volatile oil (containing thymol), resins, a bitter principle (arnicin), carotenoids, flavonoids.

Main uses *Medical* Bruises and sprains.

Arnica is both a famous herbal and homeopathic remedy for wounds, bruises, and other injuries of all kinds. Arnica extract has been reported to increase the resistance of animals to bacterial infection by stimulating the action of white blood cells to clear away harmful bacteria. It has for instance been shown to be effective against salmonella.[1] It also has a reputation used internally for reducing fevers. Goethe claimed this remedy saved his life when he was struck down with an otherwise uncontrollable high fever. Arnica also appears to stimulate the heart and circulation and cause reabsorption of internal bleeding.

CAUTION External use of this herb may cause skin rash or irritation in some people. Do not apply to broken or sensitive skin. Arnica should not be used internally except in its homeopathic form.

Artemisia absinthium
Wormwood

Green ginger

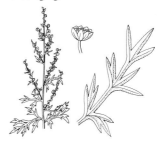

h 2–3 ft (60–90 cm). See p. 42.

Parts used Aerial parts.

Constituents Volatile oil (mainly composed of thujone, but also other compounds including chamazulene), bitter principle (absinthum), carotene, vitamin C, tannins.

Main uses *Medical* Bitter tonic, expels worms.

One of the bitterest plants, wormwood was once used to flavour absinthe, a drink which has been banned in its native France since 1915 because too much of it causes incurable damage to the nervous system. Today, wormwood is used mainly as a bitter tonic, stimulating the appetite, the digestive juices, peristalsis and the liver and gallbladder. True to its name it also expels worms, especially round and threadworms. The azulenes in the plant are anti-inflammatory and reduce fevers. The Latin name comes from the Greek goddess Artemis, who took care of women during childbirth. In ancient times this was a favourite women's herb, bringing on periods, though it is not used in this way today.

CAUTION Wormwood is classified as dangerous by the U.S. Food and Drug Administration.

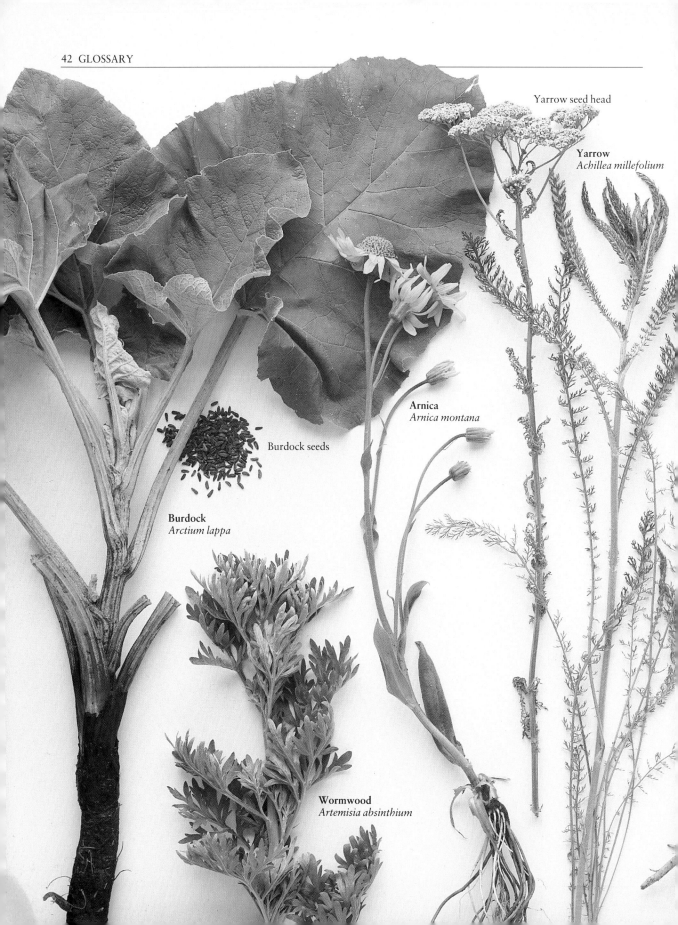

Yarrow seed head

Yarrow
Achillea millefolium

Arnica
Arnica montana

Burdock seeds

Burdock
Arctium lappa

Wormwood
Artemisia absinthium

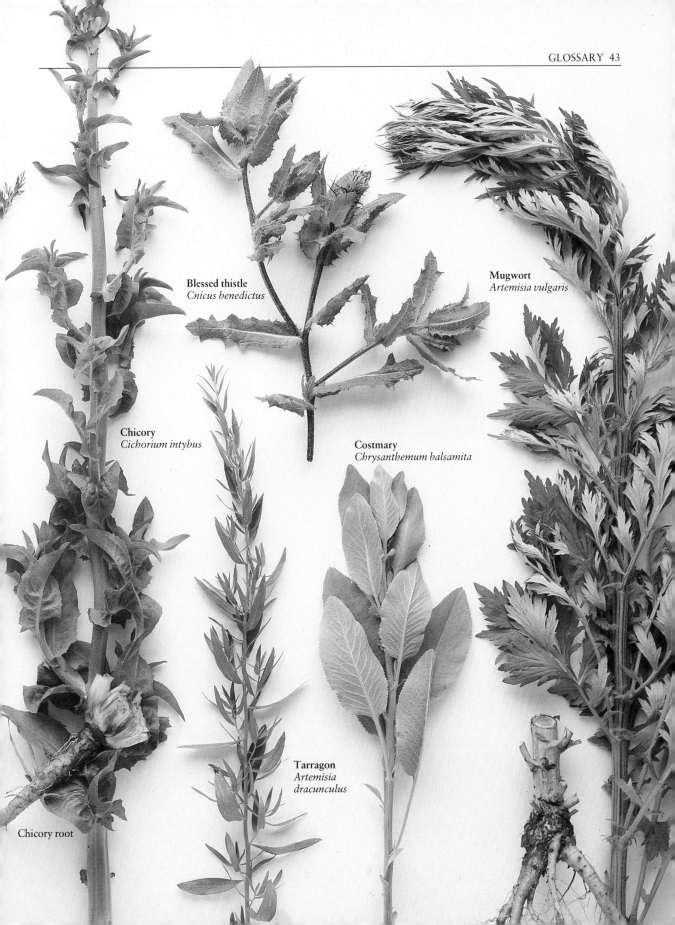

Blessed thistle
Cnicus benedictus

Mugwort
Artemisia vulgaris

Chicory
Cichorium intybus

Costmary
Chrysanthemum balsamita

Tarragon
Artemisia dracunculus

Chicory root

Artemisia dracunculus
Tarragon

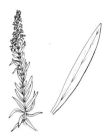

h 2 ft (60 cm). See p. 43.

Parts used Fresh or dried leaves; cultivation see pp. 274–5.

Constituents Essential oil.

Main uses *Culinary* Sauces; fines herbes (see p. 168); dressings and green salads; in vinegars (see p. 180); with cooked chicken.

Tarragon was formerly used in the treatment of toothache. But its most important property, its distinctive, appetizing taste, has assured it a lasting role as a culinary herb – especially in French cuisine.

COMPOSITAE

Artemisia vulgaris
Mugwort
Moxa, St John's herb

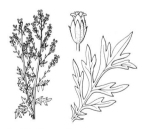

h 6 ft (2 m). See p. 43.

Parts used Aerial parts.

Constituents Volatile oil, bitter principle (absinthin), flavonoids, tannin.

Main uses *Medical* To regulate menstruation.

Used by women since ancient times, in the west mugwort is held to provoke delayed or absent periods, and is there-fore said to be contra-indicated in pregnancy. In China, however, it has been used to prevent miscarriage. Mugwort helps to regulate periods and stop pain and like wormwood was used externally as a compress to speed up the birth process and to help expel the afterbirth. Like wormwood, it also activates the digestive process and stimulates the liver. In China, in the form of moxa, it is burnt on or near the skin to alleviate rheumatic pains caused by cold and damp. Both in China and Europe it is also used externally to treat rheumatism and gout.

CAUTION Mugwort's use during pregnancy should be avoided except as prescribed by a qualified herbal practitioner. Avoid prolonged use and large doses.

Chrysanthemum balsamita
Costmary
Alecost

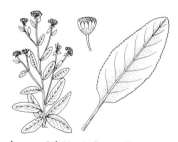

h up to 3 ft (1 m). See p. 43.

Parts used Flowers.

Constituents Volatile oil.

Main uses *Culinary* As salad; to flavour cakes; with poultry; in beers.

Used in the Middle Ages to flavour beers (hence its name alecost), costmary is now used less frequently in foods and drinks, although its balsam-like fragrance and digestive properties make it a useful culinary herb. A once-popular use of the sweet-smelling leaves was to scent rinsing water for the hair, or bath water.

Calendula officinalis
Marigold
See page 46

Cichorium intybus
Chicory
Wild succory, blue sailors

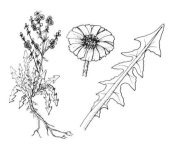

60×20 ins (150×50 cm). See p. 43.

Parts used Fresh roots and leaves.

Constituents Root and aerial parts produce a latex. Root: inulin (around 58%), a bitter compound (comprising lactucin and lactucopictin also known as intybin), cichoriin and taraxasterol, tannins, sugars, (fructose), pectin, fixed oils, small amounts of two alkaloids. Aerial parts: inulin, fructose, resin, cichoriin, esculetin.

Main uses *Culinary* Young leaves as salad (see p. 170); roasted root as coffee substitute. *Medical* As a digestive tonic and for anaemia; for gallstones; for rheumatism and gout.

Chicory resembles the dandelion in its medicinal action. It is a gentle but effective bitter tonic which increases the flow of bile.[1] It is also a specific remedy for gallstones and for this reason Galen called it "friend of the liver". Like dandelion, it also has diuretic properties and can be used for treating rheumatism and gout, because it eliminates uric acid from the body. Research has shown that an alcoholic extract of the whole plant has an anti-inflammatory activity in rats[2] and may be useful for treating rapid heart beat, heart arrhythmics, and fibrillations, since it mimics the action of one of the alkaloids in cinchona, quinidine, in depressing the heart rate.[3] Chicory also significantly lowers blood sugar, while a sesquiterpene extracted from the roasted root has anti-bacterial activities.[4]

Roast chicory root can be drunk as a coffee substitute or mixed with coffee. The freshly boiled roots are still eaten in the Middle East. The leaves can be used in salads.

Cnicus benedictus (also known as *Carduus benedictus*)
Blessed thistle

Holy thistle, St. Benedict thistle, spotted thistle

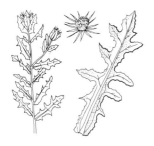

h 27 ins (70 cm). See p. 43.

Parts used Root, aerial parts and seeds.

Constituents Bitter compound (cnicine), alkaloids, mucilage, tannin, small amount of essential oil.

Main uses *Culinary* Boiled root as vegetable. *Medical* Digestive tonic; to increase the flow of breast milk.

Because of its bitter taste, blessed thistle is used as a digestive tonic which stimulates the liver, increasing gastric and bile secretions. It also is reputed to increase the flow of mother's milk. It is diuretic and induces sweating. Used as a poultice or compress, the plant has a reputation for curing chilblains.

CAUTION Strong infusions may be emetic and cause diarrhoea.

Cynara scolymus
Globe artichoke

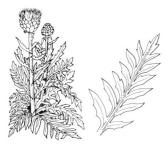

h 3–6 ft (1–2 m). See p. 50.

Parts used Flower heads, leaves, root.

Constituents A bitter principle (cynarin and sesquiterpene lactones), flavonoids including scolymoside, inulin, cynaropictin and several enzymes, taraxasterol, sugars, and a volatile oil.

Main uses *Culinary* Flower heads as vegetable. *Medical* Liver and kidney complaints; arteriosclerosis.

The flower heads of this plant are a common vegetable, but the rest of the plant provides excellent herbal medicine. Two components, cynarin and scolymoside, have been shown to stimulate bile secretion which accords with the traditional use of this remedy for treating sluggish livers and debilitated digestions.[1] Cynarin has also been demonstrated to lower both cholesterol and triglyceride levels in the blood which explains why in Europe the plant is widely used to treat arteriosclerosis.[2] The herb is also diuretic, and is used to treat kidney diseases and protein in the urine.[3]

Echinacea angustifolia, E. purpura, E. pallida
Purple coneflower

Black samson, echinacea, rudbeckia, Missouri snakeroot

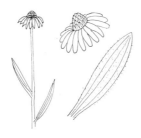

18×12 ins (45×30 cm). See p. 50.

Parts used Dried root and rhizome.

Constituents Essential oil (including humulene and caryophylene), glycoside, polysaccharide, polyacetylenes, isobutylalklamines, resin, betain, inulin, sesquiterpene.

Main uses *Medical* Immune enhancer; for skin diseases and general infections.

A herb valued by North American Indians and frontiersmen of the USA, purple coneflower became a famed remedy for snake bite and for cleansing and healing suppurative wounds. Today herbalists regard it as one of the finest blood cleansers, especially for skin problems, such as boils and abscesses, associated with impure blood.

This herb is also an excellent remedy for tonsillitis, inflamed gums, and for mucus in the nose, sinuses, lungs, and digestive tract. Externally the plant is used to treat wounds or ulcers, where it reduces putrefaction and pain.[1,2,3] A wash of purple coneflower can help relieve the unbearable itching of urticaria and this treatment is also good for stings and bites. The antibiotic effect of the plant has been scientifically verified.[4]

Purple coneflower has a deserved reputation for enhancing the immune system. Research shows that it stimulates the production of white blood cells, which fight infection,[5] and that the polysaccharide has an anti-viral activity.[6,7,8] For this reason, the plant may be useful in treating viral infections such as glandular fever (mononucleosis) and post-viral syndrome (myalgic encephalomyelitis). There is also evidence to show that it is helpful for allergies.[9]

Eupatorium perfoliatum
Boneset

Feverwort, agueweed, thoroughwort

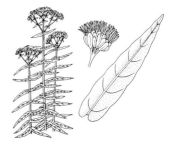

h 2–5 ft (60 cm–1.5 m). See p. 50.

Parts used Aerial parts.

Constituents Flavonoids (including quercetin, kaempferol, rutin and eupatorin), terpenoids (including sesquiterpene lactones), volatile oil, resin.

Main uses *Medical* Colds and flu; digestive tonic.

This was one of the common North American Indian remedies quickly adopted by white settlers in America.

Calendula officinalis
Marigold
Marybud, bull's eyes

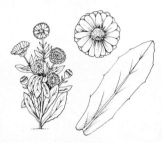

h 20 ins (50 cm)

Parts used Flowers. Cultivation see pp. 274–5.

Constituents Carotenoids, resin, essential oil, flavonoids, sterol, bitter principle, saponins, mucilage.

Main uses *General* Skin creams (see p. 144). *Culinary* Dye for butter or cheese; leaves in salads (see p.170); tea. *Medical* First aid, ulcers, painful periods.

Marigold, in the same family as arnica, displays many of its wound-healing properties. It is antiseptic and anti-bacterial promoting healing so that a compress or poultice of the flowers is excellent first aid for burns, scalds, stings and impetigo. A compress is use-ful to treat varicose veins and chil-blains, while a cold infusion may be used as an eyewash for conjunctivitis. Marigolds are also antifungal and so can help to cure thrush (*Candida albicans*). The sap from the stem has a reputation for removing warts, corns and calluses. Marigold flowers are an excellent remedy for inflamed or ulcer-ated conditions, whether used external-ly as in varicose ulcers (use a poultice) or internally to treat gastritis, gastric, or duodenal ulcers. It is a useful diges-tive remedy because it stimulates the flow of bile. Marigolds are called after the Virgin Mary, a fact which may be connected with the ability of marigold infusions to allay painful menstruation and bring on delayed periods.

CAUTION Avoid during pregnancy.

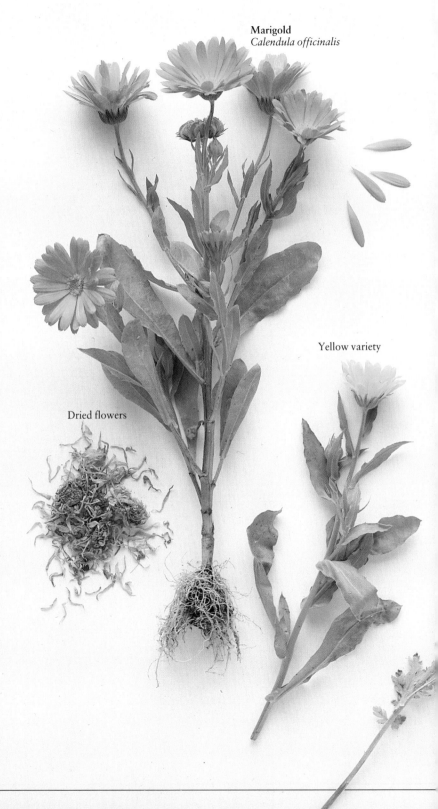

Marigold
Calendula officinalis

Yellow variety

Dried flowers

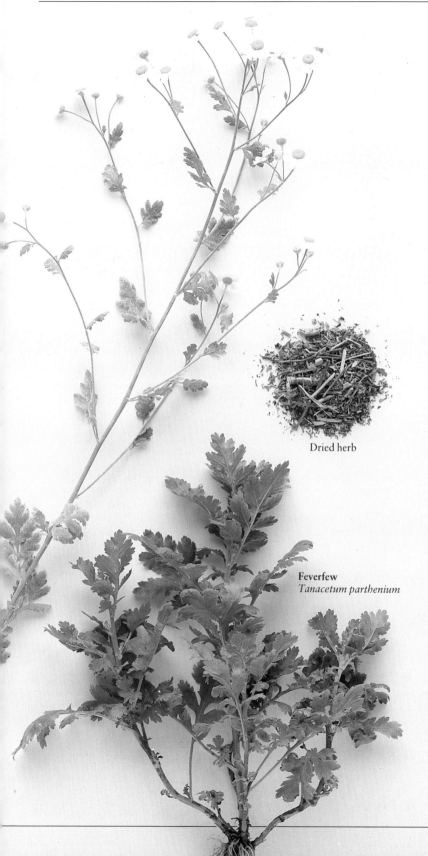

Dried herb

Feverfew
Tanacetum parthenium

Tanacetum parthenium
Feverfew

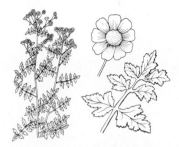

h 2–3 ft (60–90 cm)

Parts used Leaves.

Constituents Sesquiterpene lactones (including parthenolide and santamarine), volatile oil, tannins.

Main uses *Medical* Headaches and migraines, arthritis.

Feverfew is one of a handful of medicinal plants to be thoroughly scientifically investigated. In 1978 several British newspapers carried the story of a woman who had cured her severe migraine headaches with feverfew leaves. In a subsequent clinical study, seven out of ten patients taking feverfew claimed that their migraine attacks were less frequent or less painful or both. In about one in three patients, there were no further attacks. Further clinical studies have revealed that the plant can have other medicinal benefits, apparently allaying nausea and vomiting, relieving the inflammation and pain of arthritis, promoting restful sleep, improving digestion, and relieving asthma attacks. Researchers believe that sesquiterpene lactones in the plant may inhibit prostaglandins and histamine released during the inflammatory process, so preventing spasms of blood vessels in the head that trigger migraine attacks. Over half the feverfew users involved in clinical studies reported *pleasant* side effects. Some people said that feverfew helped their depression. This is in line with traditional use. Culpeper wrote that feverfew in wine might help those "troubled with melancholy and heaviness or sadness of spirits".

CAUTION One side-effect associated with feverfew is mouth ulcers. If this occurs, stop taking the herb.

Its common name, boneset, alludes to its use in treating a virulent form of flu in the USA which was called "break bone fever". Boneset in hot infusion is also an excellent remedy for colds and catarrh. It is also used to treat cases of muscular rheumatism caused by exposure to cold and damp. It is useful for stomach disorders of nervous origin. A tincture of the plant has also been demonstrated to have a weak anti-inflammatory effect.[1] In hot infusion, boneset promotes a therapeutic sweat in fevers. Its stimulation of the peripheral circulation which causes sweating, is probably due to the flavonoids and the essential oil that the plant contains.[2]

Taken in small doses as a tincture or in cold infusion, the remedy has a tonic action on the digestion, but if taken in large doses it can cause diarrhoea and vomiting.

Recent research indicates that the several sesquiterpene lactones in the plant and the flavones in both boneset and gravel root (below) may have an anti-cancer activity.[3]

Eupatorium purpureum
Gravel root

Joe-pye weed, queen of the meadow, purple boneset, kidneywort, trumpet weed, gravel weed

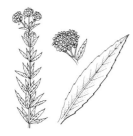

120×24 ins (300×60 cm). See p. 51.

Parts used Rhizome and roots.

Constituents Flavonoids (including eupatorin), volatile oil, resin.

Main uses *Medical* Kidney and urinary infections and stones; prostate inflammation; pelvic inflammatory disease; painful periods; rheumatism and gout.

This diuretic herb is used to treat urinary infections and stones (gravel). It tones the reproductive tract and is used to treat inflammation of the prostate, pelvic inflammatory disease and menstrual cramping. It encourages excretion of excess uric acid and so treats rheumatism and gout. For possible anti-cancer activity see Boneset (above).

Grindelia camporum
Grindelia

Gumplant, tarweed, rosinweed

Parts used Aerial parts.

Constituents Resin (around 20%), volatile oil, saponins (including grindelin), alkaloid, tannins, selenium.

Main uses *Medical* Asthma and bronchitis.

Grindelia is antispasmodic and expectorant, and particularly valuable for treating asthma and bronchitis because of its ability to relax the bronchi and expel phlegm from the airways. It should be used regularly in small doses. Grindelia slows a rapid heart rate and its antispasmodic effect also extends to the arteries so that it tends to lower blood pressure. It may also be used in asthma of cardiac origin. Grindelia can be used to relieve hayfever. Externally it is soothing to insect bites and for poison-ivy rash.

CAUTION Large doses are toxic. Use as directed by a qualified practitioner.

Inula helenium
Elecampane

Scabwort, yellow starwort, wild sunflower

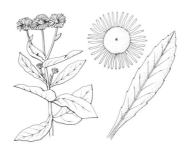

120×40 ins (300×100 cm). See p. 51

Parts used Root and rhizome; in Chinese herbal medicine the flowers are preferred; cultivation, see pp. 276–7.

Constituents Volatile oil (up to 4% including alantolactone, isoalantalactone and azulene), inulin (up to 44%), sterols, resin, pectin, mucilage.

Main uses *Culinary* To flavour bitter digestive liqueurs and vermouths; candied and used in confectionery. *Medical* Respiratory disorders; digestive tonic.

Elecampane's Latin name comes from Helen of Troy, from whose tears it is said to have sprung. The story is perhaps a clue to ancient use of this plant, because it promotes menstruation and is good for treating anaemia. However, the main use of the plant is for the respiratory system. In former times, it was a specific for TB. Recent research on 105 plant lactones found that the alantolactone and isoalantolactone in elecampane were powerful antibacterial and antifungal agents.[1] Today the warming and expectorant elecampane is used to treat asthma, bronchitis, and other pulmonary infections. Its bitter tonic properties stimulate and regulate disordered or weak digestions increasing the flow of bile. Alantolactone in the plant expels worms[2] and the plant has long been used externally for scabies, herpes and other skin diseases from which it gained its country name scabwort. Other scientific research indicates that elecampane has a sedative effect on mice.[3]

Lactuca virosa
Wild lettuce

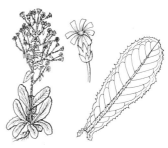

h 5 ft (1.5 m)

Parts used Dried leaves.

Constituents Bitter latex (containing

lactucin, lactucone, lactupicrin), a trace of an alkaloid, triterpenes, iron, vitamins A, B1, B2, and C.

Main uses *General* In soaps, shampoo, and bath bags. *Culinary* Relaxing tea. *Medical* Insomnia, anxiety, irritating coughs.

A wild relative of the garden lettuce, this plant contains a potent milky latex, sometimes called "lettuce opium" because it looks and to some extent acts like that extracted from the poppy. Lettuce latex has been used in cough mixtures to replace opium. The whole plant is sedative, and helps to induce sleep and calm restlessness and anxiety. It has a sedative effect on the respiratory system too, and is used for treating whooping cough and nervous and dry irritating coughs. It can also help to reduce muscle and joint pain but is not a cure for conditions that cause this.

CAUTION Overdosage may cause poisoning.

Matricaria chamomilla
German chamomile

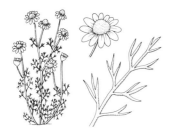

24×4 ins (60×10 cm). See p. 51.

Parts used Dried flowers; cultivation see pp. 276–7.

Constituents Volatile oil (containing chamazulene, farnesene, bisabolol), flavonoids (including rutin and quercimertrin), coumarins (including umbelliferone), plant acids (including valerianic acid), fatty acids, cyanogenic glycosides, salicylate derivatives, polysaccharides, choline, amino acids, tannin.

Main uses *Medical* Insomnia, anxiety, digestive problems of nervous origin.

Modern research substantiates the use of chamomile as a remedy for a broad range of complaints. Chamomile flowers contain a beautiful blue volatile oil (azulene). Two of its components, bisabolol and chamazule, are powerful antiseptics.[1] Chamazulene relieves pain, encourages wound healing, is anti-inflammatory and anti-spasmodic. Applied externally it promotes the recovery of burns and soothes eczema. A recent study shows that bisabolol speeds up the healing of ulcers and can prevent them occurring.[2] In addition, bisabolol has also been shown to be anti-microbial.[3,4] Another constituent, belliferone, has anti-fungal properties.[5] This and chamazulene have been shown to be effective against thrush (*Candida albicans*) and tests using chamazulene showed it to kill the bacteria *Staphylococcus aureus*.[6]

The tea has a sedative action, inducing sleep.[7] In one American hospital, chamomile tea given to a group of 12 patients put ten of them to sleep within ten minutes.[8] Herbalists use the relaxing effect of chamomile tea for restless or hyperactive children and in small amounts for teething babies. It can work in the same way by adding a strong infusion to bath water.

Chamomile is a famous remedy for digestive upsets, flatulence, heartburn, and diarrhoea. A German study shows that it acts on the smooth muscle of the intestine and uterus to relax spasms.[9] So as well as for digestive problems, herbalists sometimes use this plant to relieve painful menstruation and for premenstrual migraines.

The extracted oil diluted in a vegetable oil, rubbed on to the affected part, eases the pain of rheumatism and gout. A compress of chamomile flowers has been used to treat sciatica and ointments containing the oil are antiseptic and soothing for itchy skin conditions like eczema.[10] Steam inhalations can clear phlegm and help asthma and can cleanse the skin in cases of acne. A compress can treat cracked sore nipples and a tea is useful for sore gums and as an eyewash. Its flowers are frequently used in herbal preparations for the hair (such as shampoos and dye).

Roman chamomile (*Anthemis nobilis*) has many of the properties of German chamomile.

CAUTION Large doses may cause vomiting.

Solidago canadensis
Golden rod
Woundwort, Aaron's rod

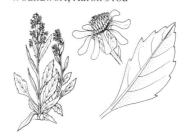

h 3 ft (1 m). See p. 50.

Parts used Flowering tops, leaves.

Constituents Saponins, flavonoids, tannins, essential oil.

Main uses *Medical* Urinary and kidney infections and stones; catarrh.

Good for kidney and urinary infections and stones, golden rod also helps to ease backache caused by these conditions. Because of its cleansing and eliminative action, it can also be used to treat arthritis. Its tannins make it a useful remedy for diarrhoea. In North America, it has a reputation for clearing upper respiratory mucus.

Tanacetum parthenium
Feverfew
See page 47

Tanacetum vulgare (also known as *Chrysanthemum vulgare*)
Tansy

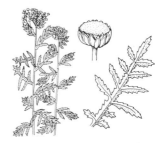

h 2 ft (60 cm). See p. 50.

Parts used Dried aerial parts; cultivation, see pp. 278–9.

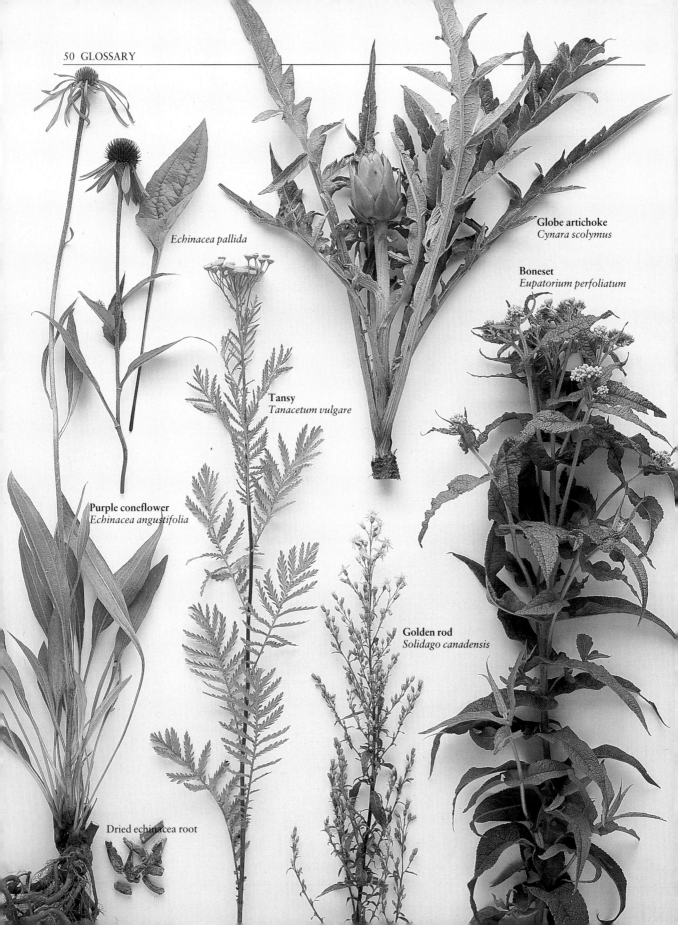

Echinacea pallida

Globe artichoke
Cynara scolymus

Boneset
Eupatorium perfoliatum

Tansy
Tanacetum vulgare

Purple coneflower
Echinacea angustifolia

Golden rod
Solidago canadensis

Dried echinacea root

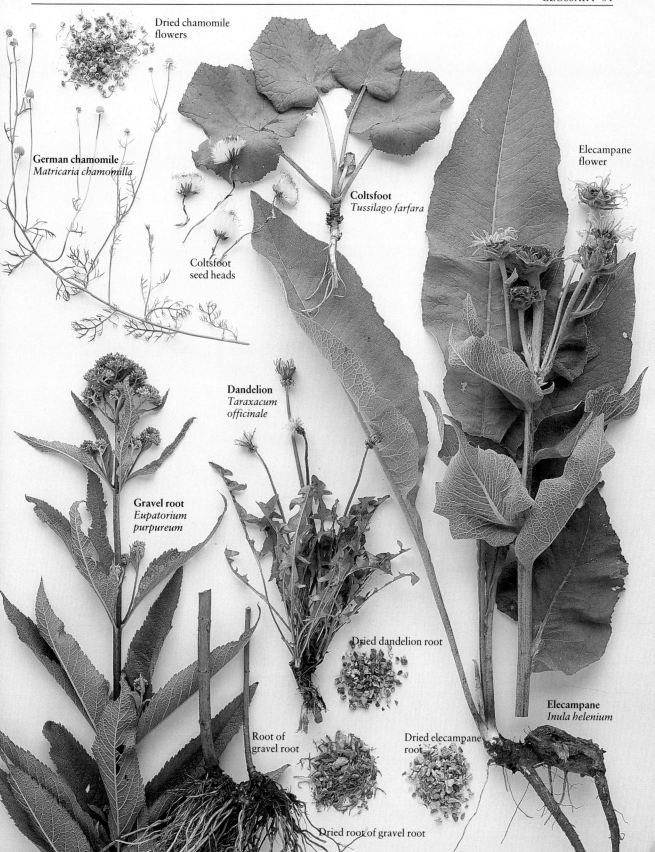

Dried chamomile flowers

German chamomile
Matricaria chamomilla

Coltsfoot
seed heads

Coltsfoot
Tussilago farfara

Elecampane
flower

Dandelion
*Taraxacum
officinale*

Gravel root
*Eupatorium
purpureum*

Dried dandelion root

Root of
gravel root

Dried elecampane
root

Elecampane
Inula helenium

Dried root of gravel root

Constituents Volatile oil (containing up to 70% thujone), bitter glycosides, sesquiterpene lactones, terpenoids including pyrethrins, tannin, resin, vitamin C, citric acid, oxalic acid.

Main uses *General* Insect repellent (see p. 160). *Medical* To expel worms.

Tansy, like wormwood, is rich in thujone which is potentially damaging to the central nervous system if taken in too large doses or for too long. However, in the hands of a trained herbalist it is useful for expelling worms (roundworm and threadworm). Externally tansy tea can be used as a wash to treat scabies and as a compress to bring relief to painful rheumatic joints. Tansy was one of the herbs strewn on the floor in the Middle Ages to deter fleas and other insects.

CAUTION Tansy is a strong emmenagogue (provoking the onset of a period) and should not be used in pregnancy. It can be fatal when taken in large doses.

Taraxacum officinale
Dandelion
Pee in the bed, lion's teeth, fairy clock

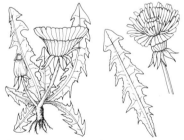

h to 1 ft (30 cm). See p. 51.

Parts used All.

Constituents Root: the bitter principle taraxacin, triterpenes (including taraxol and taraxasterol), sterols, inulin, sugars, pectin, glycosides, choline, phenolic acids, asparagine, vitamins, potassium. Leaves: lutein, violaxanthin, and other carotenoids; bitter substances; vitamins A, B, C, D (the vitamin A content is higher than that of carrots); potassium and iron.

Main uses *Culinary* Leaves in salads

(see pp. 170–1); root as coffee substitute. Flowers as wine. *Medical* As digestive tonic for constipation, liver and gallbladder disease, rheumatism, and skin diseases.

The humble dandelion is one of nature's great medicines. The root is a mildly laxative bitter tonic, valuable in dyspepsia and constipation.[1] It stimulates the liver and gallbladder (mainly due to its taraxacin content), substantially increasing the flow of bile.[2,3,4] It is useful in diseases of the liver and gallbladder. The leaves, which in spring are excellent in salads, are a powerful diuretic as attested to by one of its common English names "pee in the bed", exactly echoed in France as "pis en lit".[5] The diuretic power of the dandelion has been favourably compared with a common diuretic drug, Frusemide.[6] However, unlike conventional diuretics, dandelion does not leach potassium from the body; its rich potassium content replaces that which the body loses.[7] Dandelion cleanses the blood and tissues, and is useful in the treatment of skin diseases and rheumatism. Application of the plant's sap is said to remove warts, while the flowers make an excellent country wine.

In China, a related species, *Taraxacum mongolicum*, has been used to treat infections, particularly mastitis.

Tussilago farfara
Coltsfoot
Ass's foot, horse's hoof, hallfoot, the son before the fathers

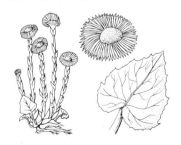

h 3–12 ins (8–30 cm). See p. 51.

Parts used Flowers and leaves.

Constituents Mucilage, alkaloid, saponins, tannin (especially in the leaf), zinc, potassium, calcium.

Main uses *Medical* Colds and coughs; as a poultice for sores.

The Latin name signifies coltsfoot's ancient use for coughs for which for centuries it has been smoked as tobacco, or taken as a tisane or as a syrup. In former times a replica of the coltsfoot flower was to be found above the door of pharmacies in Paris, an emblem of the effectiveness of their medicine.

Today, coltsfoot retains its importance for it combines an effective expectorant action with the soothing and healing qualities of the mucilage it contains. It is good for most respiratory problems as well as colds. The fresh leaves applied externally as a poultice to ulcers and sores are soothing and healing, an effect due in part to the zinc the plant contains. Coltsfoot contains a low content of the pyrrolizidine alkaloid senkirkine which by itself may damage the liver.[1] However, trials in Sweden found that a decoction boiled for 30 minutes contained no detectable pyrrolizidine alkaloids while further research indicates that the abundant mucilage in the plant made the minute amount of alkaloid in the plant safe.[2]

CAUTION There is medical controversy about this plant; it is best to avoid excessive consumption.

CRUCIFERAE

Brassica nigra
Black mustard

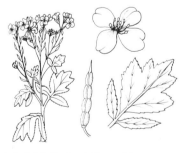

h 3–10 ft (1–3 m). See p. 54.

Parts used Seeds and leaves.

Constituents A glycoside (sinigrin) and an enzyme (myrosin); on contact with water, myrosin acts on sinigrin, setting free allyl isothiocyanate (mustard oil) responsible for mustard's pungent smell. Also: fixed oils (up to 37%), proteins, mucilage.

Main uses *Culinary* With meat, in sauces, soups, and dressings. *Medical* Coughs, colds and indigestion.

Mustard oil is strongly antibacterial and anti-fungal but it can blister the skin.[1,2] Mustard warms and stimulates the digestive system. The seeds make an excellent stimulating poultice (mixed with a soothing substance such as slippery elm powder) for stubborn coughs and arthritis joints. Mustard foot baths are good for poor circulation, chilblains, and upper respiratory mucus.

CAUTION See horseradish, right.

Capsella bursa-pastoris
Shepherd's purse
Witch's pouches, pickpocket, pepper and salt, mother's heart

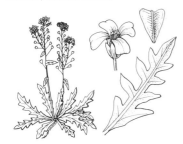

h 1 ft (30 cm). See p. 55.

Parts used Dried or fresh aerial parts.

Constituents Choline, acetylcholine and tyramine, saponins, mustard oil, flavonoids.

Main uses *Culinary* Leaves can be eaten as vegetable. *Medical* To stop bleeding; for varicose veins.

Shepherd's purse, which gains its name from the purse-like shape of its seed pods, is one of the most important herbs to stop bleeding, an effect due to the tyramine and other amines it contains. The herb is diuretic, due in part to its mustard oil. It is good for urinary infections, blood in the urine, and profuse menstruation. Such symptoms must always be investigated by a medical practitioner. It is also a useful remedy for haemorrhoids, for varicose veins and to halt nosebleeds. The leaves are eaten as a cabbage in many places.

Cochlearia armoracia (also known as *Armoracia rusticana*)
Horseradish

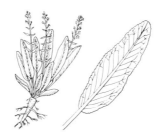

h 5 ft (1.5 m). See p. 54.

Parts used Fresh root.

Constituents Sinigrin (a glycoside which combined with water yields mustard oil), vitamin C, asparagin, resin.

Main uses *Culinary* In sauces and vinegars. *Medical* As circulatory and digestive stimulant.

Horseradish is a powerful circulatory stimulant with antibiotic properties due to the mustard oil it contains. It is effective for lung and urinary infections because mustard oil is excreted through these channels. Its diuretic effect is due to asparagin. It is taken internally for gout and rheumatism. The root must be used fresh; you should grate it outside (to avoid getting the acrid essential oil in the eyes) and combine it with cider vinegar and honey. Use it externally as a poultice for rheumatic joints and to stimulate blood flow.

CAUTION Overuse may blister the skin. Do not use it if your thyroid function is low or if taking thyroxine.

Nasturtium officinale
Watercress

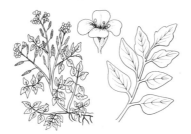

h 12 ins (30 cm). See p. 54.

Parts used Stems and leaves.

Constituents Vitamins A, C and E, nicotinamide, a glycoside, gluconasturtin, volatile oil, manganese, iron, phosphorus, iodine, copper, calcium.

Main uses *Culinary* In soups and salads (see p. 170). *Medical* Coughs, indigestion, gout, and arthritis.

Hippocrates described watercress as a stimulant and expectorant, and herbalists still make use of these properties in the plant to treat coughs and bronchitis. Its stimulating qualities and the minerals it contains make watercress important nutritionally, useful in convalescence and general debility. It invigorates the digestion and is diuretic, helping the body to unload toxic wastes from the tissues and blood. It lowers blood sugar. Chewed raw it invigorates and strengthens the gums. Pulped with sea salt, it makes a healing poultice for gout and arthritis.

CAUTION Wild watercress may be host to the deadly liver fluke. Use only plants grown commercially in watercress beds.

CUPRESSACEAE

Juniperus communis
Juniper

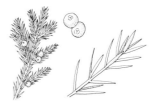

h 20 ft (6 m). See p. 55.

Parts used Berries (the female cone).

Constituents Volatile oil (major components pinene, myrcene, sabinene, also limonene, terpinene, camphene and thujone), sugars, vitamin C, flavonoids, resin, gallotannins.

Main uses *Culinary* To flavour gin and liqueurs. *Medical* Cystitis, for rheumatism and gout.

Due to their oil, juniper berries are a potent diuretic, imparting to the urine a

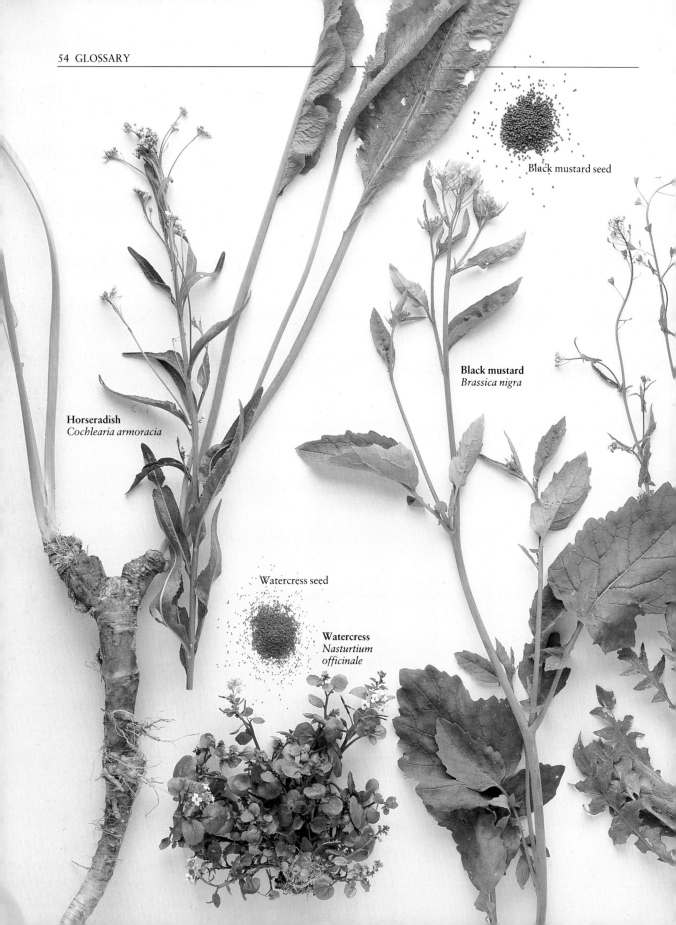

Black mustard seed

Black mustard
Brassica nigra

Horseradish
Cochlearia armoracia

Watercress seed

Watercress
Nasturtium officinale

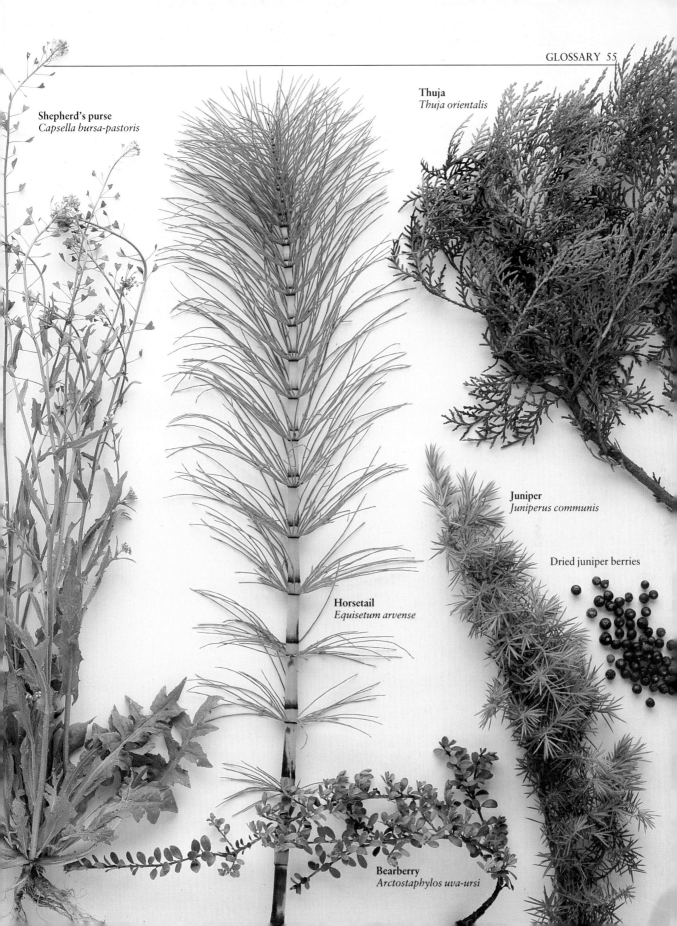

Shepherd's purse
Capsella bursa-pastoris

Thuja
Thuja orientalis

Juniper
Juniperus communis

Dried juniper berries

Horsetail
Equisetum arvense

Bearberry
Arctostaphylos uva-ursi

smell of violets. The oil is antiseptic, making the plant valuable in treating cystitis and urethritis. Juniper berries are a warming tonic for debilitated digestions and help relieve flatulence. Chewed, the berries sweeten the breath and heal infected gums. External frictions of the diluted essential oil ease neuralgia, sciatica and rheumatic pains. Steam inhalations of the berries are an excellent treatment for colds, coughs and excessive phlegm.

CAUTION Do not use juniper during pregnancy or where there is kidney disease. The internal use of the volatile oil is dangerous and only for professionals.

Thuja occidentalis
Thuja
Arbor vitae, tree of life, white cedar, yellow cedar, American cedar

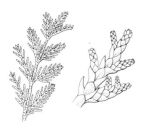

h 50 ft (15 m). See p. 55.

Parts used Leaves and young twigs.

Constituents Volatile oil (comprising up to 65% thujone, also fenchone, borneol, limonene, pinene, camphor, myrcene), flavonoid glycoside, mucilage, tannin.

Main uses *Medical* Bronchitis and excessive phlegm.

Thuja was an old North American Indian remedy for delayed menstruation; scientific research has shown that it is a stimulant to smooth muscles, such as those of the uterus and bronchial passages.[1] Its stimulating expectorant effect is useful for treating bronchitis. Externally, herbalists use an infusion as a wash for infectious skin diseases such as impetigo or scabies. An ointment is a reputed cure for warts. A hot compress eases rheumatic pains.

CAUTION Not to be used in pregnancy. Thujone, the main constituent of the volatile oil, is toxic in any quantity so the herb should only be taken in small doses and for no more than a week or two at a time. Thuja should be used as prescribed by a qualified practitioner.

DIOSCOREACEAE

Dioscorea villosa
Wild yam
Colic root, rheumatism root

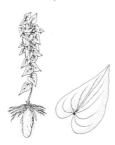

Parts used Root and rhizome.

Constituents Steroidal saponins (including dioscin and trillin which yield diosgenin), phytosterols, alkaloids including dioscorine, tannins, starch.

Main uses *Medical* Rheumatoid arthritis, colic, threatened miscarriage, menstrual cramps.

In 1943 the scientist Russell Marker astonished the world when, on a shoestring budget, he made two kilos of the female hormone progesterone from the wild Mexican yam (*Dioscorea mexicana*). Until 1970, diosgenin derived from the wild yam was the sole source of the hormonal material used to make the contraceptive pill.

Wild yam has traditionally been used for easing menstrual cramping and for threatened miscarriage. Its antispasmodic action makes it good for flatulence and colic caused by muscle spasm. The herb also promotes the flow of bile and so is sometimes used to ease the colic of gallstones. Wild yam is anti-inflammatory (again because of its steroidal saponins) and herbalists prescribe it for the inflammatory stage of rheumatoid arthritis. This plant also has a diuretic effect which, combined with its antispasmodic property, makes it benefit painful conditions of the urinary tract. Its antispasmodic action also makes it useful for treating poor circulation and neuralgia.

EPHEDRACEAE

Ephedra sinica
Ephedra

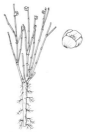

h 6–48 ins (15–120 cm)

Parts used Dried young stems.

Constituents Alkaloids (including ephedrine, norephedrine, methyl ephedrine, pseudoephedrine), tannins, saponin, flavone, essential oil.

Main uses *Medical* Asthma, hayfever.

Used in Chinese medicine for thousands of years, this herb is the source of the alkaloid ephedrine, first extracted in 1885. Ephedrine was hailed as a cure for asthma because of its power to relax the airways. Once in common use, however, the isolated drug was found to raise blood pressure markedly, and it is now hardly ever used to treat asthma. Herbalists, however, use the whole plant which contains six other related alkaloids, one of which, pseudoephedrine, actually reduces the heart rate and lowers blood pressure. This plant has been used in China for thousands of years, yet no undesirable side-effects have been recorded from the proper administration of the whole plant.

Ephedra is used to treat asthma, hayfever and other allergies. In China it is also used for the first stages of a cold or influenza (its volatile oil inhibits the influenza virus) and for arthritis and fluid retention. In the USA a related species, known as mormon tea or desert tea, has also been used for fever and for kidney and bladder problems.

CAUTION The herb should be avoided in severe hypertension, glaucoma, hyperthyroidism, prostate enlargement, and coronary thrombosis; it should not be taken by anyone using MAOI antidepressant.

RESTRICTED.

EQUISETACEAE

Equisetum arvense
Horsetail
Mare's tail, shave grass, bottlebrush, pewterwort

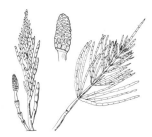

h 8–32 ins (20–80 cm). See p. 55.

Parts used Aerial parts.

Constituents Silica (up to 70% in soluble form), saponins (including equisetonin), traces of alkaloids (nicotine, palustrine and palustrinine), flavonoids, manganese, potassium, sulphur, magnesium, tannin.

Main uses *General* Cosmetics and hair shampoos (see p. 146); dried stems as metal polish (see p. 152). *Medical* Urinary infections and stones; lung complaints and arteriosclerosis.

In prehistoric times horsetail grew as high as trees; though smaller in size, the modern descendant is a potent medicinal plant. The herb is a major source of silica, and so it was regularly prescribed for lungs damaged by TB.[1,2] The plant is a storehouse of minerals and is recommended in cases of anaemia and general debility. Horsetail tea is good for broken nails and lifeless hair. It is also useful when white spotting occurs on the nails (a symptom said to indicate a calcium imbalance in the body). Its silica encourages the absorption and use of calcium by the body and also helps to guard against fatty deposits in the arteries.[3,4] Horsetail's astringent action stops bleeding, making it valuable for treating stomach ulcers. It has a mild diuretic effect but its astringency makes it useful in the treatment of bedwetting in children.[5] It is also used to treat an inflamed or enlarged prostate, cystitis and urinary stones.

ERICACEAE

Arctostaphylos uva-ursi
Bearberry
Uva ursi, beargrape, hogberry, rockberry, mountain cranberry

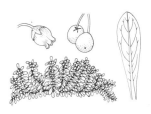

h 6 ins (15 cm). See p. 55.

Parts used Leaves.

Constituents Arbutin (about 8%), methyl arbutin, flavonoids, allantoin, tannins, phenolic acids, volatile oil, resin.

Main uses *Medical* Cystitis.

Used in traditional medicine in the Middle Ages, bearberry is a diuretic herb. In the body the arbutin in the plant converts to hydroquinone, a urinary disinfectant.[1] This is especially effective with alkaline urine, which can be achieved by observing a vegetarian diet.[2]

CAUTION Long-term use of bearberry may produce toxic effects, since large doses of hydroquinone are poisonous. Normal medicinal use, however, is perfectly safe.

Erica vulgaris (also known as *Calluna vulgaris*)
Heather
See page 58

EUPHORBIACEAE

Euphorbia hirta (and *E. pilulifera*)
Pill-bearing spurge
Asthma weed, Queensland asthma weed, catshair

Parts used Aerial parts.

Constituents Glycoside, alkaloid, triterpenoids, sterols, tannin.

Main uses *Medical* Asthma.

This common tropical plant causes relaxation of the bronchi, making it easier for asthmatics to breathe. It is also helpful for clearing upper-respiratory phlegm and hayfever. In the tropics it is used to treat amoebic dysentery.

CAUTION Although this is one of the few members of the spurge family not poisonous to humans, overlarge doses may cause nausea and vomiting.

Stillingia sylvatica
Queen's delight
Queen's root, yawroot

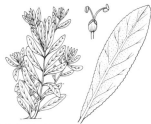

h 3 ft (1 m)

Parts used Root (not more than two years old).

Constituents Volatile oil (up to 4%), acrid fixed oil, acrid resin (sylvacrol), tannins, calcium oxalate, cyanogenic glycosides, starch.

Main uses *Medical* Respiratory complaints; skin diseases.

Once thought to be a reliable cure for syphilis (which it is not), Queen's delight is now used as a stimulating expectorant to treat bronchitis and laryngitis when the cough is harsh (the herb promotes the flow of saliva). In small doses it is laxative and diuretic; in large doses it is cathartic and emetic. It also has a considerable reputation as a blood cleanser for treating skin conditions.

CAUTION Large doses of this herb can irritate mucous membranes and it should always be used with care.

Calluna vulgaris (also known as *Erica vulgaris*)
Heather
Heath, ling

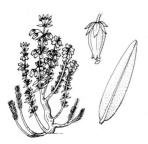

h 6 ins–3 ft (15–100 cm)

Parts used Fresh flowering tops.

Constituents Alkaloid, arbutin, citric and fumaric acids, volatile oil, tannin, flavonoids, carotene.

Main uses *Medical* Urinary disease.

Heather has a long history of use in traditional medicine. It has a reputation as a mild sedative, but its most important property for modern herbalists is its action as a urinary antiseptic, due to the arbutin it contains (see Bearberry, p.57). It is also employed to treat gout and rheumatism. A bath of heather water can help to relieve rheumatic pains. Numerous other decorative species of heather are available to the gardener.

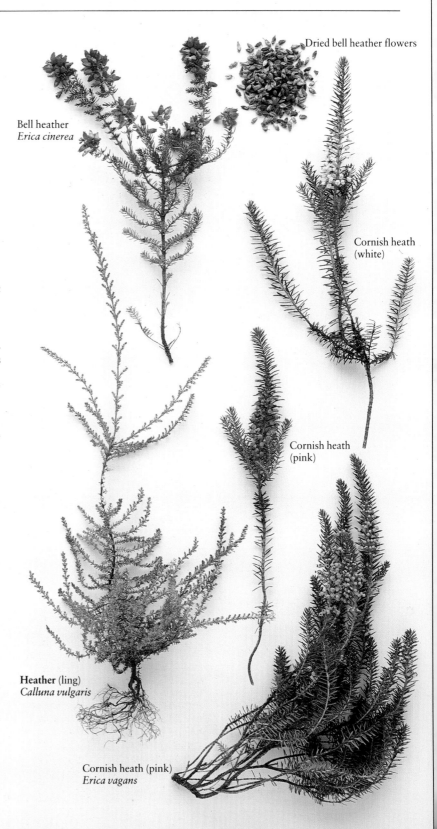

Dried bell heather flowers

Bell heather
Erica cinerea

Cornish heath (white)

Cornish heath (pink)

Heather (ling)
Calluna vulgaris

Cornish heath (pink)
Erica vagans

FAGACEAE

Quercus robur
Oak

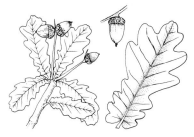

h up to 130 ft (40 m). See p. 63.

Parts used Bark.

Constituents Up to 20% tannin, gallic acid, ellagitannin.

Main uses *General* Dyeing (see pp. 158–9). *Medical* Sore throats, piles, varicose veins and bleeding.

Oak bark is a powerful astringent, possessing the therapeutic qualities of plants rich in tannins. It was once generally used in the leather industry for tanning. The powdered bark used as snuff is good for nosebleeds. As a gargle, a decoction is excellent for throat infections. Taken internally, oak bark stops the acute diarrhoea of gastroenteritis. Used as a douche it is useful for leucorrhoea, and as an ointment for piles. Externally a cold compress is good for burns and cuts.

FUCACEAE

Fucus vesiculosus
Bladderwrack
Kelp

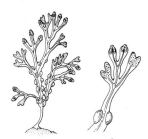

Variable in size. See p. 63.

Parts used Whole plant.

Constituents Mucilage, mannitol, volatile oil, potassium, iodine and many other minerals.

Main uses *Medical* To supply minerals to the body; for rheumatism.

This seaweed was the original source of iodine, discovered in 1812. The weight-reducing reputation of bladderwrack is probably due to its effect on an underactive thyroid.[1] The main herbal use of bladderwrack is to remineralize the body. External compresses and plasters are used to reduce the inflammation and pain of arthritis.

FUMARIACEAE

Corydalis bulbosa
Corydalis

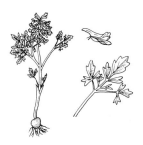

h 6–10 ins (15–25 cm)

Parts used Tuber and rhizome.

Constituents Alkaloids (corydaline, corybulbine, isocorybulbine, corycavidine, corycavamine, corydine, bulbocapriine, protopine, tetrahydropalmatine and at least ten others).

Main uses *Medical* Pain relief.

This powerful plant is the source of the alkaloid bulbocapriine which was used in orthodox medicines to treat convulsions, Parkinson's disease and Menière's disease. In Chinese traditional medicine, corydalis is a major pain reliever used particularly for menstrual cramping, gastric and abdominal pain, and headaches. According to Chinese research, Corydalis has an analgesic effect approximately 1% that of the strength of opium.

CAUTION This herb should only be used by trained herbalists.

RESTRICTED.

Fumaria officinalis
Fumitory
Earth smoke

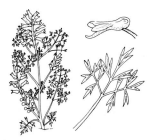

h 6–27 ins (15–70 cm). See p. 62.

Parts used Aerial parts.

Constituents 7 alkaloids (including fumarine and protopine), bitter principles, tannic acid, fumaric acid, mucilage, resin, potassium.

Main uses *General* Yellow dye from flowers. *Medical* Eczema.

The name fumitory derives from the plant's smoke-like appearance when viewed from afar. It has a long history of use for the treatment of skin diseases. It is mildly laxative, diuretic, and stimulates the flow of bile.[1]

CAUTION Large doses can cause diarrhoea.

GENTIANACEAE

Erythraea centaurium (also known as *Centaurium erythraea*)
Centaury
European centaury, bitterherb, centaury gentian

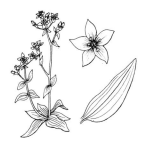

h 4 ins-1 ft (10–30 cm). See p. 71.

Parts used Dried flowering aerial parts.

Constituents Several bitter glycosides (gentiopicrin, centapicrin, swietiamarin, gentioflavoside), alkaloids (gentianine, gentianidine, gentioflavine), phenolic acids, tritepenes, wax.

Main uses *Medical* As digestive tonic; for rheumatism and gout.

Centaury, a member of the gentian family, shares several constituents with gentian, as well as its bitter tonic effect. Taken before meals, it stimulates the gastric secretions and the liver and gallbladder so it is a useful herb for the digestion. This is why it is used in vermouth and several bitter liqueurs. It is gently laxative and taken after meals is an excellent remedy for heartburn. It can also reinforce the action of antiworm herbs.

Like many bitter tonics centaury is effective in reducing fever and has been used in place of quinine. Research indicates that this action is due in part to its phenolic acid.[1] Another constituent, gentiopicrin, has been reported to have antimalarial properties.[2] Research also confirms the plant's potential for treating rheumatism and gout, for the alkaloid gentianine has exhibited strongly anti-inflammatory properties.[3]

This plant has several other healing properties. The famous German herbalist Father Sebastian Kneipp, recommended centaury for melancholy and for calming the nerves. In Egypt the plant is used to treat high blood pressure and kidney stones.[4] All over Europe it is used to remedy anaemia and liver and gallbladder disease.

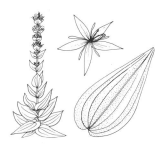

Gentiana lutea
Gentian
Yellow gentian, bitter root

h 43 ins (110 cm)

Parts used Dried root and rhizome.

Constituents Bitter glycosides (amarogentin, gentiopicrin, sweitiamarin), alkaloids (including gentianine and gentialutine), xanthones (including gentisein and gentisin), triterpenes, sugars, volatile oil.

Main uses *Medical* Digestive tonic.

Gentian root is called after Gentius, King of Illyria in the 1st century BC who is said to have discovered the plant's medicinal properties. Gentian contains one of the most bitter substances known, the glycoside amarogentin. Its bitters improve the appetite, promoting digestive juices, peristalsis and the flow of bile. Gentian is also useful for gastro-intestinal inflammation (one of its alkaloids, gentianine, has been shown to be anti-inflammatory), and for controlling fevers. The root is used in many bitter liqueurs.

CAUTION Large doses may cause vomiting.

GERANIACEAE

Geranium maculatum
American cranesbill
Spotted cranesbill, alum root, crowfoot, spotted geranium

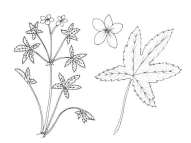

22 × 12 ins (55 × 30 cm). See p. 62.

Parts used Rhizome.

Constituents Tannic and gallic acids (up to 25%), resin.

Main uses *Medical* For diarrhoea, sore throats and stopping bleeding.

The tannins in this plant make it useful in treating diarrhoea, haemhorrage of the digestive tract, and (used locally) piles. An infusion also makes a good mouthwash for gum problems and a gargle for sore throats. Externally the powdered root can be used to stop bleeding.

GRAMINEAE

Agropyron repens
Couch grass
Twitch grass, witchgrass, dog's grass, scutch, quick grass, triticum

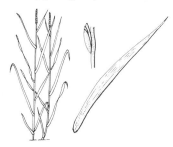

h 1–4 ft (30–120 cm). See p. 62.

Parts used Rhizome.

Constituents About 8% triticin, 3% inositol and mannitol, fixed oil, vitamins A and B, vanillin glycoside, saponin, mucilage, potassium silica, iron, a small amount of volatile oil (largely composed of agropyrone).

Main uses *Medical* Urinary tract disorders, urinary stones; prostatitis.

Couch grass is a curse to gardeners, but a blessing to herbalists. It is a soothing diuretic with antibiotic properties, making it an ideal herb for the urinary system.[1] The agropyrone in its volatile oil has been shown to have broad antibiotic properties.[2] A decoction is used to treat urinary tract infections, stones, and prostatitis. French herbalists use the leaves of couch grass to stimulate the liver and gallbladder.

Avena sativa
Oat

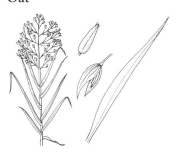

h 2–4 ft (60–120 cm)

Parts used Whole plant and seed.

Constituents Saponins, alkaloids (trigonelline and avenine), a sterol, flavonoids, starch, protein (gluten), fats, minerals (including silica, iron, calcium, copper, magnesium, zinc), vitamin B.

Main uses *Culinary* In porridge, muesli, oatmeal pastries, and oatcakes. *Medical* As a nerve tonic; for depression and insomnia.

Oats, with their vitamins, minerals, and protein, are valuable nutritionally. In addition, they provide an excellent nerve tonic. The alkaloid avenine stimulates the central nervous system – it is the component which causes horses fed on substantial quantities of oats to become highly excitable. The whole plant in medicinal doses provides a range of therapeutic and nutritional substances that feed a debilitated nervous system, making this a valuable remedy for exhaustion, convalescence, and depression.

CAUTION Over-large doses may cause headaches at the back of the head.

Zea mays
Corn
Indian corn, maize

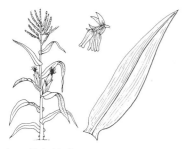

h to 12 ft (4m).

Parts used Stigma and styles.

Constituents Fats, volatile oil, gums, resin, glycosides, saponins, alkaloids, vitamins C and K, sterols, plant acids, tannin, allantoin, potassium and calcium.

Main uses *Culinary* As corn on the cob; in maize flour, for use in baking nutritious corn breads. *Medical* For urinary tract infections and stones.

The "beard" that comes with corn on the cob is corn silk, which makes an excellent soothing diuretic and so is an important herb for urinary tract infections, also helping the passage of urinary stones. French herbalists use it to thin the bile and to promote its flow. (Chinese research work also indicates that it increases the output of bile.)[1] Finally, corn silk is used by some herbalists to lower the blood pressure.

HAMAMELIDACEAE

Hamamelis virginiana
Witch hazel
Spotted alder, winterbloom, snapping hazelnut

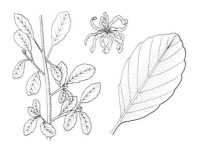

h 5–8 ft (1.5–2.5–m). See p. 63.

Parts used Leaves and bark; as distilled Witch hazel water.

Constituents Tannin (up to 10% in the leaf, consisting mainly of gallotannins, also condensed catechins and proanthocyanidins), saponins, choline, resins, flavonoids. The bark also contains a little volatile oil and fixed oil, and up to 6% tannin.

Main uses *Medical* Bruises, bleeding, haemorrhoids and varicose veins.

This is a North American Indian remedy. Ointment or suppositories containing witch hazel are effective for piles, and a compress is helpful when applied to varicose veins. Herbalists use a weak cold decoction as an eyewash to treat conjunctivitis, while as a compress it is one of the best remedies for bruises and to stop bleeding. Witch hazel water, obtained by distillation, contains no tannins, but appears equally effective.

HIPPOCASTANACEAE

Aesculus hippocastanum
Horse chestnut

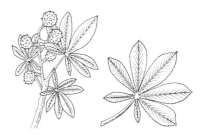

h up to 120 ft (35 m). See p. 63.

Parts used Fruit, bark.

Constituents Saponins (including aescine), flavonoids, coumarins, tannins (bark contains no saponins).

Main uses *Medical* To strengthen veins; ointment for haemorrhoids.

The astringent tannins, flavonoids, and saponins in horse chestnut combine to tone and strengthen the vein walls. In an ointment it is a first-rate remedy for haemorrhoids. It is also used to treat prostatic enlargement.

CAUTION The nuts are poisonous.

HYPERICACEAE

Hypericum perforatum
St John's wort
Common St John's wort

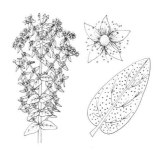

h 1–2 ft (30–60 cm). See p. 63.

Parts used Aerial parts.

Constituents Glycosides (including a red pigment, hypericin), flavonoids, tannins, resin, volatile oil.

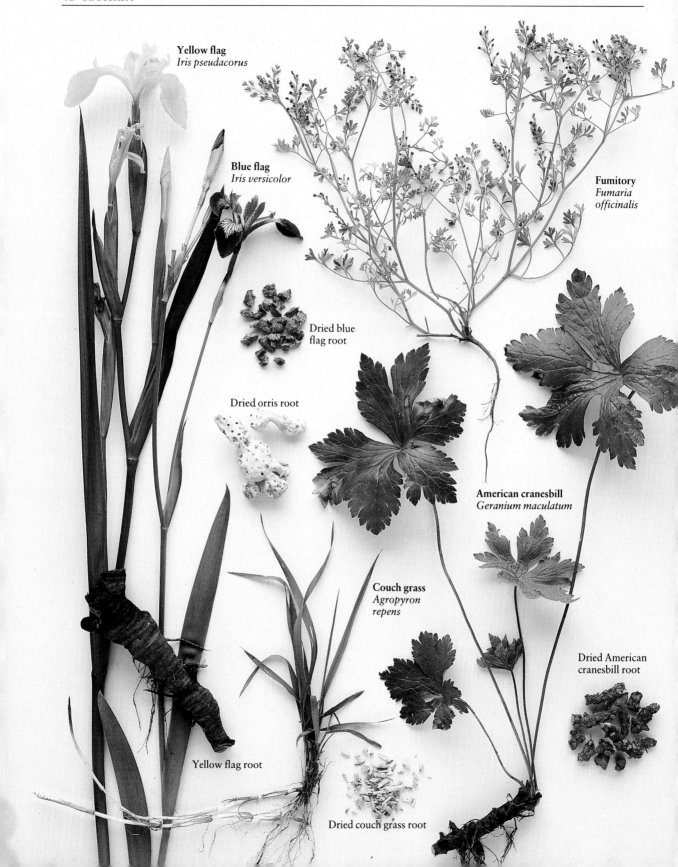

Yellow flag
Iris pseudacorus

Blue flag
Iris versicolor

Fumitory
*Fumaria
officinalis*

Dried blue
flag root

Dried orris root

American cranesbill
Geranium maculatum

Couch grass
*Agropyron
repens*

Dried American
cranesbill root

Yellow flag root

Dried couch grass root

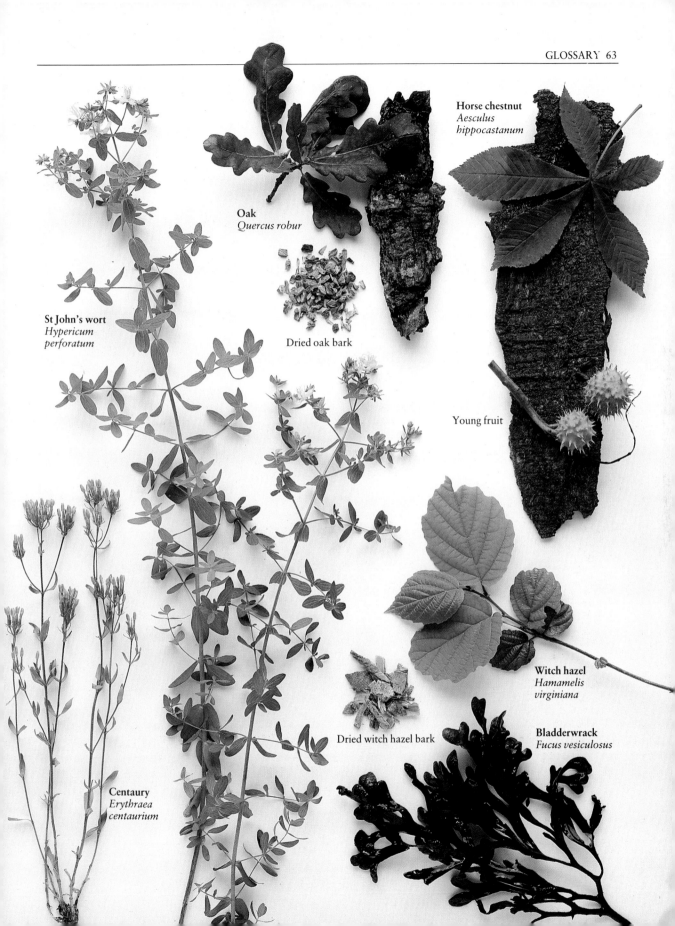

Oak
Quercus robur

Horse chestnut
Aesculus hippocastanum

Dried oak bark

St John's wort
Hypericum perforatum

Young fruit

Witch hazel
Hamamelis virginiana

Dried witch hazel bark

Centaury
Erythraea centaurium

Bladderwrack
Fucus vesiculosus

Main uses *Medical* Cuts, burns, neuralgia, depression.

St John's wort has an ancient reputation for warding off witchcraft which may be due to the plant's wide range of medicinal uses. It is effective as a compress for dressing wounds. In the Middle Ages it was commonly used to heal deep sword cuts. More recently, German research confirms the plant's antibacterial action.[1] The oil, extracted by macerating the flowers in vegetable oil, is excellent applied externally for neuralgia and can ease the pain of sciatica. This oil is also soothing for burns since it lowers the temperature of the skin and it is said to heal gastritis and stomach ulcers. St John's wort is also diuretic, helping to eliminate waste materials from the body.[2] Because of this, an infusion is recommended for gout and arthritis. The herb is used as an expectorant for treating bronchitis and a major use is to calm the nervous system and treat depression, particularly during menopause. The tea also eases menstrual cramps.

CAUTION This herb can cause sensitivity to sunlight. It is rated unsafe by the U.S. Food and Drug Administration. Avoid prolonged use.

IRIDACEAE

Crocus sativus
Saffron

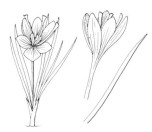

h to 18 ins (45 cm). See p. 34.

Parts used Dried stigmas and tops of styles.

Constituents Essential oil (8–10% containing terpenes, terpene alcohols and esters), crocin (a coloured glycoside), picrocrocin (a colourless, bitter glycoside).

Main uses *Culinary* In Asian and Mediterranean cuisines as dye for rice dishes, desserts and with lamb and poultry.

Saffron, one of the world's costliest spices, was prized by the ancients and is shown in Cretan paintings of 1600 BC. Quantities were exported from Persia and Asia Minor to China. In Britain, saffron's sweetish aromatic odour and orange yellow colour made it popular as an addition to traditional Cornish cakes. The French fish soup, bouillabaisse, Spanish paella, and Milanese risotto are all coloured and flavoured with saffron. It is used widely in Asian cuisine but because saffron growing is a laborious process and the price correspondingly high, turmeric is now often used as a substitute. Saffron cannot be used for fabric dyeing because it is water-soluble.

Iris florentina, Iris germanica
Orris

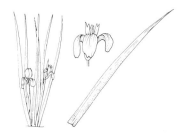

Parts used Root.

Constituents Volatile oil (0.1–0.2% containing irone which has the odour of violets), starch, resin, tannic acid, sugars.

Main uses *General* As fixative in perfumes and pot-pourris (see pp. 154–5) and generally for its perfume.

Orris is the violet-scented powdered root which has been used in perfumery since Greek and Roman times. The white Florentine iris, widely cultivated there in the Middle Ages, is still represented on the heraldic arms of that city. Powdered orris root was popular in the 18th century as a hair powder. Today, if ill health or lack of time prevents hair washing, powdered orris root is sometimes used as a dry shampoo. It removes grease and has a pleasant smell. Once used as a remedy for chest complaints, and a purgative, it is now rarely used medicinally.

Snake's head iris (*Hermodactylus tuberosa*, also known as *Iris tuberosa*) is cultivated in Europe but its use as a medicinal plant has declined. The beautiful yellow flag (*Iris pseudacorus*), was also once used medicinally but is now mainly used as a decorative garden plant. The flowers produce a yellow dye, while the rhizome yields a grey or black dye when used with an iron mordant.

Iris versicolor
Blue flag
Flag lily

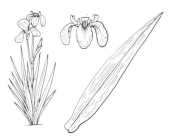

h 40 ins (1 m). See p. 62.

Parts used Dried rhizome.

Constituents Acrid resin (irisin), volatile oil, starch, salicylates, alkaloid, tannin.

Main uses *Medical* Blood purifier, skin complaints.

Blue flag was a common North American Indian remedy, once included in the United States Pharmacopeia. Amongst herbalists it still has the reputation as a blood purifier and effective cleanser of toxins, good for skin complaints. It relieves flatulence and is good for heartburn, belching, and nausea. It is used for headaches associated with digestive problems. It also acts on the liver and gallbladder to increase the flow of bile.

CAUTION The fresh root is poisonous. Small doses of the dried root are advised.

LABIATAE

Collinsonia canadensis
Stone root

Knob root, hardback, knotroot, horseweed, horsebalm

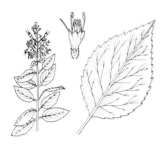

h 1–4 ft (30–120 cm). See p. 67.

Parts used Root and rhizome.

Main uses *Medical* Varicose veins, haemorrhoids, diarrhoea.

Constituents Saponin, alkaloids, tannin, resin.

This undervalued herbal remedy is often described simply as a diuretic, but its main use is to strengthen the structure and function of the veins. It is particularly good for the treatment of haemorrhoids. It is also used for treating spasmodic pain in the rectum and for anal fissures and is excellent for varicose veins taken internally. Its gentle astringent action also makes it useful to treat diarrhoea.

Hyssopus officinalis
Hyssop

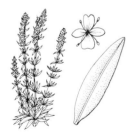

20×16 ins (50×40 cm). See p. 67.

Parts used Flowering herb; cultivation see pp. 276–7.

Constituents Volatile oil (up to 2%, comprising mainly pinocamphone, iso-pinocamphone, pinenes, camphene, and terpinene as well as over 50 other compounds), a glycoside (hyssopin), tannin (up to 8%), flavonoids, insolic acid, oleonolic acid, a bitter substance (marrubiin), resin, gum.

Main uses *Medical* Colds, flu, bronchitis, upper respiratory catarrh; bruises and burns.

Hyssop comes from the Hebrew name Esob, and the plant is mentioned many times in the Bible. Hippocrates recommended hyssop for chest complaints and today herbalists still prescribe it for a range of respiratory disorders such as influenza, colds and bronchitis. The bitter principle in the plant, marrubiin (also present in white horehound), has expectorant qualities.[1] Hyssop extracts have exhibited antiviral activities (especially against the *Herpes simplex* virus that causes cold sores).[2] Used externally, hyssop is also good for treating burns and bruises.

CAUTION Small doses only should be used: consult a qualified practitioner.

Lavandula officinalis
Lavender

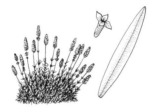

32×24 ins (80×60 cm). See p. 67.

Parts used Dried flowers; cultivation see pp. 276–7.

Constituents Volatile oil (up to 1.5%, containing linabol, linalyl acetate, lavendulyl acetate, terpinenol, cineole, camphor, borneol, pinene, limonene), tannins, coumarins (coumarin, umbelliferone, hemiarin), flavonoids, triterpenoids. Spike lavender (*L. latifolia*) contains an oil rich in cineole and camphor.

Main uses *General* In fragrant sachets (see p. 152); *Medical* Burns, stings, headache, coughs, and colds.

One of our best loved scented herbs, lavender or its oil is also one of the best remedies for burns and stings. It is excellent, too, for helping to heal cuts and has a strong antibacterial action.[1] It has many other uses. Herbalists use the oil to kill the diphtheria and typhoid bacilli as well as streptococcus and pneumococcus. Lavender has traditionally been used to treat chest infections, coughs, and colds, either as an infusion or a steam inhalation. It has sedative properties[2] and is good for calming anxiety and tension, as well as relaxing spasms of the digestive tract. An infusion is good for nervous headaches and a few drops of the oil used in a massage oil will help relax muscles and ease neuralgic and rheumatic pain. A strong infusion used as a douche is effective for leucorrhoea.

CAUTION Lavender oil should only be taken internally under supervision.

Leonurus cardiaca
Motherwort

Lion's tail, lion's ear

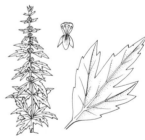

48×24 ins (120×60 cm). See p. 66.

Parts used Aerial parts.

Constituents Alkaloids (including leonurinine and stachydrine), bitter glycosides (leonurine and leonuridin), tannins, a volatile oil, vitamin A.

Main uses *Medical* To regulate menstruation.

The English name indicates an important use of this herb as a sedative particularly valuable in treating the anxiety after childbirth or at the menopause. This effect is thought to be due to the glycosides which also seem to have a short-term ability to lower blood pressure.[1]

The Latin name, cardiaca, derives from the Greek word for heart. Since ancient times, motherwort has been

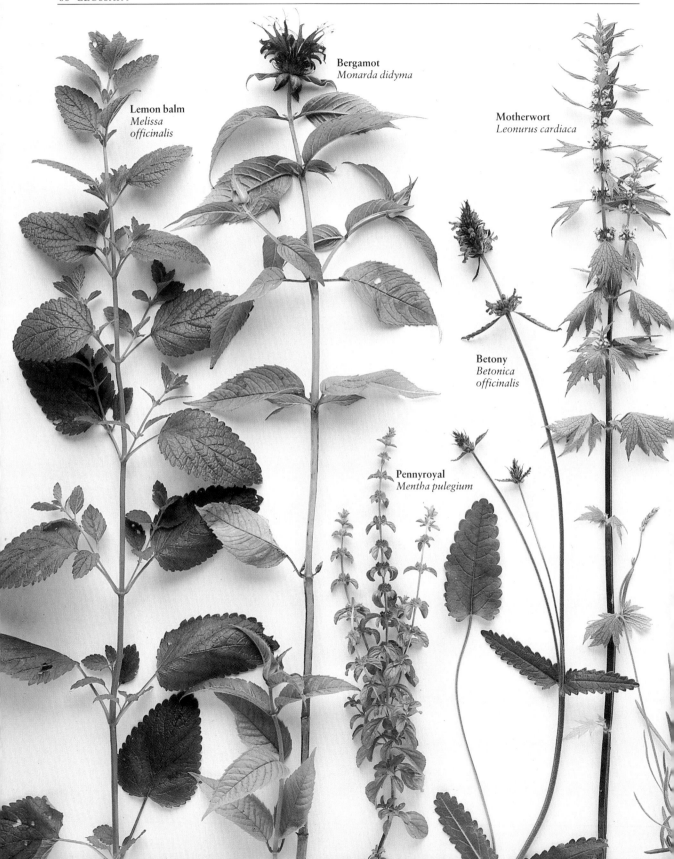

Lemon balm
Melissa officinalis

Bergamot
Monarda didyma

Motherwort
Leonurus cardiaca

Betony
Betonica officinalis

Pennyroyal
Mentha pulegium

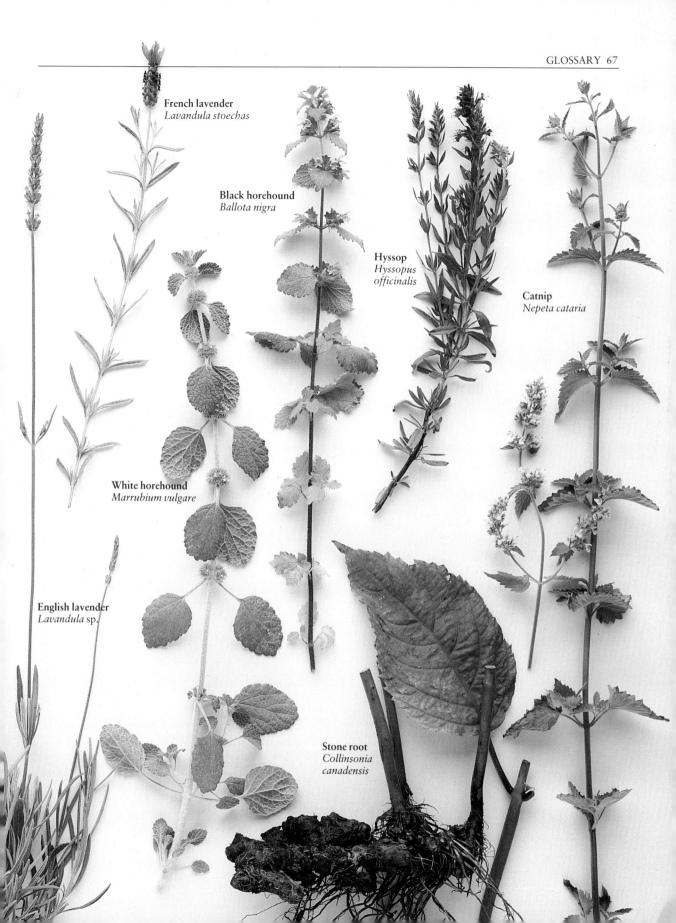

French lavender
Lavandula stoechas

Black horehound
Ballota nigra

Hyssop
Hyssopus officinalis

Catnip
Nepeta cataria

White horehound
Marrubium vulgare

English lavender
Lavandula sp.

Stone root
Collinsonia canadensis

used to treat palpitations and rapid heart beat, especially when associated with anxiety. Chinese herbalists also use motherwort for its diuretic properties. Motherwort is invaluable for treating absent or painful periods particularly when the flow is scanty. It can help regulate menstruation and treat functional infertility.

CAUTION The alkaloid stachydrine has the effect of hastening childbirth, so the herb should not be taken during pregnancy. Chinese research on *Leonurus heterophyllus*, a relative of the European motherwort, showed that decoctions of the plant were as effective as the drug ergotamine in causing the uterus to contract after delivery.[2]

Marrubium vulgare
White horehound

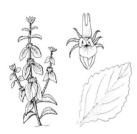

24×20 ins (60×50 cm). See p. 67.

Parts used Aerial parts.

Constituents Up to 1% marrubiin (a bitter principle), diterpene alcohols (eg marrbiol and murrubenol), small amounts of alkaloids, traces of volatile oil and a sesquiterpene, tannin, saponin, resin.

Main uses *Medical* Respiratory disorders; as a bitter digestive tonic.

This is one of the bitter herbs ordained to be eaten at Passover supper by the Jews. The plant's bitter principle, with its expectorant properties, is responsible in part for the major medicinal use of white horehound for respiratory disorders.[1] The volatile oil in the plant has the same expectorant property, as well as dilating the arteries.[2] But the effect of white horehound extends throughout the body. It also has a folk reputation for calming a nervous heart. This too has scientific backing for

marrubiin in small amounts has a normalizing effect on irregular heartbeats.[3] In hot infusion white horehound is sweat-inducing. In cold infusion it is a bitter tonic to the digestive system. Scientific evidence also shows that, as marrubiin breaks down in the body, it strongly stimulates bile production.[4] This is another property that seems to have been known for centuries since white horehound was traditionally a reliable liver and digestive remedy. The plant has also been used to reduce fevers and treat malaria.

Melissa officinalis
Lemon balm

Bee balm, melissa, sweet balm

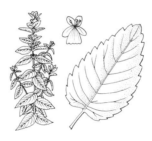

32×24 ins (80×60 cm). See p. 66.

Parts used Fresh leaves, picked just before flowering; cultivation see pp. 276–7.

Constituents Volatile oil (up to 0.2%, comprising citral, citronellal, eugenol acetate, geraniol and other components), polyphenols, tannin, flavonoids, rosmarinic acid, triterpenoids.

Main uses *Culinary* In wine cups, teas, and beers; with fish, mushrooms and soft cheeses. *Medical* For colds, flu, depression, headache and indigestion.

The great Moslem physician Avicenna recommended this plant because "it makes the heart merry" and to this day the herb and the isolated oil used in aromatherapy are recommended for nervousness, depression, insomnia, and nervous headaches. The volatile oils in the plant (particularly citronellal) have a sedative effect even in minute concentrations.[1,2,3] No wonder that the plant was an important ingredient in

Medieval cordials, distilled to strengthen the heart and lift the spirits.

Lemon balm is also an excellent infusion to take after meals, easing the digestion and relieving flatulence and colic. Scientific research now supports this use, since the oils (particularly eugenol) have antispasmodic activities.[4] Oil of balm also has an antihistaminic activity which encourages use of the plant to help allergic sufferers such as those with eczema.[5] In fact, aromatherapists and herbalists use the dilute oil as a massage for this purpose. Another important medicinal use of lemon balm is to promote menstrual periods and ease period pains.

Hot infusions of lemon balm are sweat inducing, useful for treating colds and flu. Lemon balm has antiviral properties effective against mumps, cold sores (*Herpes simplex*), and other viruses.[6] It is thought that both the polyphenols and tannin present in the plant are responsible for this effect.[7] When used in infusion, however, lemon balm is best used fresh or freeze-dried because the volatile oils in the leaves tend to disappear during the drying process. Balm oil has been reported to be antibacterial too.

Mentha piperata
Peppermint
See page 70

Mentha pulegium
Pennyroyal

European pennyroyal, pudding grass, lurk-in-the-ditch

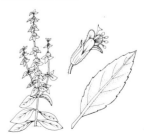

h up to 1 ft (30 cm). See p. 66.

Parts used Flowering herb.

Constituents Volatile oil (up to 1% comprising mainly pulegone, also menthone etc), tannins.

Main uses *General* As insect repellent (see p. 160). *Medical* Colds and flu.

The Latin name derives from *pulex* (flea) because of pennyroyal's power to repel fleas and other insects. The herb in a hot infusion has always been used by herbalists for colds as it promotes sweating. *Hederoma pulegoides* (American pennyroyal) has the same properties.

CAUTION Pennyroyal promotes menstruation, and should never be used by pregnant women or if pregnancy is suspected. The oil taken internally can be highly toxic and should only be used as prescribed by a qualified herbalist. There are a number of cases of the deaths of women who tried to procure abortions by taking the oil.

Monarda didyma
Bergamot
Bee balm, Oswego tea

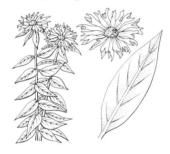

h 1–3 ft (30–100 cm). See p. 66.

Parts used Leaves, flowers, oil; cultivation, see pp. 276–7.

Constituents Volatile oil comprising compounds related to Thymol, tannic acid.

Main uses *Culinary* As tea (see p. 182).

Bergamot is named because of its fragrance, which resembles the aroma of the bergamot orange. It grew in abundance in the Oswego River district near Lake Ontario and was used by the Oswego Indians. Its popular name, Oswego Tea, reflects this locale and its popularity as a drink in many parts of the United States. The oil is sometimes used in perfumery, but should not be confused with the oil of the similarly smelling Bergamot Orange, an important aromatherapy oil and an ingredient of Earl Grey tea. Because of its distinctive fragrance, and because of the nectar its flowers secrete, bergamot is a popular plant with bees, hence its country name of bee balm.

Nepeta cataria
Catnip
Catnep, catmint

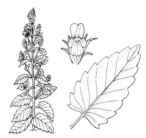

h 1–3 ft (30–100 cm). See p. 67.

Parts used Dried aerial parts.

Constituents Volatile oil (comprising carvacrol, nepetol, thymol, nepetalactone, citronellol, geraniol); tannins.

Main uses *Medical* Colds, flu, and children's illnesses.

In hot infusion this plant powerfully promotes sweating and is excellent for colds, flu, or the infectious diseases of childhood (eg measles). It soothes the nervous system and will help get a restless child off to sleep. It also helps to calm an upset stomach, countering colic, flatulence, and diarrhoea. In the USA it was used as an enema to cleanse and heal the lower bowel.

Ocimum basilicum
Sweet basil
See page 71

Origanum marjorana
Sweet marjoram
Knotted marjoram

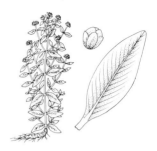

h 1–2 ft (30–60 cm).

Parts used Leaves; cultivation see pp. 276–7.

Constituents Essential oil, mucilage, bitter substances, tannic acid.

Main uses *Culinary* In bouquet garni (see p. 168); widely used with meat dishes, vegetables, and milk-based desserts.

Marjoram, which belongs to the same genus as oregano, has been used for centuries as a culinary, and to a lesser extent a medicinal, herb. It is often used in meat dishes, especially with sausage. Its success as a culinary herb may be due in part to its properties as a digestive aid.

Pot marjoram (*O. onites*) is cultivated widely in northern latitudes as a semi-hardy alternative to this herb. Additional species, including *O. dictamnus* (from Crete), *O. pulchellum*, and *O. sipyleum* are also grown.

Origanum vulgare
Oregano
Wild marjoram

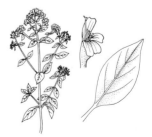

h to 30 ins (75 cm). See p. 74.

Mentha piperita
Peppermint

h 1–3 ft (30–100 cm)

Parts used Flowering herb; cultivation see pp. 276–7.

Constituents About 0.4% volatile oil (composed mainly of menthol, menthone, and menthylacetate, with smaller amounts of menthofuran, limonene, pulegone, cineole, bisabolene, isomenthol, neomenthol), flavonoids, phytol, tocopherols, carotenoids, betaine, choline, azulenes, rosmarinic acid, tannin.

Main uses *Culinary* Widely used for flavour. *Medical* Indigestion, colds.

Menthol, the main constituent of the volatile oil, is antibacterial and antiparasitic.[1,2] Dissolved in alcohol, it has proved effective against ringworm.

As well as this, peppermint has demonstrated an antispasmodic effect on smooth muscle such as that of the digestive system. The herb is an effective remedy for colic and flatulence.[3]

Because of the flavonoids it contains, peppermint stimulates the liver and gallbladder, increasing the flow of bile.[4] Azulene in the oil has anti-inflammatory and ulcer-healing effects.[5]

Externally peppermint oil or menthol is used in pain-relieving balms, massage oils, and linaments. Menthol is cooling and anaesthetic when applied to the skin, increasing blood flow to the area to which it is applied.

Inhalations of the herb or oil are effective against excessive respiratory mucus. Peppermint is a useful remedy to increase concentration.

CAUTION Avoid prolonged use of inhalants of the oil, which must never be used for babies.

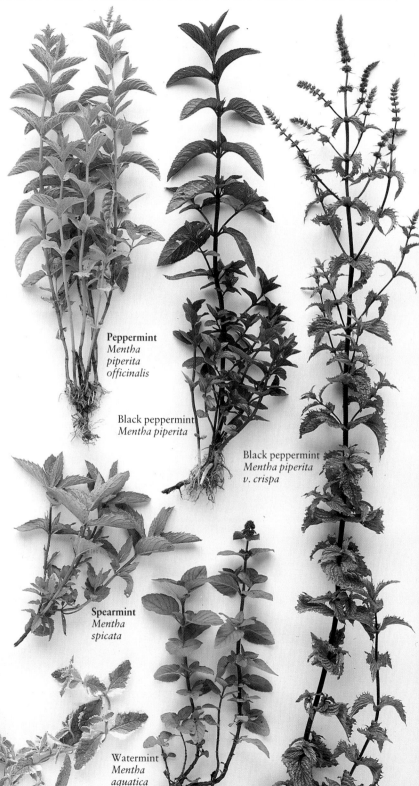

Peppermint
Mentha piperita officinalis

Black peppermint
Mentha piperita

Black peppermint
Mentha piperita v. crispa

Spearmint
Mentha spicata

Variegated apple mint
Mentha suaveolens variegata

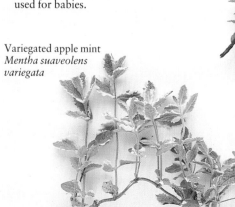

Watermint
Mentha aquatica

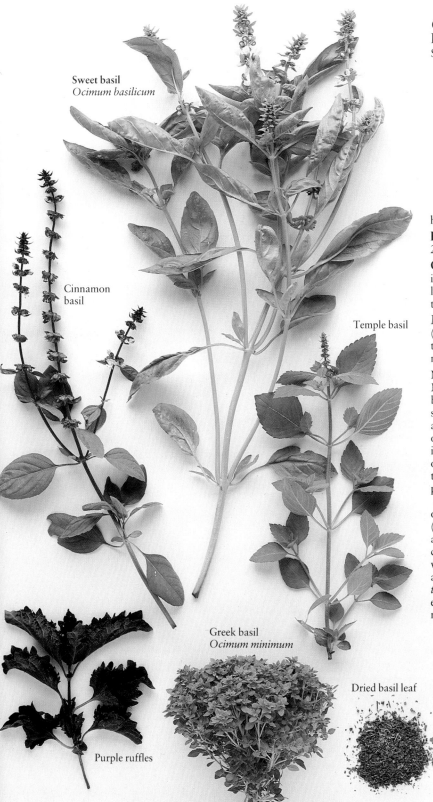

Sweet basil
Ocimum basilicum

Cinnamon
basil

Temple basil

Greek basil
Ocimum minimum

Dried basil leaf

Purple ruffles

Ocimum basilicum
Basil
Sweet basil

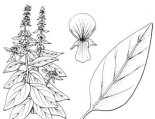

h 1–2 ft (30–60 cm).

Parts used Leaves; cultivation see pp. 276–7.

Constituents Essential oil (comprising mainly estragol but also eugenol, lineol, linalol, and sometimes thymol), tannins, basil camphor.

Main uses *General* As insect repellent (see p. 160). *Culinary* In pesto; with tomatoes; used widely in Mediterranean cuisine.

Native to India, basil has grown in the Mediterranean for thousands of years, but only reached western Europe in the sixteenth century. It is now cultivated all over southern Europe in pots placed outside houses, to repel flies. In India it is sacred to Krishna and Vishnu, gods of the Hindus. It is especially good with tomatoes and the two are companion plants (see pp. 268–9).

In addition to sweet basil, several other varieties are cultivated. Bush basil (*Ocimum minimum*) is a dwarf species about 6 ins (15 cm) tall. It has similar constituents and flavour. Decorative varieties with different foliage colours are also available. Wild basil (*Calamintha clinopodium*) is a species of northern Europe. It has a scent and flavour reminiscent of thyme.

Parts used Leaves.

Constituents Essential oil (comprising thymol, origanene, and carvacrol), bitter principles, tannic acids, resins.

Main uses *Culinary* With many meats, stuffings, and Mediterranean dishes such as pizza.

Like its close relative marjoram, oregano is widely used in cooking. It was once also used to flavour beer. Like marjoram it is an aid to digestion.

Prunella vulgaris
Heal all

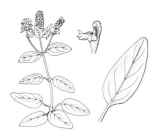

h 3 ft (1 m). See p. 75.

Parts used Dried aerial parts.

Constituents Volatile oil, bitter principles, alkaloid.

Main uses *Medical* In mouthwashes or gargles for sore throats.

Rosmarinus officinalis
Rosemary

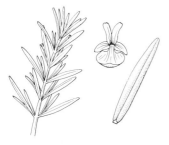

h 3 ft (1 m). See p. 75.

Parts used Leaves; cultivation see pp. 278–9.

Constituents Volatile oil (mainly comprising monoterpene hydrocarbons, cineole and borneol, also the camphors, linalool and verbenol), several flavonoids (notably diosmin), phenolic acids, carnosic acid (rosmanicine), triterpenic acids.

Main uses *General* In hair shampoos (see p.146). *Culinary* With meat dishes, especially lamb. *Medical* Headaches, for poor circulation and digestion.

Rosemary is an excellent remedy for headaches, either taken as an infusion or used externally, the oil being applied directly to the head.[1] Like many other essential oils, rosemary oil has anti-bacterial and antifungal properties.[2] The herb reduces flatulence and is stimulating to the digestion, liver and gallbladder increasing the flow of bile (as rosmanicine breaks down in the body it stimulates the smooth muscle of the digestive tract and gallbladder.[3] The herb is also used to treat painful periods. Rosemary also improves the circulation and strengthens fragile blood vessels (due to the effect of the flavonoid diosmin).[4] Rosemary oil is a component of liniments used for rheumatism.

An infusion of rosemary with borax is used as a rinse for treating dandruff. The herb is also used in many herbal hair shampoos and the plant has a long reputation as a hair tonic. Because of its pleasant, refreshing fragrance it is also used in commercially available cosmetics and perfumes.

CAUTION The undiluted oil should not be taken internally.

Salvia officinalis
Sage

Red sage

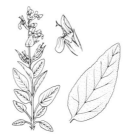

h 30–60 cm (1–2 ft). See p. 74.

Parts used Leaves; cultivation see pp. 278–9.

Constituents Up to 2.8% volatile oil (including thujone, cineole, borneol, linalool, camphors, salvene, pinine, etc), oestrogenic substances, salvin and carnosic acid, flavonoids, phenolic acids, condensed tannins.

Main uses *Culinary* Widely used with pork and poultry. *Medical* Sore throats, colds, indigestion, hot flushes, and painful periods.

The Chinese were happy to trade with the Dutch three times the amount of their best tea for European sage. The botanical name *Salvia* also suggests its importance. It comes from the latin word *Salvare*, to save. For centuries sage has been esteemed for its healing powers. It is a first-rate remedy in hot infusion for colds. The phenolic acids it contains are antibacterial, especially potent against *Staphylococcus aureus*[1,2] while thujone is a strong antiseptic. Sage tea combined with a little cider vinegar used as a gargle is excellent for sore throats, laryngitis, and tonsillitis. As a mouthwash sage tea is effective for infected gums and mouth ulcers. Due to its volatile oil, sage has both a carminative and stimulating effect on the digestion. Sage also fortifies a debilitated nervous system. Another remarkable property of this plant is its ability to stop sweating.[3] Its oestrogenic properties make it useful for the treatment of the hot flushes of the menopause.[4] Sage also has the reputation of drying up the flow of breast milk in nursing mothers. It is also useful in amenorrhoea and painful periods.

A number of other species of sage are cultivated for their medicinal and culinary properties. The oil of the decorative clary sage (*Salvia sclarea*) is used in aromatherapy. *S. lyrala* and *S. urticifolia* are common North American varieties.

CAUTION Although sage has more thujone than wormwood it seems a far safer plant. But the tea should only be taken for a week or two at a time because of the potentially toxic effects of thujone.

Satureia hortensis, Satureia montana
Summer savory, winter savory

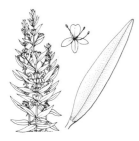

h to 16 ins (40 cm). See p. 74.

Parts used Leaves.

Constituents Essential oil (comprising mainly carvacrol and cymene), phenolic substances, resins, tannins, mucilage.

Main uses *Culinary* With vegetables, legumes, and rich meats.

These two plants are closely related. Summer savory is an annual with pink, lilac, or white flowers. Winter savory is a sturdier perennial. Both summer and winter savory are stimulating to the appetite and are commonly used culinary herbs. Their flavour is hot and peppery and goes particularly well with beans. Savory can also be used sparingly in salads. The Italians were among the first to use the herb, which in Roman times was made into a sauce with vinegar. The leaf is now used commercially to flavour salami. The flavour of winter savory is inferior to that of summer savory, being both coarser and stronger.

Stachys palustris
Marsh woundwort

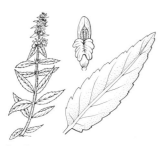

h 3 ft (1 m). See p. 75.

Parts used Aerial parts.

Constituents Not investigated.

Main uses *Medical* For gout, cramp, and other pains in the joints.

This plant had a strong reputation as a healer in the sixteenth century and adherents of traditional medicine still use a bruised woundwort leaf to stop bleeding. But the plant is used by modern herbalists for its antispasmodic properties, particularly for cramping pains. The closely related hedge woundwort (*S. sylvatica*) also has a healing reputation.

Scutellaria laterifolia
Skullcap

Helmet flower, mad-dogweed, Virginian skullcap

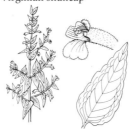

h 6–18 ins (15 to 45 cm). See p. 74.

Parts used Aerial parts (see below).

Constituents Flavonoid glycosides (including scutellonin and scutellanein), volatile oil, bitter principles, tannin.

Main uses *Medical* Nervousness, depression, insomnia, headaches.

Skullcap is an excellent tonic for the nervous system. It is good for treating anxiety, depression, insomnia, and nervous headaches. Its bitter taste is also strengthening and stimulating to the digestion. In former times, skullcap had a reputation for treating epilepsy and rabies, as one of its common names implies.

A number of other species appear in older herbals, but their medicinal properties have not been thoroughly investigated.

CAUTION Large doses may cause dizziness, mental confusion, and erratic pulse rate.

Stachys betonica
Wood betony

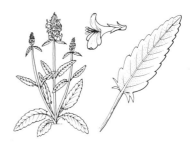

h 1–2 ft (30–60 cm).

Parts used Flowering herb.

Constituents Tannins (up to 15%), saponins, alkaloids (betonicine, stachydrine, trigonelline).

Main uses *Medical* Headaches, neuralgia, liver complaints, cuts, bruises.

The tannins in wood betony make it effective as a poultice for cuts and bruises (its three alkaloids are likewise found in yarrow, also known as a wound-healer). Taken internally, it stimulates the circulation and is useful in the treatment of headaches and migraines. The plant relaxes the nervous system and helps relieve neuralgia. In France, it is recommended for liver and gallbladder complaints. The powdered leaves were once used as snuff, and an infusion has traditionally been used to clear head colds. Trigonelline is reported to lower blood sugar levels.

Thymus vulgaris (also *T. serpyllum*, *T. pulegioides*)
Thyme

Common thyme, garden thyme

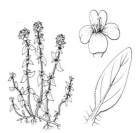

h 4–12 ins (10–30 cm). See p. 75.

Parts used Flowering aerial parts.

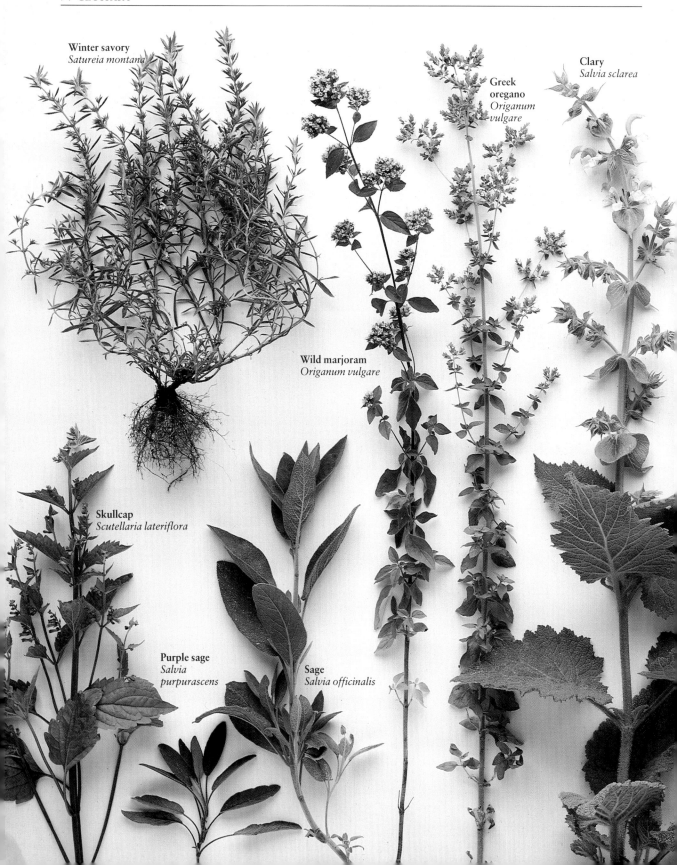

Winter savory
Satureia montana

**Greek
oregano**
*Origanum
vulgare*

Clary
Salvia sclarea

Wild marjoram
Origanum vulgare

Skullcap
Scutellaria lateriflora

Purple sage
*Salvia
purpurascens*

Sage
Salvia officinalis

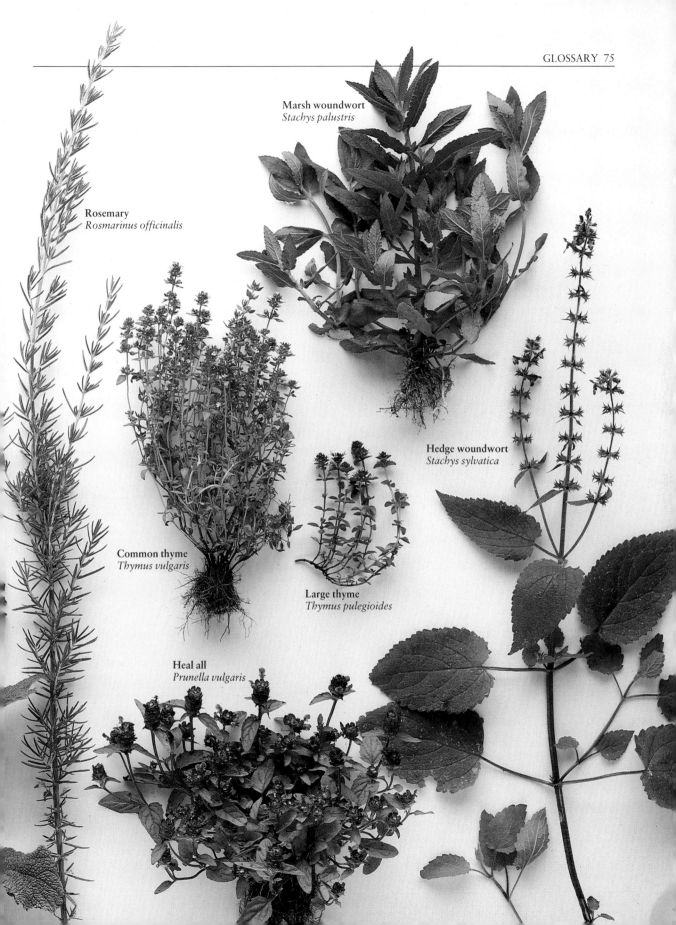

Marsh woundwort
Stachys palustris

Rosemary
Rosmarinus officinalis

Hedge woundwort
Stachys sylvatica

Common thyme
Thymus vulgaris

Large thyme
Thymus pulegioides

Heal all
Prunella vulgaris

Constituents Volatile oil (about 1%, consisting of phenol, thymol, carvacrol), monoterpene hydrocarbons (eg terpinene) and alcohols (eg linalool), tannin, flavonoids, saponins.

Main uses *Culinary* Used widely, especially with meat, poultry, in stuffings. *Medical* Sore throats, colds, coughs.

Both major components of the volatile oil, thymol and carvacrol (but particularly the former) are antibacterial and antifungal.[1] Thymol also expels worms, especially hookworms and ascarids. (It also kills mosquito larvae).[2] As a gargle or mouthwash thyme is an excellent remedy for sore throats and infected gums. In hot infusion, thyme tea is sweat-inducing and so is effective against the common cold. Because its volatile oil is partly excreted through the lungs, it is also good for bronchitis. It is often used to treat whooping cough too. Thyme has a marked expectorant effect causing the coughing up of viscid mucus.

Thyme tea eases flatulence and soothes the digestive system. This is due to the antispasmodic effect of the volatile oil on smooth muscle.

Externally baths of thyme are used to ease rheumatic pains and the oil is often used in liniments and massage oils. An ointment made from thyme is used to treat shingles (*Herpes zoster*).

Wild thyme (*T. Serpyllum*) has similar properties. Other decorative garden varieties are also available.

CAUTION Although the whole plant in medicinal doses is safe, the isolated volatile oil is toxic in any quantity and should not be used internally except by professionals. Avoid this remedy if you are pregnant.

LAURACEAE

Cinnamomum camphora
Camphor

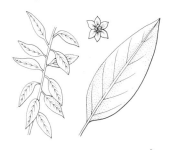

h to 36 ft (12 m). See p. 83.

Parts used Camphor, oil.

Constituents Safrole, acetaldehyde, terpineol, eugenol, phelandrene, pinene.

Main uses *Medical* Externally for rheumatic pains.

Camphor has been distilled from the wood of this tree for hundreds of years, and has been known and used in the West since the twelfth century. Its main use is as a remedy for painful joints.

CAUTION Avoid prolonged exposure to fumes.

Cinnamomum zeylanicum
Cinnamon

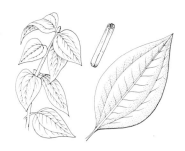

h to 30 ft (10 m). See p. 34.

Parts used Dried bark.

Constituents Volatile oil, tannins, mucilage, gum, sugars, resin, calcium oxylate, coumarin.

Main uses *Culinary* Savoury foods in Asian cuisines; with cooked fruit; in cakes. *Medical* Colds, diarrhoea.

The bark of *Cinnamomum zeylanicum*

is generally considered to be of better quality than cassia bark from *C. cassia*, a close relative. Cinnamon has been valued as an aromatic spice since ancient times and as a medicine to treat colds, to warm the digestion, and to ease flatulence. Also used to ease menstrual cramps, its astringency makes it valuable for controlling diarrhoea. Cinnamon-bark oil is antibacterial, inhibiting *E. coli*, *Staphylococcus aureus*, and thrush (*Candida albicans*).

Cinnamon is widely used in Asian cuisines. In western cooking it is employed to bring out the flavour of cakes and stewed fruit, and is added to winter drinks such as mulled wine.

Laurus nobilis
Bay
Sweet bay, sweet laurel

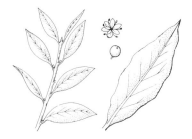

h to 6 ft (2 m) or 45 ft (30 m). See p. 78.

Parts used Leaves, oil; cultivation see pp. 276–7.

Constituents Volatile oil (1–3% comprising geraniol, cineol, eugenol terpenes), tannic acid, bitter principles.

Main uses *Culinary* In bouquet garni (see p. 168); in stocks and casseroles.

Sacred to Apollo, this plant was used to make the laurel crown of the victorious in classical times. It is most widely used as a culinary herb. Fresh leaves should be used in moderation as their flavour is much stronger than dried. They also stimulate the digestion.

CAUTION *Prunus laurocerasus*, now known as laurel, is a highly poisonous plant.

LEGUMINOSAE

Astragalus membranaceus
Astragalus
Milk-vetch root, huang qi

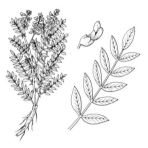

h to 9 ft (3 m)

Parts used Root.

Constituents Glycosides, choline, betaine, rumatakenin, sugar, plant acid, beta-sitosterol, vitamin A.

Main uses *Medical* To strengthen the immune system and the digestion.

First mentioned as a medicinal plant in the first century Chinese herbal the *Shen Nong Ben Cao*, this plant is one of the most famous herbs used in traditional Chinese medicine. According to the Chinese, it strengthens the digestion and the body's vital energy (called Qi in Chinese medicine). For this reason, it is used to treat lack of appetite and diarrhoea that occurs because of a debilitated digestion. It also supports the lungs and enhances the immune system. *Cancer*, the journal of the American Cancer Society, reported that this herb appeared to strengthen the immune function of a high proportion of the patients taking it.[1] Because of this astralagus may be taken by those who suffer frequently from colds.

Astragalus displays a so-called adaptogenic effect, on the one hand stopping debilitating sweating but on the other also producing a therapeutic sweat if this is appropriate. Astralagus helps discharge pus and promotes the healing of ulcers. The herb is thought more appropriate for young people than ginseng because, the Chinese say, it strengthens the outer energy while ginseng tonifies the inner energy. But these two herbs are often used together. Astragalus is also often combined with the famous Chinese blood tonic, Chinese Angelica, (Dang Gui) whenever there is poor circulation and lassitude. Astragalus is a major component of Jade Screen Powder which the Chinese use for low resistance and susceptibility to colds.

Baptisia tinctoria
Wild indigo
American indigo, yellow indigo

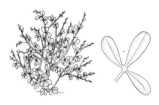

h to 3 ft (1 m). See p. 78.

Parts used Root.

Constituents Alkaloids (including baptoxin), glycosides, resin.

Main uses *Medical* Arthritis; generally for inflammation (see below).

Wild indigo is useful to treat sepsis and inflammation throughout the body. The American herbalist Ellingwood used it in "the treatment of long protracted and sluggish forms of fever with great depression of the vital forces". It is also used by herbalists to counter inflammation of the lymph glands. Externally an ointment is good for infected ulcers and sore or ulcerated nipples.

CAUTION Strong doses of wild indigo may have a purgative and emetic effect.

Cassia senna
Alexandrian senna
(or *Cassia angustifolia*, Indian senna)

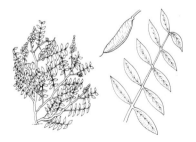

h to 30 ins (75 cm). See p. 83.

Parts used Leaves and pods.

Constituents Anthraquinone glycosides (up to 3% consisting mostly of sennosides A and B), flavonoids, resin, tartaric acid.

Main uses *Medical* Constipation.

The sennosides in this plant are cathartic. Like all anthraquinones they irritate the bowel wall, stimulating evacuation. Because of this action, the habitual use of this herb is inadvisable since the bowel can quickly become dependent on it. The remedy should not be used in cases of spastic constipation. Chronic constipation should anyway be investigated by a qualified practitioner. Senna causes griping pains when used on its own and is therefore usually combined with aromatics or digestive herbs such as ginger, cloves, dill, fennel, coriander, orange peel, or licorice.

CAUTION Avoid prolonged use.

Glycyrrhiza glabra
Licorice

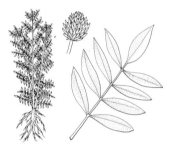

h 20–60 ins (50–150 cm). See p. 78.

Parts used Roots and runners.

Constituents Glycyrrhizin, flavonoids, isoflavonoids, chalcones, coumarins, triterpenoid saponins, sterols, starch, sugars (up to 14%), amino acids, amines (asparagine, betaine, choline), gums, wax, a volatile oil.

Main uses *Culinary* As flavouring in confectionery. *Medical* Sore throats, coughs, heartburn, ulcers, colic.

Licorice is one of the most commonly used herbal remedies because it has the ability to harmonize and blend all the other herbs in a prescription and is useful to mask the taste of many bitter remedies (glycyrrhizin is 50 times sweeter than sugar). However, licorice is itself a

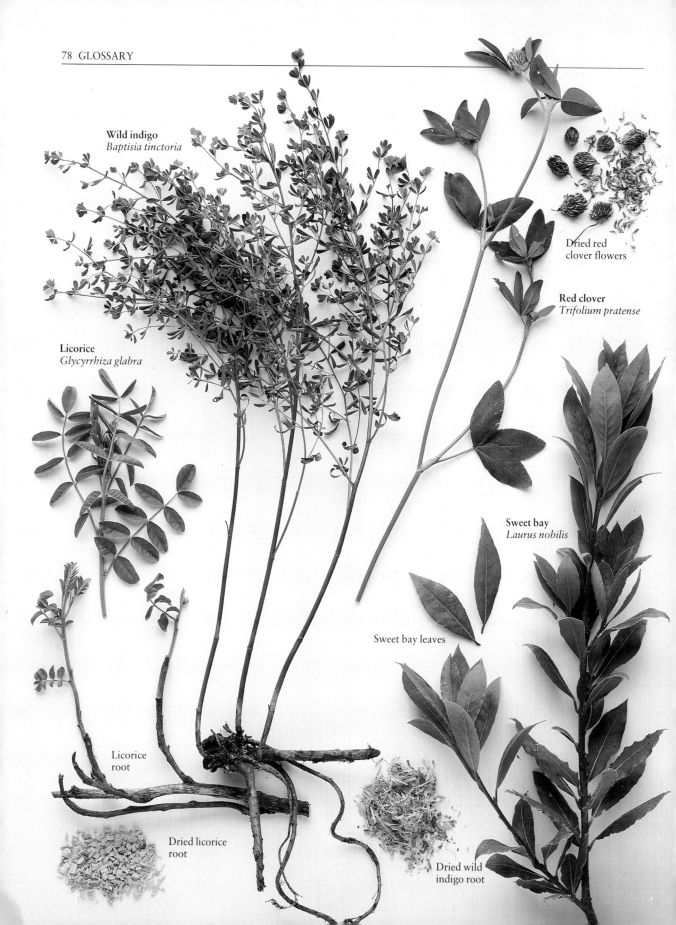

Wild indigo
Baptisia tinctoria

Licorice
Glycyrrhiza glabra

Dried red
clover flowers

Red clover
Trifolium pratense

Sweet bay
Laurus nobilis

Sweet bay leaves

Licorice
root

Dried licorice
root

Dried wild
indigo root

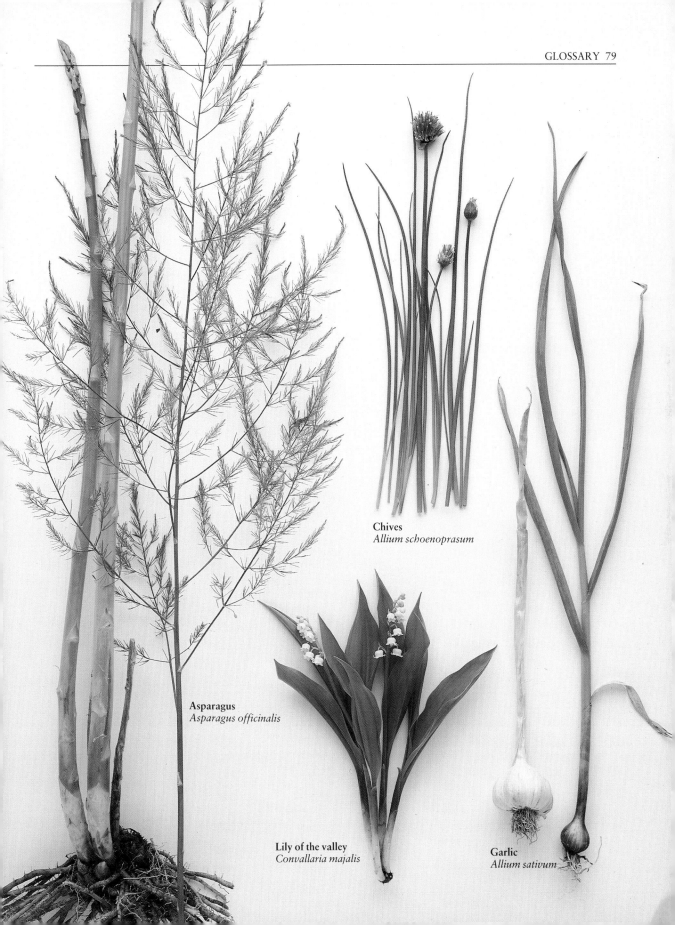

Chives
Allium schoenoprasum

Asparagus
Asparagus officinalis

Lily of the valley
Convallaria majalis

Garlic
Allium sativum

most valuable medicine. In the body glycyrrhizin yields glycyrhetinic acid, which has a similar structure to the hormones of the adrenal cortex. This may explain why licorice demonstrates potent anti-inflammatory and antiarthritis effects similar to cortisone.[1] There is a case on record of a woman with failure of the adrenal cortex who was supported solely on a regular intake of licorice.[2] The adrenal-like effect of licorice also makes it anti-allergic.

Licorice is a valuable remedy for the digestive system. It is gently laxative and lowers stomach-acid levels, so relieving heartburn. It has a remarkable power to heal stomach ulcers because it spreads a protective gel over the stomach wall and, in addition, it eases spasms of the large intestine.[3] Licorice can neutralize many toxins such as those of diphtheria and tetanus. It also increases the flow of bile, and lowers blood cholesterol levels. In addition it has a marked ability to reduce irritation of the throat (similar to codeine) and yet has an expectorant action. It is also effective in helping to reduce fevers (glycyrrhetinic acid has an effect like aspirin).[4] In addition, evidence now exists that licorice is antibacterial, and has a possible oestrogenic effect.[5]

CAUTION The action of licorice is like that of the hormone ACTH, causing retention of sodium and potassium and a rise in blood pressure. Although the plant contains asparagine which acts to counter this tendency, avoid licorice if you have high blood pressure or kidney disease or are pregnant. Avoid prolonged use of large doses.

Trifolium pratense
Red clover
Wild clover, trefoil

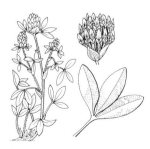

h 20 ins (50 cm). See p. 78.

Parts used Dried flowerheads.

Constituents Phenolic glycosides, flavonoids, salicylates, cyanogenic glycosides, coumarins.

Main uses *Medical* Respiratory and skin disorders.

Red clover is relaxant and expectorant, making it useful in treating coughs, bronchitis, and whooping cough. It is also used for treating skin conditions such as eczema and psoriasis and herbalists use it for children with eczema/asthma syndrome. It has been employed in the herbal treatment of cancer, but there is no scientific evidence for this.

LILIACEAE

Allium sativum
Garlic

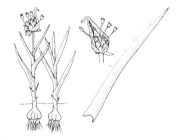

h 12 ins (30 cm). See p. 79.

Parts used Cloves; cultivation see pp. 274–5.

Constituents Volatile oil, vitamins A, B, and C, fats, amino acids. The oil contains alliin which once the cloves are cut or crushed, is converted to allicin. Once exposed to air, allicin is converted to diallydisulphide which is the component responsible for the antibacterial (gram-negative and positive) effect of garlic.

Main uses *Culinary* Used widely, especially in Mediterranean and eastern cuisines; in butters, vinegars, and garlic salt. *Medical* Colds, coughs, to aid digestion, for high blood pressure, arteriosclerosis.

Garlic has been used as a food and medicine since at least the time of the ancient Egyptians. The Greek historian Herodotus tells us that the slaves who built the Great Pyramid ate great quantities of it. Modern science has confirmed many of garlic's reputed healing properties.[1] Experiments conducted in India show that eating garlic can significantly lower blood cholesterol and other fats.[2] Research at George Washington University, USA, shows that garlic can also reduce blood-clotting, so making it useful in cardiovascular disease. Since garlic has also been shown to reduce blood pressure in both animals and humans, it is evidently useful in guarding against strokes which can occur when blood pressure is raised or the blood clots in the cerebral arteries.[3]

In both World Wars, garlic was applied to wounds to prevent septic poisoning and gangrene. Garlic has also been used successfully to control diarrhoea, dysentery, pulmonary TB, diphtheria, whooping cough, typhoid and hepatitis. It is effective against many fungal infections and trichomonas. It can be used to expel worms. Garlic has been shown to lower blood sugar levels, indicating its use in controlling mild diabetes.

Herbalists consider garlic to be a first-rate digestive tonic, and also use it to treat toothache, earache, coughs, and colds (regular intake can prevent colds and reduce excess phlegm). Garlic's folk reputation for treating cancer has received scientific support from two Japanese researchers who showed in 1963 that injections of garlic extract killed tumour cells in rats.

Allium schoenoprasum
Chives

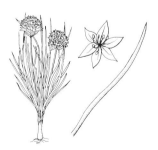

h 8–12 ins (20–30 cm). See p. 79.

Parts used Leaves.

Constituents Essential oil (containing sulphur).

Main uses *Culinary* In savoury dishes from salads, soups, and soft cheese to grilled meats.

Chives are used extensively in cooking. In Europe they are layered on top of a thick bacon omelette. They have no medicinal use.

Aloe vera (also known as *Aloe barbadensis*)
Aloe
Aloe vera, first-aid plant, medicine plant *Aloe ferox* gives cape aloe

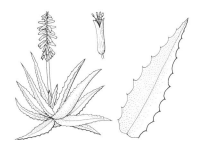

h 1–5 ft (30–150 cm). See p. 82.

Parts used Bitter juice and gel.

Constituents Bitter juice (drug aloe): Anthraquinone glycosides and free anthraquinones, resins. Gel: glucomannan, a polysaccharide similar to guar and locust-bean gums; also said to occur are steroids, organic acids, enzymes, antibiotic principles, amino acids, saponins, minerals.

Main uses *Medical* Burns, cuts, and wounds.

Aloe yields two distinct medicinal substances. The juice (drug aloe), which is obtained by cutting the leaves at their base, and a gel extracted by breaking the leaves themselves. The juice is a powerful cathartic, which is hardly suitable for medicinal use.

The gel, on the other hand, is one of the most remarkable healing substances known. Applied locally it encourages skin regeneration and may be used directly on burns, cuts and wounds. It also has emollient properties. The gel is now available commercially but harsh solvents used in its extraction, and fre-

quent adulteration, make many of these products unreliable. But aloe is easy to grow as a houseplant.

Asparagus officinalis
Asparagus
Garden asparagus, sparrow grass

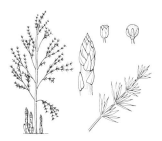

h 3–9 ft (1–3 m). See p. 79.

Parts used Stem, tips, root.

Constituents Asparagin, saponins, flavonoids, volatile oil, glucoside, gum, resin, tannic acid.

Main uses *Culinary* Tips as vegetable. *Medical* Root for urinary and bowel disorders.

Wild asparagus was eaten by both the Greeks and the Romans as a vegetable. We now eat the cultivated variety. This species has diuretic and laxative properties, especially if the fresh juice is taken. The root is also used for its diuretic properties.

Chamaelirium luteum (also known as *Helonias dioica*)
False unicorn root
Helonias, blazing star

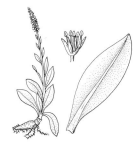

h 1–3 ft (30–90 cm)

Parts used Rhizome and root.

Constituents Steroidal saponins (including chamaelirin).

Main uses *Medical* As tonic to the reproductive system.

False unicorn root contains hormone-like saponins, which account in part for its considerable reputation as an ovarian and uterine tonic. Herbalists use it to encourage fertility in women and to treat impotence in men. They also employ the plant to treat disturbances of menstruation accompanied by a bearing-down sensation. It has a reputation for preventing miscarriage and is sometimes effective against morning sickness. Such treatments, however, should be left to the professional. The herb's tonic properties also benefit the appetite and digestion. This plant is sometimes confused with *Aletris farinosa*, or *true* unicorn root. *Aletris* also contains steroidal saponins (diosgenin) and is reported to have oestrogenic properties.[1]

CAUTION Use only as prescribed by a qualified practitioner.

Convallaria majalis
Lily of the valley
May lily

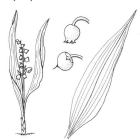

h 4–8 ins (10–20 cm). See p. 79.

Parts used Leaves.

Constituents Cardiac glycosides (including convallatoxin, convalloside, and gluconvalloside), saponins, flavonoids, asparagin.

Main uses *Medical* Heart disease.

This herb, like the foxglove (see p. 112), contains cardiac glycosides which increase the strength of the heart beat while slowing and regularizing its rate without putting extra demand on the coronary blood supply. But in lily of the

Exotic herbs

Many of the herbs used in medicine grow in remote parts of the globe or will only survive in hot climates. They are therefore most familiar in dried or prepared forms, which are widely available from herbal suppliers in the West. The range is great, from oriental ginseng to Jamaican dogwood, kola from Africa and Brazil to senna from the Middle East and India. This variety reflects the medical herbalism of many different countries.

Key to photograph

1 Kola seed pods 2 Kola powder
3 Aloe vera plant 4 Aloe powder
and gum 5 Dried red ginseng root
6 Dried white ginseng root 7 Fresh
white ginseng root 8 Dried skunk
cabbage root 9 Dried sarsaparilla
root 10 Jamaican dogwood root
11 Camphor 12 Camphor gum
13 Dried pleurisy root 14 False Balm
of Gilead 15 True Balm of Gilead
buds 16 Dried buchu leaves
17 Myrrh gum-resin 18 Senna
leaves and flowers 19 Dried senna
leaves 20 Dried senna pods
21 Dried grindelia 22 Dried kava
kava root 23 Dried boldo leaves
24 Guaiacum bark 25 Astragalus
root 26 Tragacanth bark 27 Gutu
kola plant 28 Dried gutu kola leaves

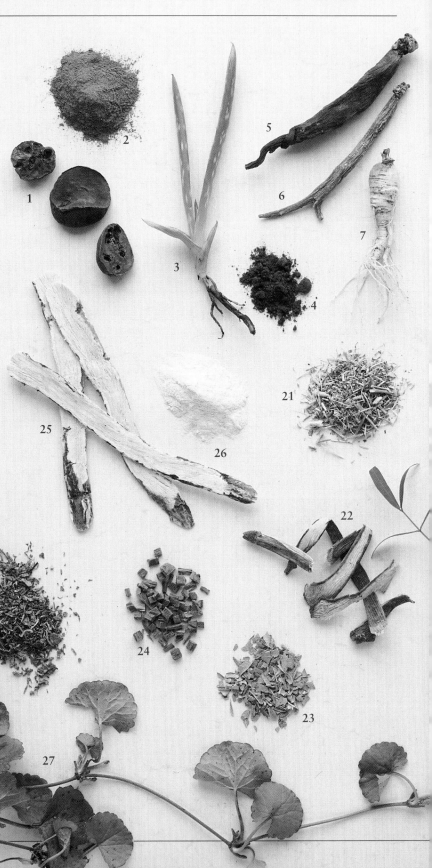

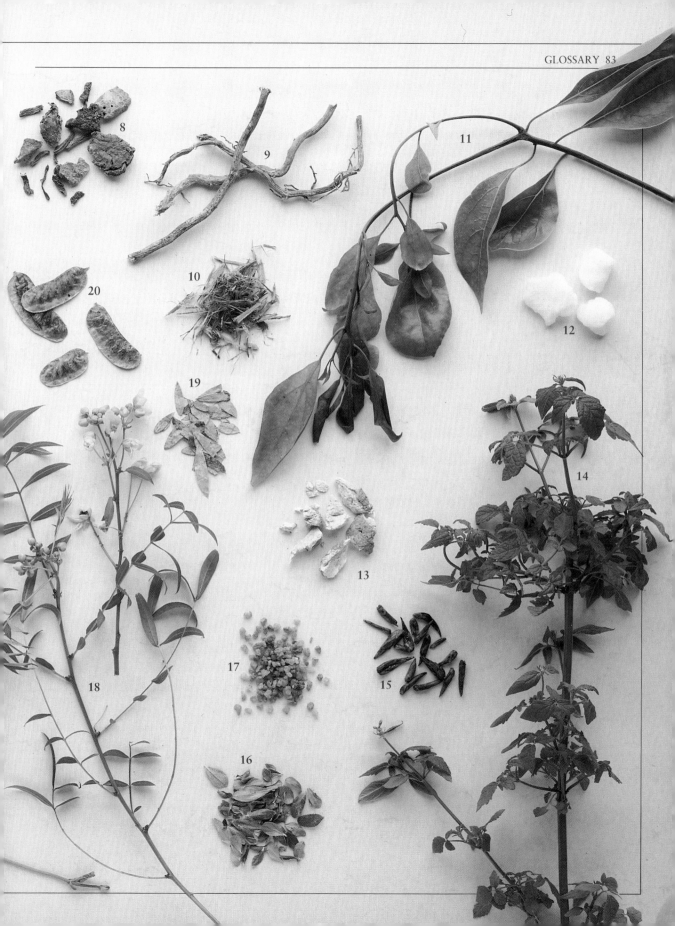

valley, the active cardiac glycosides are released sequentially rather than all at once and are readily excreted by the kidneys, so avoiding the kind of toxic build up that can happen when taking foxglove or its isolated glycoside, digoxin.[1]

The flavonoids in the plant encourage the arteries to dilate while the asparagin acts as a diuretic, helping the body to void excess fluid. Thus the herb can be used safely if there is high blood pressure.

RESTRICTED The U.S. Food and Drug Administration has classified this plant as poisonous.

Smilax officinalis (and spp.)
Sarsaparilla

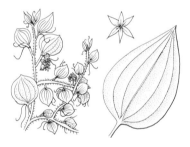

Size variable. See p. 83.

Parts used Root.

Constituents Steroids and steroidal saponins, sarsapic acid, starch, resin, volatile oil.

Main uses *Medical* Rheumatism and skin complaints.

In Europe, sarsaparilla came to prominence in the sixteenth century as a potential cure for syphilis and remained a main remedy for this disease until this century although its effectiveness has never been established. However, a Chinese species, *Smilax glabra*, has been found to be highly effective for this disease and has also been used to treat mercury poisoning.[1] Today herbalists consider sarsaparilla to be a blood purifier, useful in treating rheumatism and skin complaints such as psoriasis.

Sarsaparilla is also used to flavour soft drinks. This use is popular in the Caribbean.

Trillium erectum (also known as *T. pendulum*)
Beth root

Birth root, wake-robin

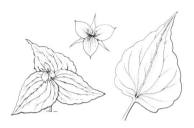

h to 20 ins (50 cm)

Parts used Dried rhizome and root.

Constituents Steroidal saponins (including diosgenin), fixed oil, gum, volatile oil.

Main uses *Medical* Menstrual disorders.

For many generations herbalists have used this North American Indian herb to stop post-partum haemorrhage. It also has the reputation (in professional use only) for preventing over-profuse menstruation and leucorrhoea. Its astringent action has been put to use to treat gastro-intestinal bleeding, diarrhoea, and dysentery, and the plant has also been employed externally as an antiseptic poultice. The saponin diosgenin in the plant has a close relationship to human sex hormones, cortisone, Vitamin D, and cardiac glycosides.

Urginea maritima
Squill

White squill, sea squill

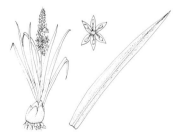

h to 5 ft (150 cm)

Parts used Dried fleshy inner part of the bulb.

Constituents Cardiac glycosides, flavonoids, mucilage, tannin, volatile oil, a carbohydrate.

Main uses *Medical* Catarrhal bronchitis.

Squill, like foxglove and lily of the valley, contains cardio-active glycosides, but in the case of squill, these are broken down so quickly in the body that they have little or no effect on the heart. The main use of this remedy is as a stimulating expectorant useful in bronchitis and other lung disorders. It is especially applicable if there is lung disease leading to a right-sided heart problem. The herb is also diuretic.[1]

CAUTION Large doses of white squill can cause vomiting. Red squill contains scilliroside, a powerful emetic used as a rat poison. This squill is not used in medicine.

LINACEAE

Linum usitatissimum
Flax

Linseed

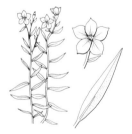

h 12–50 ins (30–130 cm). See p. 87.

Parts used Oil and seeds.

Constituents Fixed oil (up to 40%, including linoleic and linolenic acid), mucilage (6%) protein (25%), a cyanogenic glycoside (linamarine).

Main uses *Medical* As a laxative, for coughs, as a poultice for burns.

Flax is one of the most ancient cultivated plants. It is most widely known for the fibres obtained from its stems. The plant was grown and used by early Mesopotamians, Egyptians and Greeks to make cloth.

The oil from the seeds is known as

linseed oil. It is used widely in paints and varnishes. Linseed oil is also used in cooking and recently has been recommended to help leach toxic heavy metals such as aluminium from the body. The oil, mixed with slippery elm powder, makes a good poultice for burns.

The ground seeds also make an excellent drawing and healing poultice. The seeds are an effective bulk laxative, while a decoction of linseed is good for coughs and urinary infections.

CAUTION 3½ oz (100 g) of the seeds eaten at once have been known to cause poisoning. Do not exceed 2 oz (60 g) internally. Do not use immature seeds. Only use oil sold for human consumption.

LORANTHACEAE

Viscum album
Mistletoe
European mistletoe, birdlime

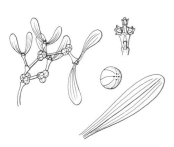

h to 3 ft (1 m). See p. 87.

Parts used Twigs and leaves.

Constituents May vary according to the host plant. Eleven proteins, viscotoxin (a cardioactive polypeptide), triterpenoid saponins, resin, mucilage, histamine, traces of an alkaloid.

Main uses *Medical* To lower blood pressure; as sedative.

Mistletoe acts to slow the heart rate and dilate the arteries, so lowering blood pressure.[1,2] It also has a sedative effect on the nervous system. Some controversy exists as to this remedy's supposed toxic effects on the liver[3] but to date these have remained unsubstantiated.[4] Indeed, there is evidence that mistletoe may have anti-tumour activities.[5]

CAUTION The berries are highly poisonous. This herb should only be prescribed by a qualified practitioner. RESTRICTED The U.S. Food and Drug Administration has classified American Mistletoe as unsafe.

MALVACEAE
Althea officinalis
Marsh mallow
See page 86

MENYANTHACEAE

Menyanthes trifoliata
Bogbean
Buckbean, water shamrock, marsh trefoil, water trefoil

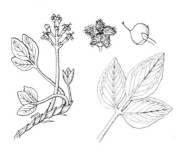

h to 10 ins (25 cm). See p. 87.

Parts used Leaves and rhizome; cultivation see p. 248.

Constituents Bitter glycosides, alkaloids, saponin, essential oil, flavonoids; the rhizome contains the bitter sweroside found in century.

Main uses *Medical* Indigestion and rheumatism.

The bitters in this plant give it a tonic action similar to century and gentian (see pp. 59 and 60), useful in indigestion and anorexia. It also has a reputation for easing rheumatic pains and being mildly sedative.

CAUTION Large doses may be emetic. Avoid in inflammatory bowel disease.

MONIMIACEAE

Peumus boldo
Boldo
Boldus

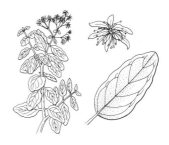

h 16–20 ft (5–6 m)

Parts used Leaves.

Constituents Alkaloids (including lamotetanine, boldine, isoboldine), volatile oil (including cymene, asconiodole, linalool, flavonoid glycosides, resin, tannins.

Main uses *Medical* Urinary infections and gallstones.

Boldo is a diuretic and urinary antiseptic remedy, useful in the treatment of cystitis. It also stimulates the liver and gallbladder. It increases the flow of bile, and is often prescribed by herbalists to treat gallstones.[1,2]

MYRICACEAE

Myrica cerifera
Bayberry
Wax myrtle, waxberry, candleberry

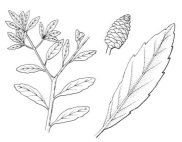

h to 33 ft (10 m)

Parts used Dried root bark.

Constituents Tannins, triterpenes (including myricadiol), flavonoid glycoside (myricitrin), resin, gum.

Althea officinalis
Marshmallow

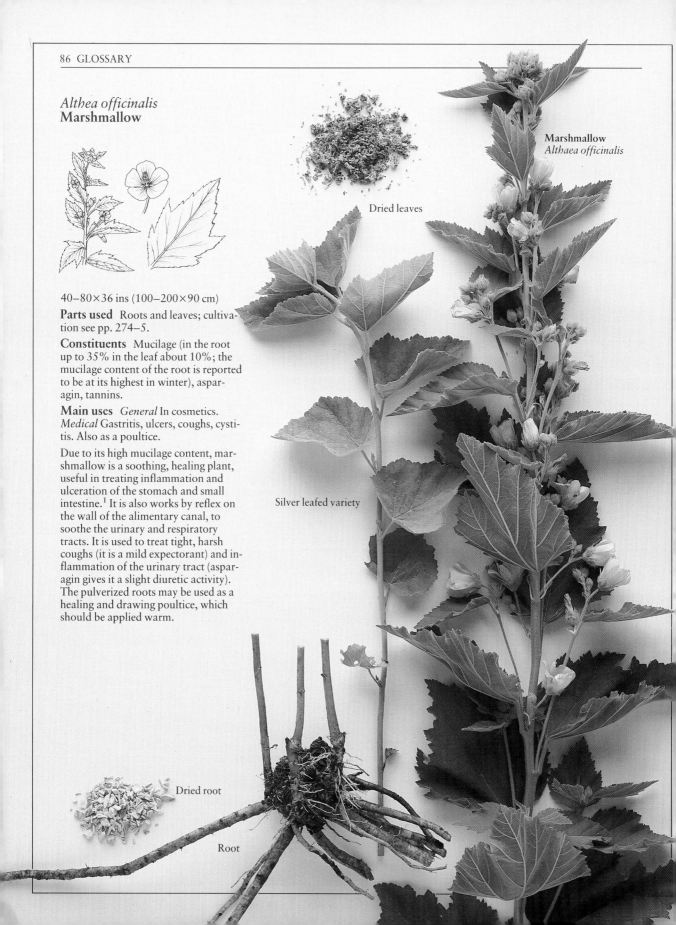

40–80×36 ins (100–200×90 cm)

Parts used Roots and leaves; cultivation see pp. 274–5.

Constituents Mucilage (in the root up to 35% in the leaf about 10%; the mucilage content of the root is reported to be at its highest in winter), asparagin, tannins.

Main uses *General* In cosmetics. *Medical* Gastritis, ulcers, coughs, cystitis. Also as a poultice.

Due to its high mucilage content, marshmallow is a soothing, healing plant, useful in treating inflammation and ulceration of the stomach and small intestine.[1] It is also works by reflex on the wall of the alimentary canal, to soothe the urinary and respiratory tracts. It is used to treat tight, harsh coughs (it is a mild expectorant) and inflammation of the urinary tract (asparagin gives it a slight diuretic activity). The pulverized roots may be used as a healing and drawing poultice, which should be applied warm.

Dried leaves

Marshmallow
Althaea officinalis

Silver leafed variety

Dried root

Root

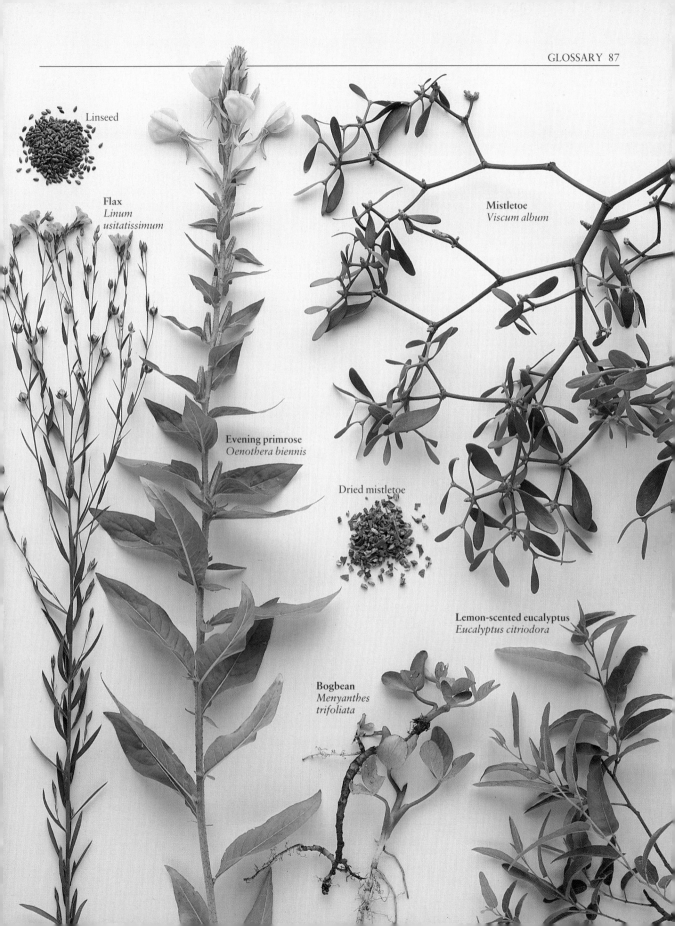

Linseed

Flax
*Linum
usitatissimum*

Mistletoe
Viscum album

Evening primrose
Oenothera biennis

Dried mistletoe

Lemon-scented eucalyptus
Eucalyptus citriodora

Bogbean
*Menyanthes
trifoliata*

Main uses *Medical* A stimulating astringent with a wide range of uses.

This plant produces an edible fat which is still used to make candles. The herb was a key astringent used by the North American Physiomedical herbalists and was a major component of Samuel Thomson's famous composition powder. Bayberry is used to treat the inflammation and infection of the gastrointestinal tract. It has been used to treat post-partum haemorrhage and taken internally and used as a douche is recommended for excessive menstruation and leucorrhoea. A hot decoction is employed to treat colds and fevers. The powdered bark has been used as a snuff for congested nasal passages and a decoction makes a good gargle for throat infections. A compress is effective for healing cuts and ulcers. Myricitrin is bactericidal and encourages the flow of bile.[1] Another constituent, myricadiol is reported to cause retention of salt and potassium excretion.

CAUTION Avoid prolonged use.

MYRTACEAE

Eucalyptus globulus
Eucalyptus

Tasmanian blue gum

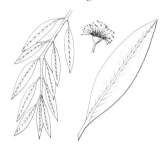

h to 230 ft (65 m). See p. 87.

Parts used Oil of leaves.

Constituents Oil comprising 70% cineole, pinenes, sesquiterpene alcohols, aromadendrene, cuminaldehyde.

Main uses *Medical* Colds and coughs.

Eucalyptus oil is strongly antiseptic and is used externally in inhalations for colds and excess phlegm and diluted as a chest rub for coughs. It also eradicates lice and fleas. A lemon-scented species,

E. citriodora, is a popular ingredient in dry pot pourris.

CAUTION Do not use internally.

Eugenia aromatica (also known as *Syzygium aromaticum*)
Clove

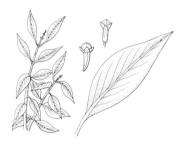

30–45 ft (10–15 m). See p. 34.

Parts used Dried buds.

Constituents Volatile oil (15%), gallotanic acid (13%), caryophyllin.

Main uses *General* In pot-pourris and pomanders. *Culinary* Used widely, especially with ham, fruit, mulled winter drinks; in garam masala and five-spice powder (see p. 169).

Cloves are the dried flower buds of the clove tree, which were used in China as early as 266 BC. Their strong, spicy odour and pungent taste are a particular feature of Asian cuisine. Oil of cloves is strongly antiseptic due to the high percentage of phenols (84–95%). It has long been employed as an effective remedy for toothache.

Pimenta officinalis
Allspice

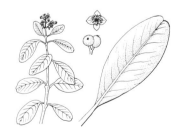

h to 40 ft (12 m). See p. 34.

Parts used Berries.

Constituents Volatile oil (to 4.5% comprising mainly eugenol, plus cineole, phellandrene, caryophyllene).

Main uses *Culinary* In pickles, preserves, cakes, and biscuits.

Most supplies of allspice come from Jamaica. The name was coined in the seventeenth century to describe the flavour, which was like a mixture of cinnamon, nutmeg, and cloves. Because of its hybrid flavour, allspice blends very well with other spices and is therefore an ingredient in many spice mixtures. The part of the berry with the strongest flavour is the shell, so it is best to use whole berries and grind them immediately before use to obtain the best flavour. Allspice can be used in a wide range of foods, both sweet and savoury – from pâtés to biscuits, curries to winter drinks such as mulled wine. Like many herbs used in cooking, it has the reputation of easing flatulence. Allspice may also be added to pot pourris.

MYRISTICACEAE

Myristica fragrans
Nutmeg

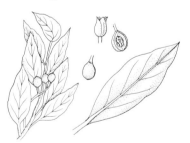

h to 40 ft (12 m). See p. 35.

Parts used Seed and covering.

Constituents Volatile oil (5–15% comprising eugenol and iso-eugenol), fixed oil (25–40%) yielding fat and comprising myristic acid (60%), oleic, palmitic, lauric and linoleic acids, also terpineol, borneol, terpenes.

Main uses *Culinary* In milk and cheese dishes; in sweet desserts; with green vegetables.

Nutmegs were introduced by the Arabs into the eastern Mediterranean in the middle of the twelfth century. In 1191 nutmeg was one of the aromatics strewn in the streets of Rome for its fumigant properties, on the occasion of Emperor Henry VI's coronation. The pendulous, globular fruit of this tree splits to release the nutmeg kernel. It is covered by the scarlet mace, which can also be bought separately and used as a spice. The flavours of nutmeg and mace are similar, but mace is stronger. As well as its culinary uses, nutmeg helps to relieve flatulence, vomiting and nausea.

CAUTION Nutmeg is toxic in anything but small amounts and should be used very sparingly. Side effects include disorientation, double vision, hallucination and convulsions.

OLEACEAE

Chionanthus virginicus
Fringe-tree
Snowdrop tree, snowflower, white fringe, old man's beard, poison ash tree, chionanthus

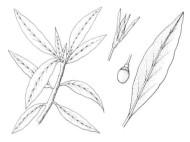

h to 27 ft (8 m)

Parts used Dried root bark, bark.

Constituents Saponins, phyllyrin (a lignan glycoside).

Main uses *Medical* For liver and gallbladder disease.

This North American tree, which is cultivated for its snow-like appearance when in flower, is an excellent bitter tonic. It is used to treat liver and gallbladder disease. It promotes the flow of bile from the gallbladder, stimulates the appetite and gastric secretions, and has a laxative action. It is also used for the treatment of intermittent fevers and to strengthen the constitution after chronic debilitating diseases such as glandular fever (mononucleosis). The bark is used as a poultice for healing wounds.

ONAGRACEAE

Oenothera lamarkiana
O. biennis
Evening primrose

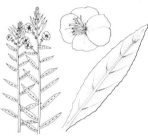

60×24 ins (150×60 cm). See p. 87.

Parts used Extracted oil.

Constituents Essential fatty acids, especially gammalinoleic acid (GLA).

Main uses *Medical* PMS and many other disorders.

Were it not for an increasingly substantial body of scientific evidence backing the extraordinary therapeutic range of the oil extracted from the evening-primrose plant, the claims made on its behalf would seem mere quackery. Evening primrose oil can have startling effects in the treatment of the premenstrual syndrome (PMS).

In 1981, at St Thomas's Hospital, London, 65 women with PMS were treated with oil of evening primrose. Of these 61% experienced complete relief, and 23% partial relief. One symptom, breast engorgement, was especially improved. 72% of the women reported feeling better.[1]

In November 1982, the prestigious British medical journal, the *Lancet* carried the results of the double blind crossover study on 99 patients with ectopic eczema.[2] This showed that when high doses of evening primrose oil were taken about 43% of the patients in the trial experienced an improvement.

Studies of the effect of evening primrose oil on hyperactive children also indicate that this form of treatment is beneficial in calming the children down. About two-thirds of the children treated responded favourably.[3] Evening primrose oil, it appears, is also useful to counteract alcoholic poisoning. It is highly effective in preventing hangovers. A study in Inverness, Scotland, demonstrated that the oil will encourage a liver damaged by alcohol to regenerate.[4] Other work indicates that oil of evening primrose can help withdrawal from alcohol and ease post-drinking depression.[5]

Another Scottish study has shown that evening primrose oil can help dry eyes and brittle nails.[6] When combined with zinc the oil may be used to treat acne. More controversially, oil of evening primrose is also claimed to be of benefit to sufferers of multiple sclerosis. Its use for MS sufferers has been recommended by Professor Field who directed MS research at the UK Medical Research Council's Demyelinating Diseases Unit.

Oil of evening primrose is also effective in guarding against coronary artery disease. Its active ingredient, gammalinoleic acid (GLA), is a powerful anti-blood-clotter.[7] It has also been shown to reduce blood pressure in animals with high blood pressure. A New York hospital discovered that people more than ten percent above their ideal body weight lost weight when taking the oil.

Perhaps the most remarkable study of all was completed at Glasgow Royal Infirmary in 1987 using evening primrose oil to treat patients with rheumatoid arthritis. 60% of patients taking the oil were able to stop their normal anti-arthritis drugs, and those taking fish oil in addition to evening primrose oil fared even better.

There is scientific explanation for these extraordinary results. GLA is a precursor of a hormone-like substance called PGEI which has a wide range of beneficial effects in the body. The production of this substance in some people may be blocked. GLA has been found in oil extracted from blackcurrant seeds and borage seeds, both of which are now commercial sources of this substance.

CAUTION Side effects of headache, skin rashes, and nausea have been reported. Use for epileptics is not recommended.

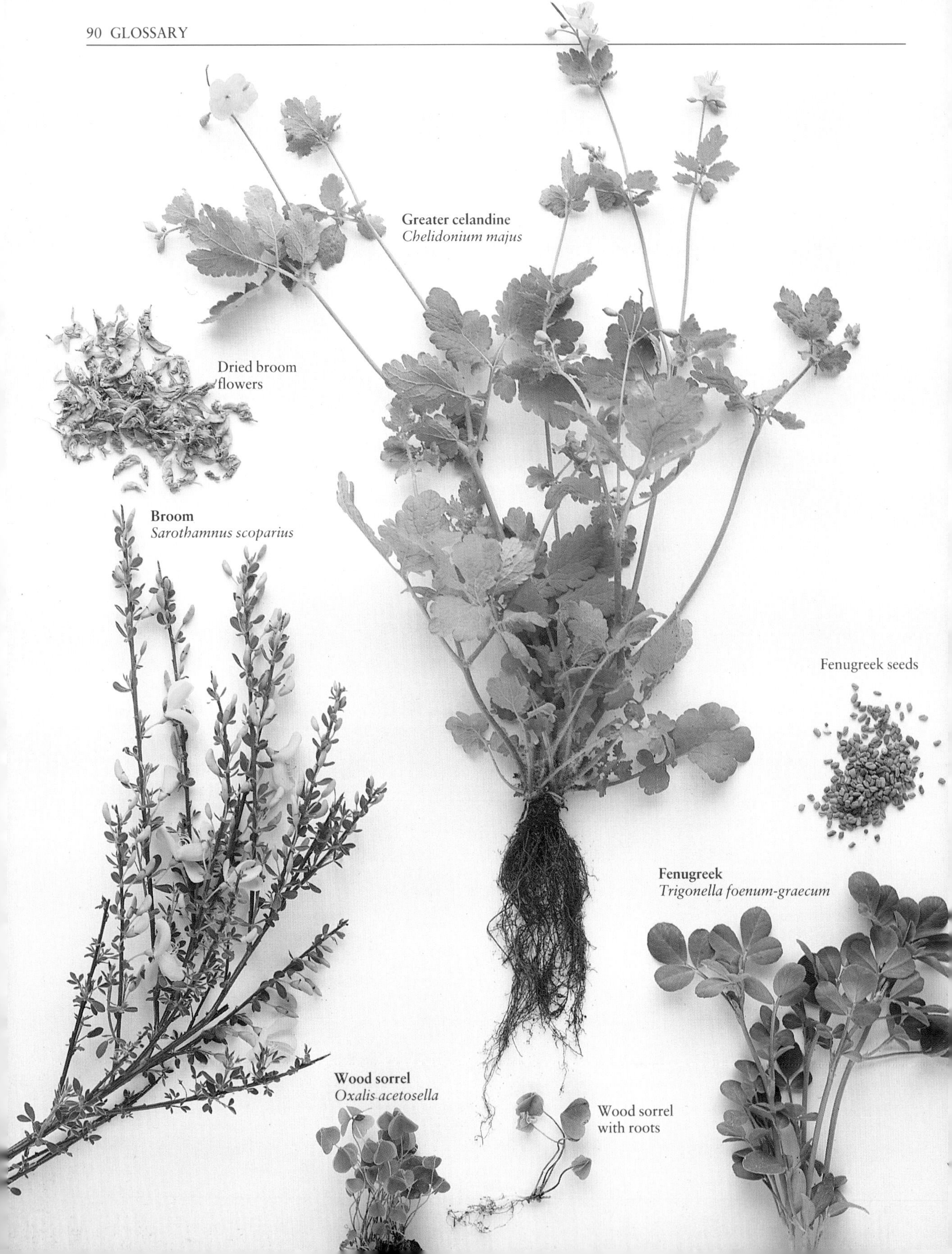

Greater celandine
Chelidonium majus

Dried broom
flowers

Broom
Sarothamnus scoparius

Fenugreek seeds

Fenugreek
Trigonella foenum-graecum

Wood sorrel
Oxalis acetosella

Wood sorrel
with roots

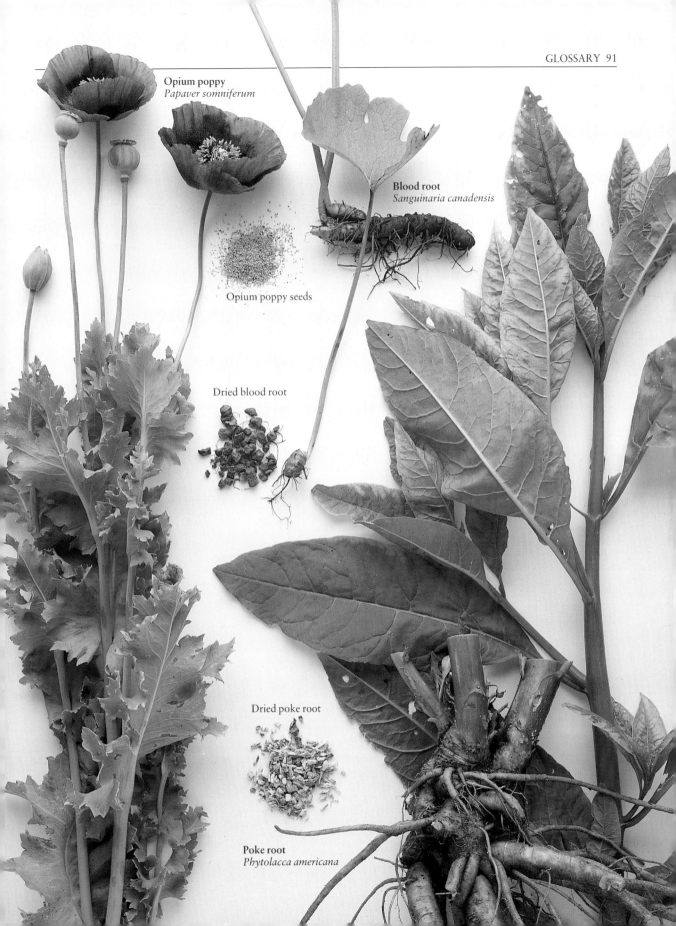

Opium poppy
Papaver somniferum

Opium poppy seeds

Blood root
Sanguinaria canadensis

Dried blood root

Dried poke root

Poke root
Phytolacca americana

ORCHIDACEAE

Cypripedium pubescens
Lady's slipper

Yellow lady's slipper, nerve root

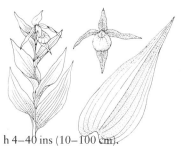

h 4–40 ins (10–100 cm).

Parts used Dried root.

Constituents Volatile oil, glucosides, resins, tannins.

Main uses *Medical* To calm nervous tension, for headaches, cramps.

The North American Indians used this root for nervous diseases and to allay pain. It relaxes and calms nervousness and tension. The plant provides a gentle and effective treatment for nervous headaches; it quiets anxiety, and promotes sleep. It also eases muscle and menstrual cramping. Recently lady's slipper has become difficult to obtain. It is a protected species.

CAUTION Large doses can cause headaches and disorientation. The fresh plant can cause contact dermatitis.

OXALIDACEAE

Oxalis acetosella
Wood sorrel

Wood sour, three-leaved grass, stubwort

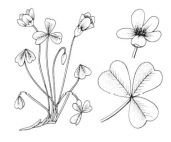

h 2–4 ins (5–8 cm). See p. 90.

Parts used Leaves and root

Constituents Oxalic acid, potassium oxalate, mucilage, vitamin C.

Main uses *Culinary* In salads and sauces (small amounts only).

This plant was widely used in sauces in the Middle Ages, but was largely replaced in culinary uses by buckler-leaf sorrel (*Rumex scutatus*). The sharp acidic taste of the leaves gave the plant its Latin name, which is derived from the Greek word for "sour". The taste also made the leaves a substitute for vinegar.

CAUTION This plant is poisonous in large quantities. It should be avoided by sufferers of kidney stones, rheumatism, or gout.

PALMAE

Serenoa serrulata var *S. Repens*
sabal serrulata
Saw palmetto

Sabal

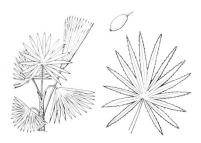

h 3–6 ft (1–2 m)

Parts used Berries.

Constituents A green volatile oil, fixed oil, steroidal saponins, resin, tannins.

Main uses *Medical* Reproductive disorders, colds, catarrh, and urinary diseases.

In his book on saw palmetto, the American doctor, Hule, noted the fattening properties of the berries after the summer drought. The North American Indians and white settlers recognized that the berries had the same nutritive properties for humans, stimulating the appetite and encouraging assimilation, so increasing fat, flesh and strength.

The berries' nourishing qualities are reputed to extend to the sexual organs (the steroidal saponins are probably significant here). The remedy has been prescribed for atrophy of the testes, low libido, and impotence in men. The herb is also recommended for inflammation of the prostate and enlarged prostate. According to the eclectic doctor Ellingwood, saw palmetto is also effective for functional infertility in women and to increase the supply of mother's milk. Saw palmetto may be used to relieve painful periods associated with lack of tone of the reproductive organs.

The berries have a toning and soothing influence on mucous membranes throughout the body as well as an expectorant property, making this a useful remedy for colds and catarrh (the isolated oil is an effective inhalant). It has a traditional use for asthma and bronchitis. The herb is also used to treat urinary disorders and enuresis. It is reputed to be mildly sedative to the nervous system.

PAPAVERACEAE

Chelidonium majus
Greater celandine

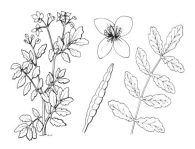

h 12–36 ins (30–90 cm). See p. 90.

Parts used Aerial parts; cultivation, see pp. 274–5.

Constituents Orange latex containing about ten alkaloids including chelidonine, chelerythrin, protopine, sanguinarine, saponin.

Main uses *Medical* Gallbladder disease and stones.

Greater celandine is an excellent remedy for stimulating the liver and gallbladder as well as being specific for infections of the gallbladder and gallstones. The plant has narcotic properties and is reputed to have an anticancer activity. The external application of the orange latex to warts is an old and often successful folk remedy.

CAUTION Poisonous in large doses. RESTRICTED.

Papaver somniferum
Opium poppy

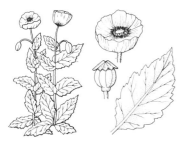

h 2–4 ft (60–125 cm). See p. 91.

Parts used Seeds.

Constituents Some 25 alkaloids (including morphine, codeine, papaverine, thebaine, narceine), meconic acid.

Main uses *Culinary* In baking.

The unripe seed capsules of the opium poppy are used for the extraction of morphine and the manufacture of codeine. It is the ripe seeds of the poppy that we use in cooking.

Sanguinaria canadensis
Blood root
Red root, Indian paint

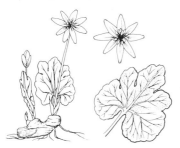

h 12 ins (30 cm). See p. 91.

Parts used Dried rhizome and root.

Constituents Many alkaloids (including sanguinarine, sanguidimerine, cholerythrine, protopine, berberine, copticine), also red resin.

Main uses *Medical* Bronchial catarrh.

The North American Indians used this plant to make a body paint. It is a fairly harsh stimulating expectorant. Sanguinarine has been reported to have a possible antibacterial and anti-cancer activity.[1]

CAUTION Large doses can be poisonous. Blood root is classified by the U.S. Food and Drug Administration as unsafe.

PAPILIONACEAE

Sarothamnus scoparius (also known as *Cytisus scoparius*)
Broom
Broomtops, scotch broom

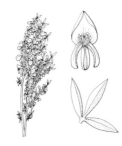

10×7 ft (3×2 m). See p. 90.

Parts used Flowering tops.

Constituents Alkaloids (sparteine, genisteine and sarothamnine), amines, amino acids, volatile oil, tannin.

Main uses *Medical* To regulate the heart; diuretic.

The Mediaeval name, *planta genista*, of this shrub was adopted by Henry II of England as his family name, Plantagenet. As today's names indicate, this plant makes an effective broom. Sparteine has a cardio-depressant action and herbalists use broom to regulate and strengthen the heartbeat.[1] It causes constriction of the peripheral blood vessels and thus a rise in blood pressure. Its use should be avoided in cases of high blood pressure. Broom is an effective diuretic and is used for fluid retention because of an incompetent heart. In France, the ashes of the whole plant are macerated in white wine, which is then strained and taken as a diuretic.

CAUTION Use only as prescribed by a qualified herbal practitioner. Broom must never be used during pregnancy or when there is high blood pressure. It is classified by the U.S. Food and Drug Administration as unsafe.

Trigonella foenum-graecum
Fenugreek
Bird's foot, Greek hay-seed

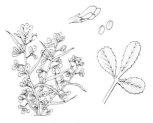

20×12 ins (50×30 cm). See p. 90.

Parts used Seed.

Constituents Alkaloids (trigonelline, choline, gentianine, carpaine), steroidal saponins (mainly diosgenin), flavonoids, oils (up to 8%), mucilage (up to 30%), protein (up to 20%), vitamins A, B, and C, calcium, iron, other minerals.

Main uses *Culinary* For flavouring in confectionery; as a spice in curries, chutneys. *Medical* Reproductive disorders and as a drawing poultice.

Fenugreek has been used as a spice and medicine since ancient times. The Arabs roast the seeds and use them as a kind of "coffee". The plant has exciting therapeutic possibilities because of its steroidal saponins which closely resemble the body's own sex hormones. This may account for the folk reputation of fenugreek as an aphrodisiac and for its substantial reputation for increasing the flow of milk in nursing mothers. In China fenugreek is prescribed for impotence in men and is also recommended for menopausal sweating and depression. It is a useful source of vitamins and minerals particularly calcium (again important after the menopause).

In addition, fenugreek is a soothing remedy for bronchitis and the pulve-

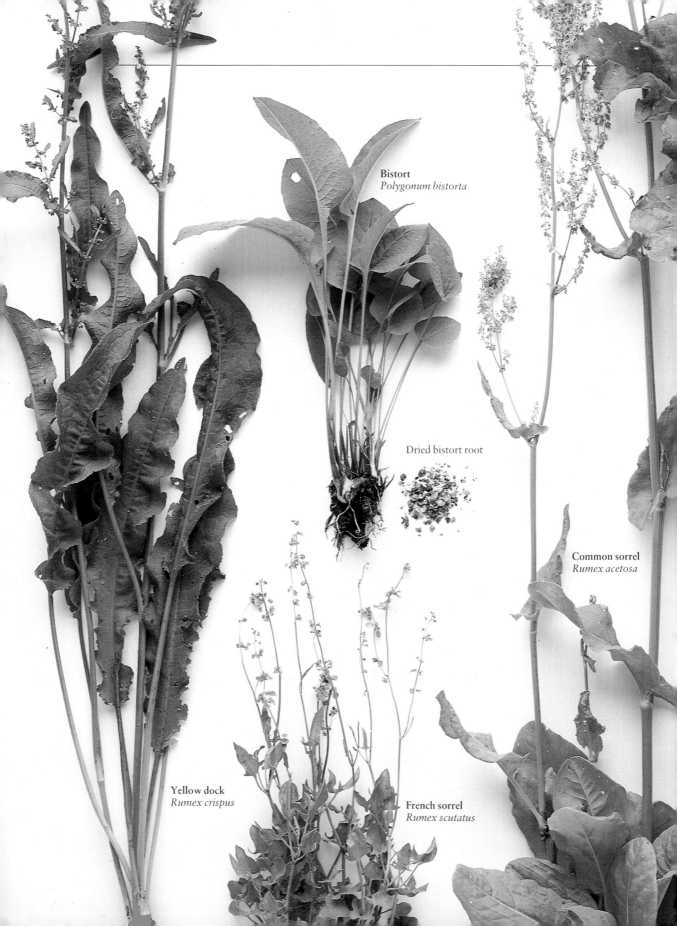

Bistort
Polygonum bistorta

Dried bistort root

Common sorrel
Rumex acetosa

Yellow dock
Rumex crispus

French sorrel
Rumex scutatus

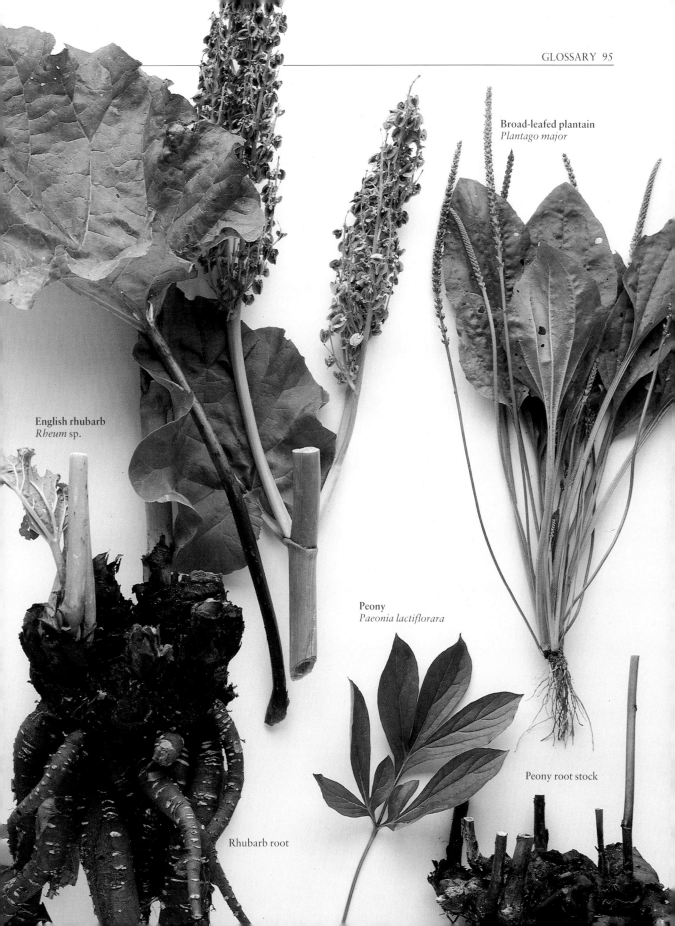

Broad-leafed plantain
Plantago major

English rhubarb
Rheum sp.

Peony
Paeonia lactiflorara

Rhubarb root

Peony root stock

rized seeds make an excellent poultice for rheumatic pains or boils which benefit from its drawing power.

In culinary use, fenugreek seeds are valued for their taste, which is similar to celery, and their vitamin and mineral content. They are used most frequently in spice mixtures for curries and in preserves. An additional species, *T. purpurascens*, is sometimes grown for culinary use.

CAUTION Fenugreek has a stimulating effect on the uterus and should not be used as a medicine during pregnancy.[1]

PARMELIACEAE

Cetraria islandica
Iceland moss

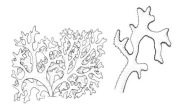

h 1–5 ins (3–12 cm)

Parts used Dried whole lichen.

Constituents Mucilage (up to 70% including lichenin and isolichenin), bitter fumaric acids, usnic acid, iodine.

Main uses *Medical* Respiratory disorders.

Iceland moss is a lichen with antibiotic properties. It used to be prescribed for TB because it was reputed to kill the tubercle bacillus and clear phlegm in the lungs. Herbalists still use it for asthma and other respiratory disorders. Its bitter taste and mucilage makes it both stimulating and soothing to the digestive tract.[1] It is used to quell nausea and vomiting. Iceland moss has nourishing properties and has been used as a food after the bitterness was removed by boiling.

PASSIFLORACEAE

Passiflora incarnata
Passionflower

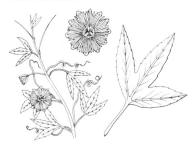

h 20–32 ft (6–10 m)

Parts used Flower and vine.

Constituents Alkaloids (harmane, harmol, harmaline, harmine and harmalol), flavonoids, sugars, sterols, gum.

Main uses *Medical* As a tranquillizer.

Passion flower relaxes the nervous system and has non-addictive sedative properties.[1] It is an important remedy for anxiety, tension, and insomnia. It is also used to reduce high blood pressure. Its alkaloids and flavonoids are reported to have tranquillizing effects.

Harpogophytum procumbens
Devil's claw

Parts used Tuber.

Constituents Iridoid glycosides, (harpogoside, harpagide and procumbine), sugars, gum-resin, Beta sitosterols.

Main uses *Medical* Arthritis.

This African plant gains its rather forbidding common name from its large hooked, claw-like fruit which has been known to trap and injure livestock grazing where it grows. It is, however, the tuber which is used in herbal medicine. Since the first scientific tests in 1958 at the University of Jena in Germany showed that this plant has strong anti-inflammatory properties,[2,3] compared to cortisone and phenylbutazone.[4] its healing reputation for treating arthritis and myalgia has spread far and wide. Recent French and German studies confirm the anti-inflammatory and pain-relieving potential of devil's claw comparable to that

of cortisone and phenylbutazone.[5,6] The plant also appears to be diuretic, to stimulate the liver and gallbladder and the lymphatic system and to lower blood sugar. Two components of the plant, harpogoside and Beta sitosterol, have anti-inflammatory properties but experiments indicate that the whole plant, not an isolated chemical, works best. Devil's claw also has a reputation, used externally, for treating skin disease.

CAUTION It has been suggested that devil's claw stimulates uterine muscle and should therefore be avoided in pregnancy.

PHYTOLACCACEAE

Phytolacca americana (also known as *P. decandra*)
Poke root
Coakum, pigeonberry, poke

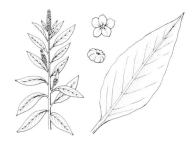

40×24 ins (100×60 cm). See p. 91.

Parts used Dried root.

Constituents Triterpenoid saponins, alkaloid (phytolaccine), resins, phytolaccic acid, tannin.

Main uses *Medical* Tonsillitis, swollen glands, and mastitis.

Poke root has a considerable reputation for stimulating the lymphatic system. Herbalists use it for tonsillitis, swollen glands and mumps. It is also used in rheumatism because it stimulates elimination from the tissues. As a poultice it is used to treat mastitis.

CAUTION The fresh plant is poisonous. In large doses the dried root is emetic and cathartic. Overdoses can be fatal.

PIPERACEAE

Piper methysticum
Kava kava

h 6 ft (2 m). See p. 82.

Parts used Dried rhizome and roots.

Constituents Oleo-resin including lactones, alkaloid, starch, mucilage.

Main uses *Medical* Urinary disorders.

In the south-sea islands an alcoholic drink made from kava kava was employed for inducing hallucinogenic states during religious ceremonies. The plant at first stimulates, then depresses the nervous system. It achieved wide fame as a possible cure for gonorrhoea. Today herbalists use it as a diuretic, urinary antiseptic and anti-inflammatory, making it useful for cystitis and prostatitis. It is also employed to treat gout and rheumatism. Externally it has been used as an analgesic in liniments.

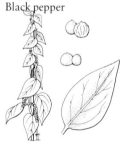

Piper nigrum
Pepper
Black pepper

Size variable. See p. 34.

Parts used Dried peppercorns.

Constituents Volatile oil (up to 2.5% containing the alkaloids piperine, piperettine), hydrocyanic acid, resins, starch.

Main uses *Culinary* For seasoning.

Pepper has been one of our most highly prized spices since earliest trade with the east. It was used as a currency during the siege of Rome in AD 408 and "peppercorn rents", now meaning very low rents, were commonly paid to land-lords. The high cost of pepper and other spices motivated the Portuguese to find a sea route to India. Black pepper and white pepper come from the same shrub. Instead of picking the unripe berries and drying them to produce black pepper, the fruit is allowed to ripen and then soaked to remove the dark outer skin, producing the white variety, which is milder than black. Whole peppercorns are used in pickles, marinades, stews, and stocks while ground pepper is included in savoury dishes. Because pepper loses its flavour quickly when ground, the whole corns should be kept in a mill and ground when required. Pepper stimulates the taste buds and helps to promote gastric secretions.

PLANTAGINACEAE

Plantago major
Broad-leafed plantain
Common plantain, snakeweed
Also *P. lanceolata* (long or lance-leaved plantain); *P. psyllium* (psyllium plantain or fleaseed)

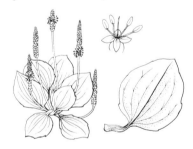

h 2–16 ins (5–40 cm). See p. 95.

Parts used Leaves of *P. major* and *P. lanceolata*; the seeds of *P. psyllium*.

Constituents *P. major* and *P. lanceolata* Mucilage, glycosides, tannins, silica. *P. psyllium* Mucilage up to 30%, monoterpene alkaloids, glycosides, sugars, triterpenes, fixed oil, fatty acids (eg linoleic), tannins.

Main uses *Medical* Cuts, stings, and insect bites. Psyllium seeds as bulk laxative.

Broad-leafed and lance-leafed plantain have similar properties. The crushed leaves can be applied directly to the skin to stop bleeding and allay the pain of bee stings and insect bites. Internally, an infusion of the leaves has a soothing, expectorant property making them good for the treatment of bronchitis and other lung problems.[1] Plantain's astringent action is useful in treating diarrhoea and cystitis. The plant is also said to be diuretic. Its silica and tannin content make it useful in treating varicose veins and haemorrhoids. Silica is beneficial for damaged lungs too.

Psyllium seeds (*Plantago psyllium*) are derived from two related species. Pale or blond psyllium seeds are inferior to the black seeds which are a gentle bulk laxative. Two teaspoons of the unground seeds should be put into a cup of warm water and stirred. After five minutes the contents should be swallowed and the dose repeated once to three times a day.

CAUTION Inhaling psyllium powder can cause asthma. Unsoaked seeds can cause gastrointestinal problems.

POLYGONACEAE

Polygonum bistorta
Bistort
Snake root

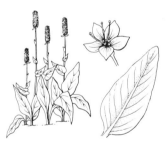

h 10–20 ins (25–50 cm). See p. 94.

Parts used Fresh leaves, dried rhizome.

Constituents Tannins, vitamin C, starch, oxalic acid.

Main uses *Culinary* Leaves boiled as vegetable in spring. *Medical* Diarrhoea, haemorrhoids, cuts, and sores.

This plant is rich in tannins, accounting for its astringent action. As well as being used in medicine it has a long history of use for food in northern Europe.

Rheum officinale
Chinese rhubarb

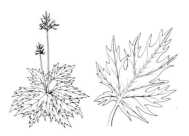

h to 6 ft (2 m). See p. 95.

Parts used Root and rhizome.

Constituents Anthraquinone glycosides (up to 5% including sennosides A, B, C, D, E and F), free anthraquinones including emodin, tannins.

Main uses *Medical* Constipation.

Rhubarb has apparently contradictory effects that are due to its variety of constituents. In small doses, the astringent tannins in the root make it effective for diarrhoea and also tonic to the digestive system. In larger doses, the irritative action on the bowel due to the anthraquinones give it a decidedly cathartic effect. In China, rhubarb root is an important ingredient in many prescriptions to treat high fevers.

CAUTION Avoid if suffering from arthritis, kidney disease, or urinary problems; and during pregnancy. The root of English rhubarb (*R. rhaponticum*) has similar properties but its leaf blades are poisonous.

POLYGONACEAE

Rumex crispus
Yellow dock

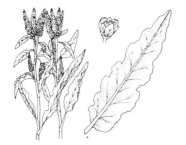

h 20–40 ins (50–100 cm). See p. 94.

Parts used Root.

Constituents Anthraquinone glycosides, tannins, iron.

Main uses *Medical* Skin diseases.

Although yellow dock, like rhubarb, contains anthraquinone glycosides, it has a gentle laxative rather than cathartic effect. This action is encouraged by its stimulating effect on bile production. It is a valuable cleansing remedy to help treat skin eruptions. A compress can help to soothe itchy skin. The plant's high iron content makes it valuable for correcting anaemia.

Rumex scutatus
French sorrel

Buckerleaf sorrel, garden sorrel

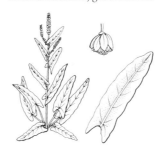

16×16 ins (40×40 cm). See p. 94.

Parts used Leaves›.

Constituents Oxalates, in small quantities, vitamin C.

Main uses *Culinary* In salads, egg dishes, sauces, soups; with fish.

Young green sorrel leaves have a slightly acid, lemony taste. Sorrel contains vitamin C and is a nutritious cleansing herb in spring. The leaves can be eaten raw in salads, cooked in butter, or incorporated into sauces and soups.

R. acetosa is a related species with leaves that may be eaten either raw, boiled or cooked like spinach and eaten with turnips or light meats such as lamb.

CAUTION Due to the oxalic acid content of this plant, avoid sorrel if you are suffering from arthritis or kidney disease. Avoid large doses.

PRIMULACEAE

Primula veris
Cowslip

Keyflower, palsywort

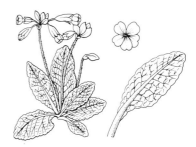

10×8 ins (25×20 cm). See p. 99.

Parts used Flowers and root; cultivation, see pp. 278–9.

Constituents Up to 10% saponins and glycosides (primulaveroside and primveroside containing salicylates), a volatile oil, and flavonoids.

Main uses *Culinary* Flowers in cowslip wine. *Medical* Insomnia and nervous tension. Arthritis (the root).

This is a plant with a wide range of uses. The flowers, which carry most of the essential oil (known as primula camphor) are a simple remedy for insomnia and nervous tension. Cowslip syrup was a country remedy for palsy (paralysis), hence its alternative name, palseywort. A tea of the flowers is commonly used for headache. Cowslip flowers also have a reputation for treating measles and an ointment made from them is good for sunburn. Cowslip wine strengthens the nervous system when taken in medicinal doses.

The high saponin content in the root probably accounts for the reputation of this part of the plant for treating whooping cough and bronchitis (both the flowers and root have an expectorant effect). The salicylates present in the root explain the widespread use in Europe of this part of the plant in the treatment of arthritis. For this reason in many old herbals the roots are called *radix arthritica*.

This once common grassland flower has now become relatively rare. Although it is beginning to establish itself on roadside verges away from damaging pesticide spraying, care should be taken not to over-collect it.

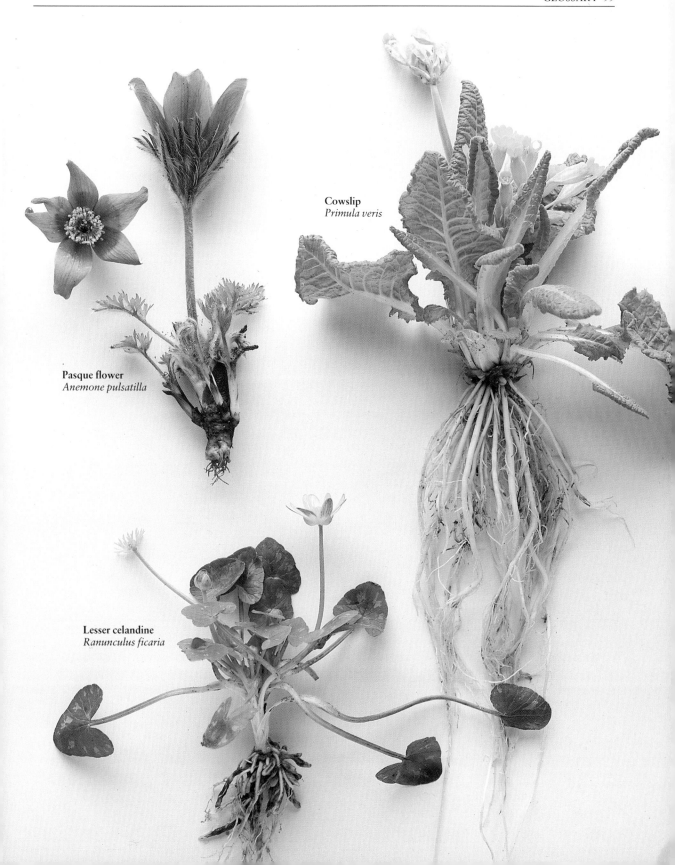

Cowslip
Primula veris

Pasque flower
Anemone pulsatilla

Lesser celandine
Ranunculus ficaria

RANUNCULACEAE

Anemone pulsatilla
Pasque flower

Pulsatilla, windflower, prairie or meadow anemone

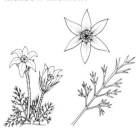

4–12×8 ins (10–30×20 cm). See p. 99.

Parts used Aerial parts; cultivation, see pp. 274–5.

Constituents The fresh plant contains the glycoside, ranunculin, which in the dried plant converts to anemonin; also saponins and a resin. The dried plant should not be stored for longer than a year.

Main uses *Medical* Nervous tension, neuralgia, earache, inflammation of the reproductive system.

This plant is called pasque flower because it blooms at Easter. According to Greek legend, it sprang from the tears of Venus, and Dioscorides mentions its use for ophthalmia, advice echoed by Gerard and Culpeper. In homeopathy tearfulness is one of the chief symptoms for which pulsatilla is prescribed.

Herbalists make judicious use of this apparently frail but powerful plant, using it in small doses. As in homeopathy, it is particularly applicable to women, being useful for neuralgia, headache, and nervous exhaustion. It is also useful for pain and inflammation of the reproductive system, alleviating menstrual cramps especially useful when the woman is anxious or irritable. It is employed for treating male reproductive disorders too. But reproductive ailments need professional attention. The tincture is also prescribed for earache. Herbalists use the plant externally to treat skin infections because of its antibacterial properties.

CAUTION This plant should only be used as prescribed by a qualified herbal practitioner. The fresh plant is poisonous.

Cimicifuga racemosa
Black cohosh

Black snakeroot, bugbane, squawroot

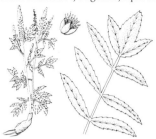

h 3–6 ft (1–2 m).

Parts used Dried root and rhizome.

Constituents Triterpene glycosides (actein and cimigoside), resin (cimicifugin), salicylates, isoferulic acid, tannin, ranunculin (which yields anemonin), volatile oil.

Main uses *Medical* Nerve and muscle pain; arthritis.

This is another valuable remedy inherited from the North American Indians. It is widely used for treating neuralgia. Its sedative effect is probably due in part to anemonin which depresses the central nervous system. Black cohosh is employed for treating headaches and tinnitus. A resinous compound insoluble in water lowers blood pressure and dilates the blood vessels.[1,2] This ability to dilate the blood vessels is in character with another major activity of black cohosh, which is antispasmodic, easing cramping and muscle tension. The herb has been used to treat arthritis where there is muscular as well as joint pain. The salicylates in the plant are anti-inflammatory and research confirms that the whole plant has this effect, which is helpful to the respiratory system.

Black cohosh's antispasmodic action makes it a remedy for asthma and whooping cough. The herb is also effective in treating menstrual cramps and is useful during childbirth. According to the eclectic physician Dr Felter, the remedy is "an ideal regulator of uterine contractions during labour".

CAUTION A powerful remedy only to be used by those experienced in herbal medicine. Overdose can result in intense headache, dizzyness, visual disturbances, a slow pulse rate and nausea and vomiting. Avoid in pregnancy.

Hydrastis canadensis
Golden seal

Yellow root, orange root, Indian turmeric, eye root

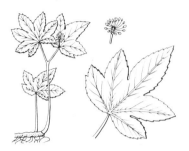

12×10 ins (30×25 cm).

Parts used Rhizome and root.

Constituents Alkaloids (hydrastine and berberine, also canadine and others), resin, volatile oil.

Main uses *Medical* Inflammation of the digestive system.

Golden seal is a famous North American Indian medicine. It is one of the most effective herbal remedies for inflamed and catarrhal conditions of the mucous membranes. It is invaluable in treating peptic ulcers and strongly stimulates the secretion of bile. An infusion makes an effective douche for trichomonas and thrush (*Candida albicans*). A mouthwash or gargle of golden seal is good for infected gums and sore throats. It is an ingredient in many soothing and healing eye lotions and eardrops. An external wash is highly effective in eradicating skin infections or sores, particularly impetigo or ringworm, although it stains the skin yellow. Modern research confirms the plant's potential. The plant's major alkaloids hydrastine and berberine are sedative and tend to lower blood pressure. Both exhibit a strong antibacterial and even an anti-viral action.[1,2]

CAUTION Berberine stimulates the uterus. Do not use golden seal during pregnancy (see also Barberry, p. 29).

Paeonia lactiflora
Peony

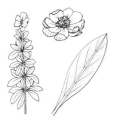

h to 3 ft (1 m). See p. 95.

Parts used Root.

Constituents Benzoic acid, asparagin, essential oil, alkaloid.

Main uses *Medical* Kidney and gallbladder disease.

This plant has a long history of medicinal use from China to western Europe, but its use has now declined.

CAUTION This plant is poisonous.
RESTRICTED.

Ranunculus ficaria
Lesser celandine
Pilewort

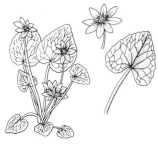

h 2–10 ins (5–25 cm). See p. 99.

Parts used Whole plant.

Constituents Anemonin, protoanemonin, tannin.

Main uses *Medical* Piles.

This is one of the earliest of spring flowers whose tubers give the plant its Latin name *ficaria* – from the Latin for a fig, *ficus*. To adherents of the Doctrine of Signatures, the tubers looked like piles. In former times, herbalists re-

commended the plant to be taken both internally and externally for piles, hence its alternative name, pilewort, but its acrid nature makes it more suitable for use as a pile ointment which is made from the plant.

The English name celandine is confusing because the plant is not related to greater celandine (*Chelidonum majus*).

RHODOPHYTA

Chondrus crispus
Irish moss
Carragheen

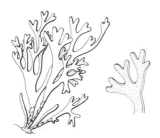

fronds 4–12 ins (10–30 cm).

Parts used Dried fronds (thalli).

Constituents Five polysaccharide complexes known as carageenans (up to 80%) containing sulphur, iodine, bromine, iron.

Main uses *General* In cosmetic hand gel (see p. 145). *Culinary* As gelling and thickening agent. *Medical* Respiratory disorders; as a nourishing food for invalids.

Irish moss swells and partially dissolves in cold water, producing a viscous solution. It forms a gel on cooling after being decocted and reacts strongly with milk protein to form a thick gel. Irish moss has traditionally been used for its demulcent and emollient properties. It has frequently been prescribed to soothe a TB cough or bronchitis and to heal and ease the pain of gastric and duodenal ulcers. Carrageenan, a constituent of the plant, is reported to reduce gastric secretions.

Irish moss is traditionally given as a nourishing food for invalids. It can be boiled with milk and made into a dessert.

ROSACEAE

Agrimonia eupatoria
Agrimony
Church steeples, cockeburr, cocklebur

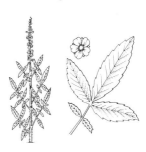

Parts used Aerial parts

Constituents Tannins, bitter principles, essential oil, silica.

Main uses *Medical* To stop bleeding.

Named after Mithridates Eupator, king of Pontus, who was a famous herbalist, agrimony retains its importance today as a healing herb with a wide range of uses. The plant is tonic to the digestive system, the gentle astringency of its tannins toning the mucus membranes, improving their secretion and absorption. Agrimony is a useful remedy for healing peptic ulcers and for controlling colitis. The bitter principles in the plant regulate the function of the liver and gallbladder. In Germany, agrimony has been used to treat gallstones and cirrhosis of the liver. It is also employed to counter high uric-acid levels in rheumatism and gout (it is said to have diuretic properties).

In traditional Chinese medicine, agrimony is a major herb for stopping bleeding and it is used to treat profuse menstruation. Chinese research indicates that agrimony can increase coagulation of the blood by up to 50%.[1] In Europe, too, agrimony is valued for this property – internally for blood in the urine (a symptom which requires medical investigation) and externally for wounds and cuts. Agrimony is a favourite herb for inflamed gums and sore throats (mouthwash or gargle). As a douche it treats leucorrhoea and it is beneficial as an eyewash for conjunctivitis.

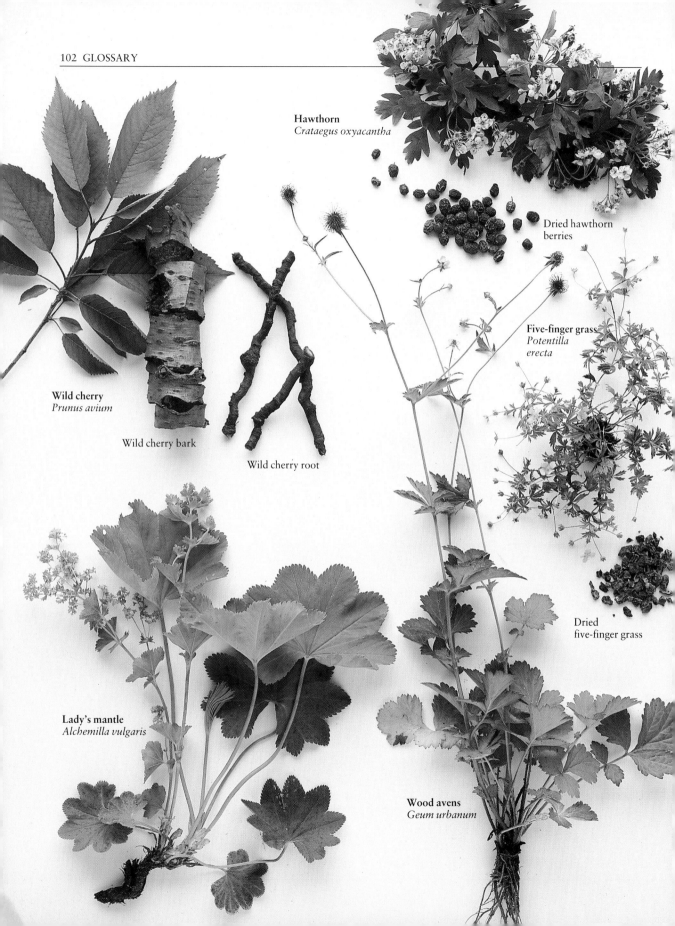

Hawthorn
Crataegus oxyacantha

Dried hawthorn
berries

Wild cherry
Prunus avium

Wild cherry bark

Wild cherry root

Five-finger grass
*Potentilla
erecta*

Dried
five-finger grass

Lady's mantle
Alchemilla vulgaris

Wood avens
Geum urbanum

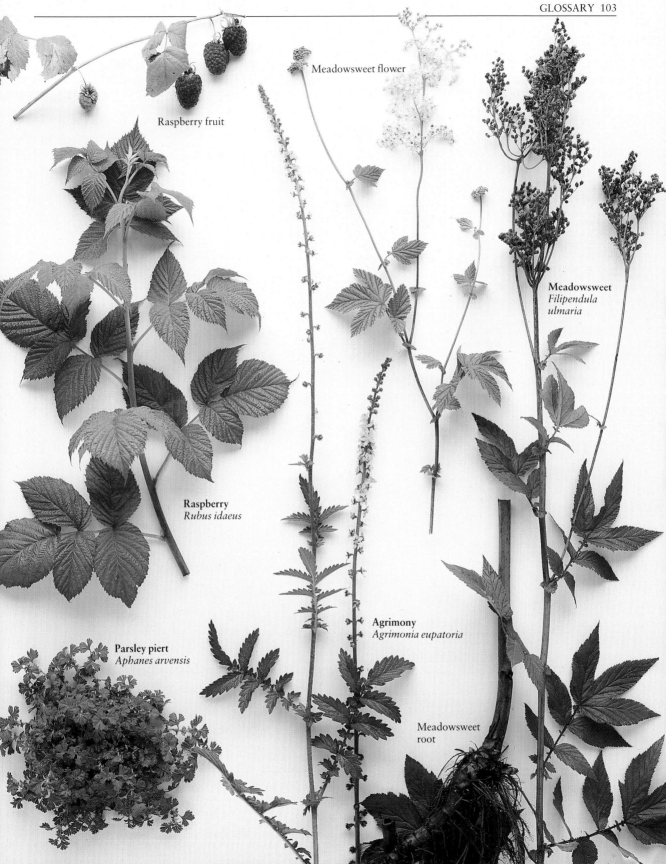

Raspberry fruit

Meadowsweet flower

Meadowsweet
*Filipendula
ulmaria*

Raspberry
Rubus idaeus

Agrimony
Agrimonia eupatoria

Parsley piert
Aphanes arvensis

Meadowsweet
root

Alchemilla vulgaris
Lady's mantle
Lion's foot, bear's foot

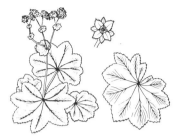

h 4–20 ins (10–50 cm). See p. 102.

Parts used Herb and root; cultivation, see pp. 274–5.

Constituents Tannins.

Main uses *Medical* Menstrual disorders.

The Latin name comes from the word alchemy, since this herb was once believed to have magical properties. In former times it was used externally on wounds and cuts – Culpeper called it "one of the most singular wound herbs". Like agrimony herbalists use it to treat heavy periods and as a douche for leucorrhoea. It is also an astringent tonic to the digestive tract, useful in stemming diarrhoea caused by gastroenteritis.

Alchemilla arvensis (p. 103) is parsley piert (also known as field lady's mantle) which is a well known traditional remedy for gravel, kidney stones and urinary infections.

Crategus oxyacantha (or *C. monogyna*)
Hawthorn
Mayblossom, whitethorn

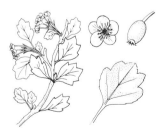

h to 30 ft (9 m). See p. 102.

Parts used Flowers, leaves, berries.

Constituents Flavonoid glycosides, saponins, procyanidines, trimethylamine, condensed tannins.

Main uses *Medical* Heart and circulatory disease.

Hawthorn is one of our most valuable remedies for the heart and circulation. It contains flavonoids which dilate the coronary and peripheral arteries,[1] and procyanidines which appear to slow the heart beat.[2] A report in the *British Medical Journal* showed that the berries reduced high blood pressure caused by hardening of the arteries and kidney disease, while research work published on the effect of the flowers showed that they significantly improved the health of patients suffering from an "ageing heart" and those who had heart-valve disease. The extraordinary feature of this herb is its ability both to lower high blood pressure and to restore low blood pressure to normal. It is also valuable in treating angina, irregular heartbeat, spasm of the arteries (eg Reynaud's disease), and insomnia of nervous origin.[3] In China, hawthorn berries are used to aid digestion and in France similarly, they have a reputation for treating dyspepsia and diarrhoea.

Filipendula ulmaria
Meadowsweet
Queen of the meadow, bridewort

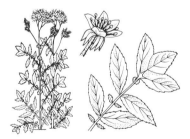

2–3 ft×1 ft (60–90 cm×30 cm). See p. 103.

Parts used Flowers and leaves; cultivation see pp. 274–5.

Constituents Salicylates (opiraein, salicin, gaultherine), tannin (up to 10%), mucilage, flavonoids, volatile oil, vitamin C, sugar.

Main uses *Medical* Rheumatism, fevers, and children's diarrhoea.

In 1838, an Italian professor first produced salicylic acid from the flowerbuds of the graceful meadowsweet as well as from willow bark (*Salix alba*). In 1899, the drug company, Bayer, formulated a new drug (acetylsalicylic acid) and called it aspirin, a name derived from the old botanical name for meadowsweet *Spirea ulmaria*.

Meadowsweet exemplifies the herbal principle that the whole plant is greater than the sum of its constituent parts. The anti-inflammatory action of the salicylates in the plant makes it effective against rheumatism. But its tannin and mucilage content appear to buffer the adverse effect of isolated salicylates, which can cause gastric bleeding. In fact, the whole plant is a traditional remedy for acid stomach. Because of its tannin content, it is also useful for children's diarrhoea. In addition, meadowsweet has an antiseptic diuretic action (salicylic acid is antiseptic) promoting the excretion of uric acid.[1] In hot infusion it is sweat-inducing, and its salicylate content points to its use in controlling fevers – it is a sort of herbal aspirin, in fact.

Geum urbanum
Wood avens
Herb bennet, colewort, goldy stone, clove root

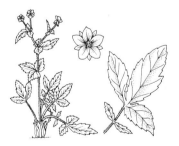

h 1–3 ins (3–7 cm). See p. 102.

Parts used Herb and root.

Constituents Tannins, volatile oil (comprising mainly eugenol), bitters, resin.

Main uses *Medical* Digestive disorders, piles, bleeding.

Avens is undoubtedly an underrated medicinal plant. It combines bitter-tonic properties with the healing astringent effect of its tannins and the antiseptic action of its volatile oil which has a clove-like aroma (its constituent eugenol is found in clove and allspice oil). Paracelsus recommended this plant for stomach and intestinal disorders (eugenol increases the activity of the digestive enzyme, trypsin) and diarrhoea. Due to its bitter component, it also regulates liver and gallbladder function. Avens is considered an excellent tonic for fevers and has been substituted for quinine. The plant is used to treat piles, for leucorrhoea, and to stop both internal and external bleeding.

Potentilla erecta
Five-finger grass
Red root, tormentil, cinquefoil

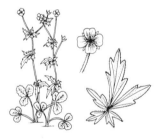

h 4–16 ins (10–40 cm). See p. 102.

Parts used Root.

Constituents Catechol-tannins (up to 20%), glycoside (tormentilline), bitter quinovic acid, red pigment, resin, gums.

Main uses *General* The roots produce a red dye. *Culinary* Extract of the root used in certain types of schnapps. *Medical* Diarrhoea, sore throats and gums.

This plant is a powerful astringent formerly used in tanning. It is excellent for treating gastroenteritis and its resulting diarrhoea. It is also tonic to the large intestine. It is employed as a gargle for sore and infected gums. It has a reputation for treating intermittent fevers which is interesting in the light of the reported constituent quinoric acid, also present in Cinchona bark. As a douche, it is effective for leucorrhoea. Externally, it is styptic and healing for

cuts and wounds. It can be used as an ointment or wash for haemorrhoids. A weak decoction is good for conjunctivitis.

Prunus serotina
Wild cherry
Wild black cherry, choke-cherry

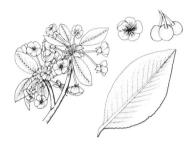

h 32–65 ft (10–20 m). See p. 102.

Parts used Bark (that collected in the fall yields the highest prussic acid content, while that collected in the spring gives less).

Constituents Cyanogenic glycosides (including prunasin), an enzyme (prunase), coumarins, volatile oil, tannins, resin.

Main uses *Medical* Irritating, nervous or continuous coughs.

Wild cherry bark is an important cough remedy. Once ingested, the cyanogenic glycosides are hydrolized to glucose, bensaldehyde, and hydrocyanic acid, otherwise known as prussic acid. Prussic acid is excreted rapidly, largely via the lungs where it at first increases respiration and then sedates the sensory nerves which provoke the cough reflex. Although prussic acid is highly poisonous, if wild cherry bark is used in medicinal doses, the low prussic acid content (0.07–0.16%) ensures that the remedy is quite safe. Both the cyanogenic glycosides and volatile oil in wild cherry bark improve the digestion.

CAUTION The leaves and pits are poisonous.

Rosa spp
Rose
See page 106

Rubus idaeus
Raspberry
European red raspberry

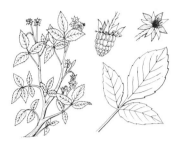

h 3–5 ft (90–150 cm). See p. 103.

Parts used Leaves and fruit.

Constituents Leaves: fragarine, tannin. Fruit: sugars, citric and malic acid, vitamins A, B, C and E, pectin, volatile oil, iron, calcium, phosphorus.

Main uses *Culinary* Fruit widely used. *Medical* For childbirth.

Raspberry leaf is a good astringent remedy, useful for children's diarrhoea. A cold infusion makes an effective gargle or mouthwash. This herb's most famous application, however, is in preparing mothers-to-be for childbirth. Raspberry-leaf tea appears to tone the uterine and pelvic muscles. Dr. Violet Russel in a letter to *The Lancet* said of raspberry-leaf tea: "somewhat shamefacedly I have encouraged expectant mothers to drink this infusion. In a great many cases labour has been free and easy from muscular spasm". Raspberry-leaf tea can be taken during the last three months of pregnancy. This infusion also enriches and encourages the flow of mother's milk.

The fruit is rich in nutrients and helps to combat anaemia. In Chinese medicine, Chinese raspberries (the fruit) are used to strengthen the kidneys and to treat enuresis.

Raspberries have long been cultivated for their culinary, as well as their medicinal, virtues. There are many ways of serving these fruits as a dessert to take advantage of their high iron and vitamin C content. The French make a liqueur from raspberries, called Framboise.

The related North American wild raspberry, *Rubus strigosus*, has the same medicinal properties. Many other species are grown for fruit.

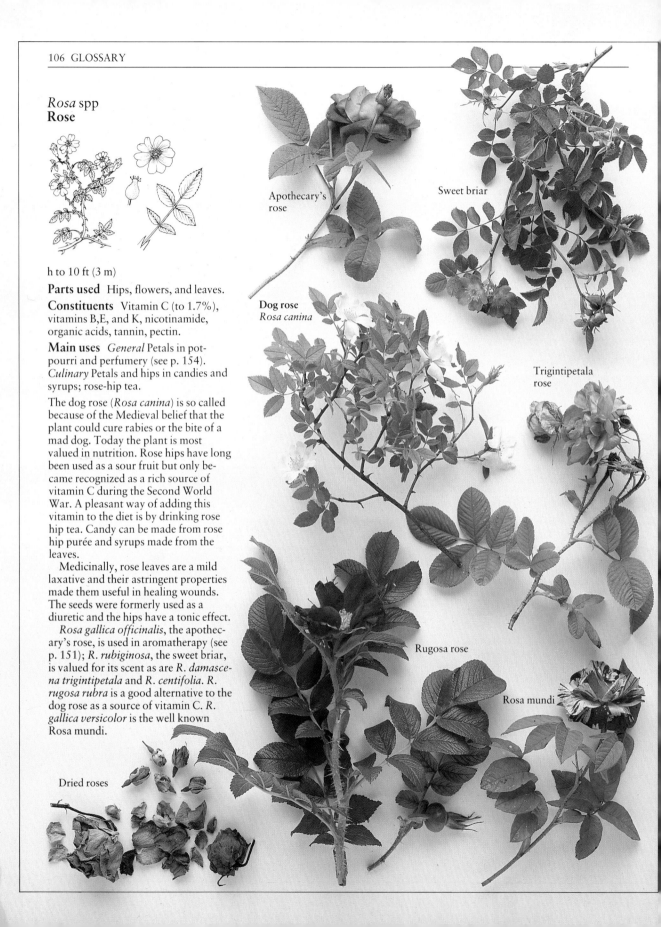

Rosa spp
Rose

h to 10 ft (3 m)

Parts used Hips, flowers, and leaves.

Constituents Vitamin C (to 1.7%), vitamins B,E, and K, nicotinamide, organic acids, tannin, pectin.

Main uses *General* Petals in pot-pourri and perfumery (see p. 154). *Culinary* Petals and hips in candies and syrups; rose-hip tea.

The dog rose (*Rosa canina*) is so called because of the Medieval belief that the plant could cure rabies or the bite of a mad dog. Today the plant is most valued in nutrition. Rose hips have long been used as a sour fruit but only became recognized as a rich source of vitamin C during the Second World War. A pleasant way of adding this vitamin to the diet is by drinking rose hip tea. Candy can be made from rose hip purée and syrups made from the leaves.

Medicinally, rose leaves are a mild laxative and their astringent properties made them useful in healing wounds. The seeds were formerly used as a diuretic and the hips have a tonic effect.

Rosa gallica officinalis, the apothecary's rose, is used in aromatherapy (see p. 151); *R. rubiginosa*, the sweet briar, is valued for its scent as are *R. damascena trigintipetala* and *R. centifolia*. *R. rugosa rubra* is a good alternative to the dog rose as a source of vitamin C. *R. gallica versicolor* is the well known Rosa mundi.

Apothecary's rose

Sweet briar

Dog rose
Rosa canina

Trigintipetala rose

Rugosa rose

Rosa mundi

Dried roses

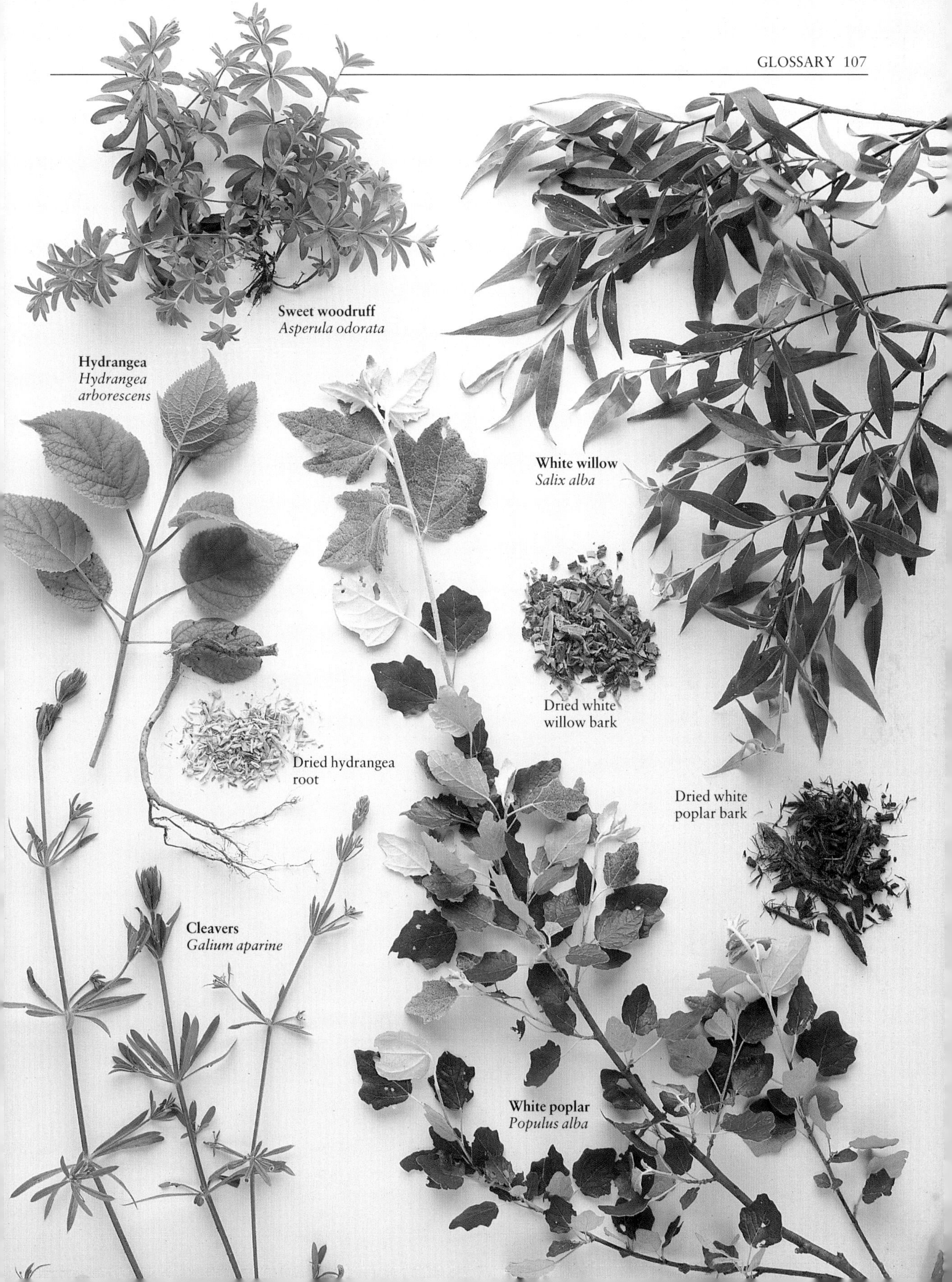

Sweet woodruff
Asperula odorata

Hydrangea
Hydrangea arborescens

White willow
Salix alba

Dried white
willow bark

Dried hydrangea
root

Dried white
poplar bark

Cleavers
Galium aparine

White poplar
Populus alba

RUBIACEAE

Asperula odorata
Woodruff
Sweet woodruff

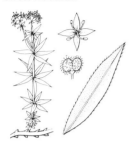

h 10 ins (25 cm). See p. 107.

Parts used Leaves, stems, flowers; cultivation see p. 274–5.

Constituents Coumarin, tannin, citric acid, rubichloric acid.

Woodruff was widely used as a strewing herb for home and church, carpeting the floor and scenting the air. It was also used to stuff beds, and to perfume bed linen. Its sweet scent (like new-mown hay) is due to its coumarin content. The flowers and leaves make a delicious tea. In Germany woodruff is added to Rhine wine and drunk on the first of May.

CAUTION Large doses can cause dizziness and vomiting.

Cinchona succiruba and *Cinchona calisaya*
Red cinchona and yellow cinchona
Peruvian bark, Jesuit's bark, fever tree

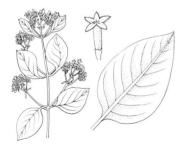

h 20–83 ft (6–25 m)
Parts used Bark.
Constituents Over 36 alkaloids (up to 16%) comprising mostly quinine, quinidine, cinchonine, and cinchonidine; tannins, glycosides, quinic acid, starch, resin, wax.

Main uses *Medical* Malaria.

Cinchona bark and its extracted alkaloid quinine are perhaps the most famous anti-malarial medicines. Cinchona was first introduced into Europe in the seventeenth century by the Jesuits. In recent years, malarial parasites which have become resistant to synthetic drugs have once more succumbed to this tried and trusted herbal remedy. Cinchona is used to treat fever in general and as a bitter digestive tonic. Both quinidine and quinine depress the action of the heart and cinchona bark has been used to treat cardiac arrhythmias. Quinine sulphate, an orthodox drug, is employed to treat cramping.

CAUTION The alkaloids are potentially toxic and stimulate uterine contractions. Avoid during pregnancy. Overdoses may cause headaches, fever, vomiting, blindness, deafness, loss of consciousness, and even death. RESTRICTED.

Galium aparine
Cleavers
Clivers, goosegrass, gripgrass, sticky-willie, catchweed, hedgeburs

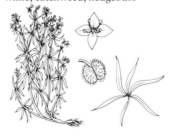

h up to 4 ft (120 cm). See p. 107.

Parts used Aerial parts.

Constituents Coumarins, a glycoside red dye, tannins, citric acid.

Main uses *General* In deodorant (see p.147). *Medical* Urinary stones, skin disease.

Cleavers is a reliable diuretic used to help clean gravel and urinary stones and to treat urinary infections. It also stimulates the lymphatic system and relieves swollen lymph glands. The body relies on the lymphatic system to drain away toxins and wastes, these, under the influence of cleavers, will be voided in the urine, and so it is understandable that the herb has been described as an alterative and blood purifier. It is useful, therefore, in treating diseases such as eczema, psoriasis and arthritis in which the body requires cleansing. It is also traditionally used for cancer, particularly that of the lymphatic system. It is reputed to help lower blood pressure and cool the body during fevers and is used as an external wash for sores and wounds.

Cleavers has a number of uses in herbal cosmetics and body care. An infusion of the herb applied to the skin is said to clear the complexion and can also be used as a hair rinse to treat dandruff. In addition, a reliable natural deodorant can be made from the plant.

The fresh leaves and tips can be boiled and eaten like spinach.

Mitchella repens
Squawvine
Partridgeberry, checkerberry, deerberry

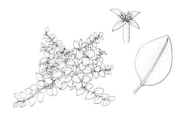

Size variable.

Parts used Leaves.

Constituents Saponins, mucilage, tannins.

Main uses *Medical* To prepare for childbirth, painful periods.

North American Indian women used this herb to prepare themselves for childbirth, for which purpose it is still used today because, like raspberry leaves, it is reputed to promote an easy labour. Not only is the herb a uterine tonic but it also has a calming effect on the nervous system and in addition improves the digestion.

RUTACEAE

Agathosma betulina (also known as *Barosma betulina*)
Round buchu

Agathosma cremulata
Long buchu

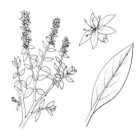

h 3–5 ft (1–1.5 m). See p. 83.

Parts used Leaves.

Constituents Volatile oil (about 2% containing pulegone, isopulegone, bucum camphor, menthone, limonone, and over 100 other compounds), flavonoids, resin, mucilage.

Main uses *Medical* Cystitis

These two deciduous shrubs grow in the Cape Province of South Africa. Black South Africans use the leaves as a body perfume, mixing them with oil. The species are distinguished by the shape of their leaves, but have similar constituents, and medicinal properties.
  The oil in the buchu plant is responsible for its reputation as a diuretic and urinary antiseptic, useful in treating urinary-tract infections (but see caution). The plant is also used in its homeland, South Africa, for its carminative properties.
CAUTION May irritate diseased kidneys. Avoid in kidney infections.

Citrus spp
Orange
See page 110

Ruta graveolens
Rue
See page 111

Zanthoxylum americanum
Northern prickly ash
(And *Z. clava-herculis*, Southern prickly ash)
Toothache tree

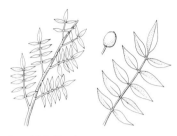

h to 10 ft (3 m)

Parts used Bark and berries.

Constituents Northern prickly ash bark: several coumarins (including zanthyletin), 6 benzophenanthridine alkaloids (consisting mainly of lauritoline and nitidine), resins, tannins, an acrid volatile oil. Southern prickly ash bark lacks the coumarins but also contains alkaloids (including chelerythrine and magnoflorine), asarinin (a lignan), resins, tannins, volatile oil. Berries: known to contain a resin and volatile oil.

Main uses *Medical* arthritis, poor circulation.

Herbalists use these two related trees in the same way. The bark and berries are both stimulating to the circulation, the latter being reputedly the more active. Such stimulation causes blood to flow to the periphery and promotes sweating which helps to bring down the temperature in fevers. In days when dentists were few and far between, the bark was chewed to allay the pain of toothache because of its counter-irritant properties. Prickly ash warms the stomach and stimulates the salivary glands and mucous membranes. It reduces colic and flatulence and is strengthening to a debilitated digestion, especially if the pulse is weak and the tongue is pale and flabby. Prickly ash has a considerable reputation for allaying rheumatic pain[1] and is also reputed to have some anti-cancer activity.[2] The isolated bensophenanthridene alkaloids are reported to be destructive to cells. There are, however, no accounts of any adverse side-effects from taking this herb in medicinal doses.

SALICACEAE

Populus candicans. See p. 36

Populus tremuloides
White poplar

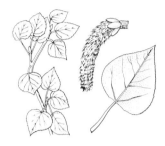

h to 100 ft (30 m) See p. 107.

Parts used Bark.

Constituents Glycosides, populin, essential oil, tannin.

Main uses *Medical* Rheumatism.

Its anti-inflammatory action makes this plant a good remedy for arthritis and rheumatism. Herbalists also use it for fevers and infections.

Salix alba
White willow

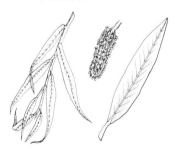

h to 83 ft (25 m).

Parts used Bark.

Constituents Salicylic glycosides (including salicin), tannins.

Main uses *Medical* Fevers, arthritis.

This tree and others of its genus are a natural source of the chemicals that form the basis for aspirin. Hardly surprisingly, for thousands of years willow bark has been used to treat fevers and arthritis. Now we know that salicin contained in the bark has antipyretic, antirheumatic and analgesic properties.

Citrus aurantium and *Citrus vulgaris*
Orange

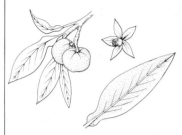

Parts used Fruit, peel, and flowers.

Constituents Flowers: Volatile oil (oil of neroli). Fruit and peel: Volatile oil (containing limonene), vitamin C, flavonoids, bitter principles.

Main uses *General* In perfumery. *Culinary* In conserves and for flavouring a variety of dishes.

Several different species of oranges are used in cooking, perfumery, and medicine. The bitter orange (*Citrus aurantium*, also known as *C. bigarardia*) is most familiar as the main ingredient in marmalade. Its flowers also yield oil of neroli, used in aromatherapy for treating anxiety and nervous depression. The sweet orange (*C. vulgaris*) and the many commercially grown varieties of tangerine are widely eaten for their flavour and vitamin C content. In Chinese medicine the dried peel is used as a diuretic and for its digestive properties.

CAUTION Migraine sufferers and those with arthritis should avoid oranges if they aggravate the symptoms.

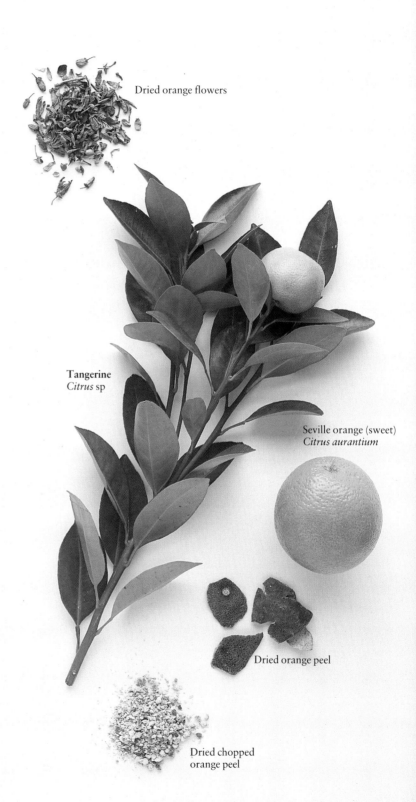

Dried orange flowers

Tangerine
Citrus sp

Seville orange (sweet)
Citrus aurantium

Dried orange peel

Dried chopped
orange peel

Rue
Ruta graveolens

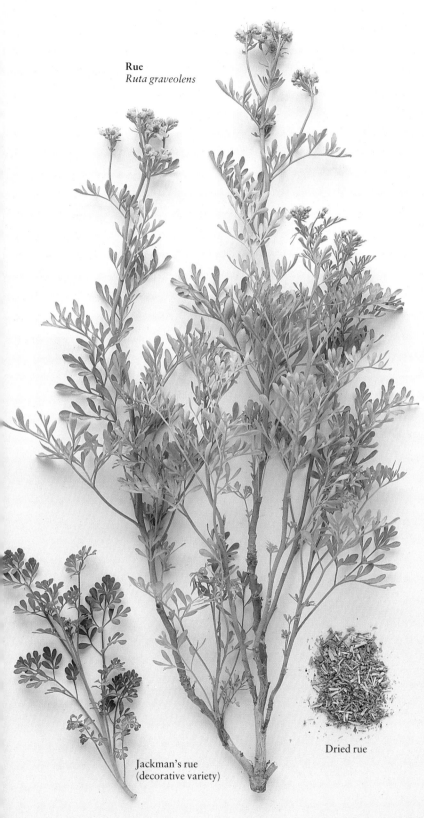

Jackman's rue
(decorative variety)

Dried rue

Ruta graveolens
Rue
Herb of grace

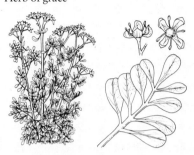

2 ft×16 ins (60×40 cm).

Parts used Aerial parts; cultivation see pp. 278–9.

Constituents Volatile oil (containing up to 90% methylnonylketone, also limonene, cineole etc); several alkaloids including fagarine and arborinine, coumarins (bergapten, xanthotoxin, psoralen).

Main uses *Medical* Strains and sprains. Absent periods (professional use only).

Rue is a powerful remedy and low doses are the rule. It has a special place in the treatment of strained eyes and headaches caused by eyestrain. It is also useful for nervous headaches and heart palpitations. The antispasmodic action of its oil and alkaloids explain its use in treating nervous indigestion and colic. The tea also expels worms.[1] Its alkaloids, arborinine and fagarine as well as the oil and coumarins all stimulate the uterus and because of this rue strongly promotes menstruation. The rutin strengthens fragile blood vessels and varicose veins. An ointment containing rue is good for gouty, rheumatic pains and for sprained or bruised tendons as well as chilblains. In Chinese medicine rue is specific for snake and insect bites.

CAUTION Not to be used in pregnancy. The coumarins may cause photosensitivity and skin contact can cause a rash. Large doses may be poisonous.

But like meadowsweet this herb is also said to be good for heartburn and stomach disorders. This may be due to the tree's tannin content. Willow bark makes a useful gargle for sore throats.

Black willow (*S. nigra*), a tree native to North America has the same properties.

SAXIFRAGACEAE

Hydrangea arborescens
Hydrangea

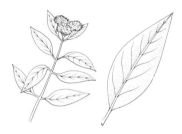

See p. 107.

Parts used Root.

Constituents Glycoside (hydrangin), saponin, resin, rutin, volatile and fixed oils.

Main uses *Medical* Urinary stones, prostatitis.

Hydrangea has a reputation as a diuretic said to be especially useful for preventing and moving urinary stones.

SCROPHULARIACEAE

Chelone glabra
Balmony
Turtlebloom, snakehead, shellflower

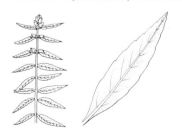

h 2–4 ft (60–120 cm)

Parts used Leaves.

Constituents Not investigated.

Main uses *Medical* Expelling worms, liver and gallbladder disease.

In general, balmony is a bitter tonic which stimulates the appetite and debilitated digestions. It has two specific uses. Firstly, it regulates the liver and gallbladder, and is used to treat gallstones and gallbladder infections. Secondly, it rids the body of round and thread worms, having a gentle action particularly appropriate for treating children. It is a mild laxative. Externally, balmony ointment is said to be good for healing mastitis, ulcers, and haemorrhoids.

Euphrasia officinalis
Eyebright

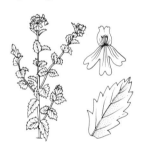

2–12 ins (5–30 cm).

Parts used Aerial parts.

Constituents Glycosides (including aucubin), saponins, tannins, resin, volatile oil.

Main uses *Medical* Eye disorders, hayfever, catarrh.

Eyebright, as its name suggests, is a specific remedy for eye problems. It is particularly suited to sore, itchy eyes which may have a discharge. It may be used on the eyes as a compress or eyewash or taken internally as an infusion. Eyebright is also a remedy for nasal congestion and catarrh. It is especially appropriate when there is a profuse watery nasal discharge. It is good for treating hay fever and colds as well as measles when accompanied by these symptoms. As a mouthwash or gargle, eyebright may be employed for inflammations of the mouth and throat.

Digitalis purpurea
Foxglove

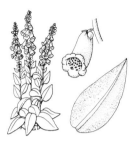

h up to 6 ft (2 m). See p. 114.

Parts used Leaves.

Constituents Several glycosides including digitoxin, gitoxin, and gitaloxin, which act on the heart muscle.

Main uses *Orthodox medicine* Heart disease.

Since the eighteenth century this plant has been used in orthodox medicine to treat heart disorders. Today the related *Digitalis lanata* is used.

CAUTION This extremely poisonous plant can cause paralysis and sudden death. RESTRICTED.

Leptandra virginica,
Veronicastrum virginicum, Verona virginicum
Black root
Culver's root, bourman's root, physic root

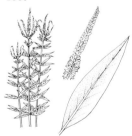

h up to 7 ½ ft (2.25 m). See p. 114.

Parts used Dried root.

Constituents Bitter principle (leptandrin), saponin, glycoside, volatile oil, tannins, resin.

Main uses *Medical* Liver disease.

This is a bitter root which when dried acts as a gentle laxative and liver tonic, stimulating the flow of bile. It has been used to ease the symptoms of hepatitis:

for pain around the liver area, jaundice, and accompanying depression. It was formerly used to treat malaria and other fevers.

CAUTION Use only the dried root: the fresh root is cathartic and emetic.

Scrophularia nodosa
Figwort
Carpenter's square, scrofula plant

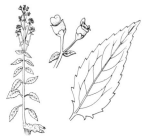

h 16–48 ins (40–120 cm).

Parts used Aerial parts

Constituents Saponins, flavonoids, resin.

Main uses *Medical* Skin diseases.

Herbalists have labelled figwort an alterative because of its cleansing properties. It is thought to stimulate the lymphatic system. As its name implies, it was once used to treat scrofula (TB of the cervical lymph nodes). Because of its eliminative power, figwort is useful for eruptive skin diseases.

CAUTION Poisonous in large doses. RESTRICTED.

Verbascum thapsus
Mullein
Aaron's rod, lady's foxglove, donkey's ears

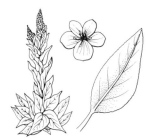

h 7 ft (200 cm). See p. 115.

Parts used Leaves and flowers; cultivation see p. 278–9.

Constituents Saponins, mucilage, gum, volatile oil, flavonoids, glycosides (including aucubin).

Main uses *Medical* Respiratory disorders.

Mullein combines the expectorant action of its saponins with the soothing effect of its mucilage, making this a most useful herb for the treatment of hoarseness, tight coughs, bronchitis, asthma, and whooping cough. A tea of the flowers is reputed to be sedative and can be used for insomnia. Mullein is also diuretic, helping to allay inflammation of the urinary system and counter the irritating effect of acid urine. Olive oil in which the flowers are macerated for several days has been used for earache as eardrops and rubbed in to rheumatic joints to ease the pain. Mullein leaves make an excellent poultice for boils and sores.

Infusions of the leaves should be strained through a cloth to remove the fine hairs which cover the plant as these may irritate the throat.

Veronica beccabunga
Brooklime
Water pimpernel

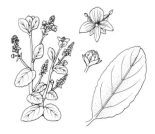

h to 2 ft (60 cm). See p. 114.

Parts used Aerial parts.

Constituents Tannins, glucoside; other constituents not known.

Main uses *Culinary* Shoots as spring green.

Now used rarely in medicine, this plant can be used in salads in the same way as watercress, to which it has a similar taste.

SOLANACEAE

Capsicum frutescens (also known as *C. minimum*)
Chillies
Cayenne, bird pepper

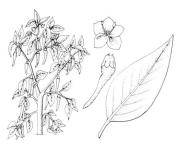

h 1–3 ft (30–90 cm). See p. 35.

Parts used Pods.

Constituents An alkaloid (capsaicin), up to 1.5% pungent principles, carotenoids, flavonoids, vitamins A and C, of volatile oil.

Main uses *Culinary* As seasoning in Asian and Central American cuisines. *Medical* A heart and circulatory stimulant.

This familiar condiment is a powerful local stimulant, producing a burning sensation on contact with the skin. It is used externally in ointments, liniments, and plasters as a counter-irritant to treat muscular pains, arthritis, neuralgia, lumbago and unbroken chilblains.

Internally, cayenne is a major circulatory stimulant. The American herbalist Dr T. J. Lyle wrote "it is the most powerful and persistent heart stimulant known . . . its influence reaches every organ". Cayenne is an excellent remedy to ward off chills and is useful at the onset of a cold. It causes sweating and supports the body's defence system (it is rich in vitamin C and is antibacterial). Small quantities will also stimulate a debilitated appetite.

In the kitchen, chillies are used in hot dishes, particularly in South and Central America, home of the well known chilli con carne. Cayenne pepper is ground from the dried fruit. It is the main ingredient in tabasco sauce. Central American people use cayenne as a seasoning because of its healing actions.

CAUTION Avoid excessive consumption, which may cause digestive, liver, or kidney disorders.

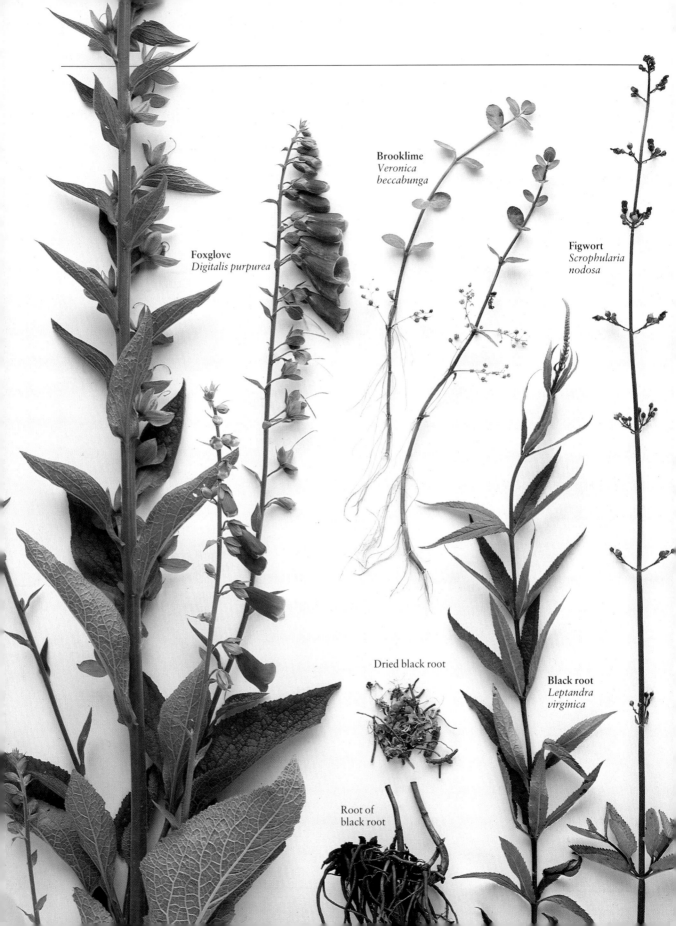

Foxglove
Digitalis purpurea

Brooklime
Veronica beccabunga

Figwort
Scrophularia nodosa

Dried black root

Black root
Leptandra virginica

Root of
black root

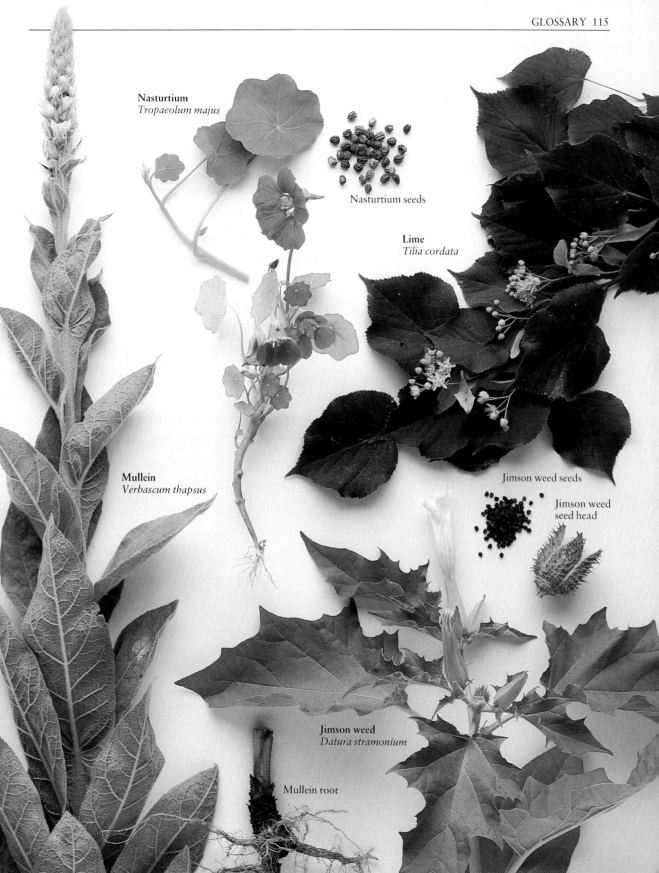

Nasturtium
Tropaeolum majus

Nasturtium seeds

Lime
Tilia cordata

Mullein
Verbascum thapsus

Jimson weed seeds

Jimson weed
seed head

Jimson weed
Datura stramonium

Mullein root

Datura stramonium
Jimson weed

Thornapple, Jamestown weed, devil's apple, mad apple

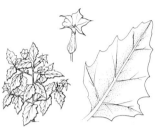

h 1–5 ft (30 cm-1.5 m). See p. 115.

Parts used Dried leaves.

Constituents Tropane alkaloids (including hyoscine, hyoscamine, traces of atropine).

Main uses *Medical* Asthma.

Jimson weed is a highly toxic plant. Its main use is in the treatment of asthma (for which it is also smoked). The alkaloids in the plant relax spasms of the bronchioles during an asthma attack.[1] In therapeutic doses, it has been used to control the spasm of Parkinson's disease. Externally an ointment relieves the pain of rheumatism and sciatica.

CAUTION An overdose will cause double vision, thirst, an urge to urinate but an inability to do so, palpitations, restlessness, confusion and hallucinations. Jimson weed is classified by the U.S. Food and Drug Administration as poisonous. It must not be used in pregnancy, prostatic disease, tachycardia, glaucoma or taken by those on antidepressant drugs. RESTRICTED.

STERCULIACEAE

Cola vera (also known as *C. nitida*), and *C. acuminata*
Kola nut

h to 50 ft (15 m). See p. 82.

Parts used Dried seed (with the seed coat removed).

Constituents About 2% caffeine, small quantities of theobromine, a red pigment (kola red), glycoside, tannin, protein, starch, fats, sugars.

Main uses *General* Red dye. *Medical* Central nervous stimulant.

The caffeine and theobromine in kola explain its use as a central nervous stimulant. It is traditionally recommended for headaches but is unlikely to bring relief to those who regularly drink coffee or other caffeinated drinks.

TILIACEAE

Tilia europaea
Lime

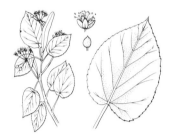

h 50–133 ft (15–40 m)

Parts used Flowers, inner bark.

Constituents Volatile oil (containing farnesol which gives the flowers their characteristic smell), flavonoid glycosides (including hesperidin and quercitrin), saponins, condensed tannins, mucilage, manganese salts. The bark contains coumarins.

Main uses *Medical* Nervous tension, insomnia.

Tilia europaea is a hybrid between *T. platyphillos* and *T. cordata*. The flowers of all three have the same uses.

Limeflowers in hot infusion are an excellent sweat-inducing remedy for colds, flu and catarrh. They also relax the nervous system and are a good remedy for overactive children. In France, irritable children are traditionally given afternoon tea in the shade of the tree. Limeflower tea helps to alleviate headaches and insomnia.

The bioflavonoids in limeflowers may account for their reputation to lower blood pressure. They are also a remedy for arteriosclerosis. The inner bark of the tree is used for its diuretic effect and to treat kidney stones and gout. The sapwood of the inner bark is antispasmodic and dilates the coronary arteries, making it useful in the treatment of coronary artery disease.

TROPAEOLACEAE

Tropaeolum majus
Nasturtium

Indian cress

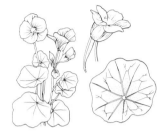

h up to 10 ft (3 m). See p. 115.

Parts used Seed, flowers, leaves.

Constituents Glycoside, (glucotrapaeoline which hydrolyzes to yield antibiotic sulphur compounds).

Main uses *General* In hair rinses. *Culinary* Salads; substitute for capers. *Medical* Bronchitis, urinary infections.

Nasturtium was introduced to Europe from Peru by the conquistadores. It is said that on hot summer days sparks are emitted from the heart of the flower due to its high phosphoric acid content. Nasturtium is a natural antibiotic which, unlike orthodox antibiotics, does no damage to our intestinal flora.[1] An infusion of the leaves is used for bronchitis and for genito-urinary infections. In addition, nasturtium is reputed to promote the formation of red blood cells. The seeds have a purgative action.

TURNERACEAE

Turnera diffusa var. *aphrodisiaca*
Damiana

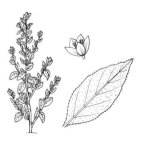

h to 2 ft (60 cm)

Parts used Dried aerial parts.

Constituents Volatile oil (up to 1% which includes alpha and beta pinene, cineole, thymol, cymene, alpha copaene, beta cadinene, calamenene, beta sitasterol), a cyanogenic glycoside, a bitter amorphous substance (damianin), resins, gum.

Main uses *Medical* Debility, depression, and lethargy.

The Latin variant for this plant, *aphrodisiaca*, perpetuates an old belief that this plant is a sex tonic. The truth is that it is a stimulating nerve tonic used for debility, depression and lethargy.[1] It has mild laxative properties.

CAUTION Too much damiana can cause insomnia and headaches.

ULMACEAE

Ulmus fulva
Slippery elm
Indian elm, moose elm, sweet elm

Parts used Dried inner bark.

Constituents Mucilage (a mixture of polyuronides), starch, tannin.

Main uses *Medical* As a nourishing food and for inflammation.

Constituents Mucilage (a mixture of polyuronides), starch, tannin.

Slippery elm is both a food and a medicine. The inner bark is one of the best soothing remedies useful wherever there is inflammation. It lubricates and relieves gastro-intestinal irritation. It is good for diarrhoea (for which it has also been prescribed as an enema) because it is also mildly astringent. The finely powdered bark makes a nourishing food, easily assimilated during convalescence. It can be flavoured with a little cinnamon or nutmeg, it makes a wholesome food for children. A slippery elm poultice is one of the most effective healing agents for ulcers, wounds, and boils. Collection of the inner bark usually leads to destruction of the tree. Because of the worldwide demand for slippery elm, the fine powdered inner bark is in short supply and the coarser outer bark is substituted. This lacks the healing power of the inner bark.

UMBELLIFERAE

Anethum graveolens
Dill

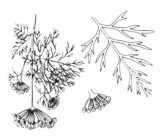

h to 3 ft (1 m). See p. 118.

Parts used Aerial parts.

Constituents Oil of dill (containing, d-carvone, d-limonene, phellandrine).

Main uses *Culinary* With fish, salads, cream; seeds in pickles and vinegars.

Dill is a culinary herb which improves the appetite and digestion. It is still a constituent of gripe water and other children's medicines because of its ability to ease flatulence and colic.

Angelica archangelica
Angelica

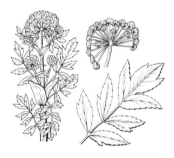

5–8 ft×3 ft (1.5–2.5 m×90 cm). See p. 119.

Parts used Roots, stems and seeds.

Constituents 1% volatile oil (including phellandrene, pinene, limonene, caryophyllene, linalool etc), a large number of coumarins (including umbelliferone, bergapten, xanthotoxol), plant acids, resin, starch, sugar.

Main uses *Culinary* Stems candied; leaves with fruit, fish. *Medical* Indigestion, anaemia, coughs, colds.

Angelica is said to have gained its name because the medicinal qualities of the plant were revealed to a monk by an angel who told him it was a cure for the plague. The herb's aromatic, bittersweet taste commends itself to the stomach, easing indigestion, griping, colic, and flatulence.[1] It is stimulating and warming to the digestion.

Angelica also stimulates the circulation, warming cold hands and feet. It is recommended in anaemia. Angelica is antibacterial and antifungal (the coumarin, umbelliferone, is a proven antifungal agent). Pinene, a component of the oil, is antimicrobial[2] and expectorant, and the whole plant is a warming expectorant useful for asthma and bronchitis made worse by damp, cold conditions. Angelica in hot infusion is sweat-inducing and eases colds. It also has antiseptic, diuretic properties, again due to its oil, so that it is a useful agent for urinary infections. Its antispasmodic action[3] makes it effective in treating painful periods.

Chinese angelica (*Angelica sinensis*), called dang gui and sometimes termed "women's ginseng", is a blood tonic used in Chinese herbal prescriptions.

CAUTION Wild angelica has several poisonous lookalikes. The coumarins bergapten and xanthotoxol can cause photosensitivity. Avoid large doses and prolonged use.

Anthriscus cerefolium
Chervil

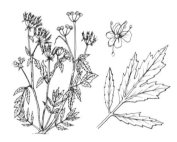

2×1 ft (70×30 cm). See p. 119.

Parts used Fresh leaves.

Constituents Volatile oil.

Main uses *Culinary* In fines herbes (see p. 68); with soups, salads, omelettes, dressings.

Chervil is used mainly for culinary purposes and is popular in France.

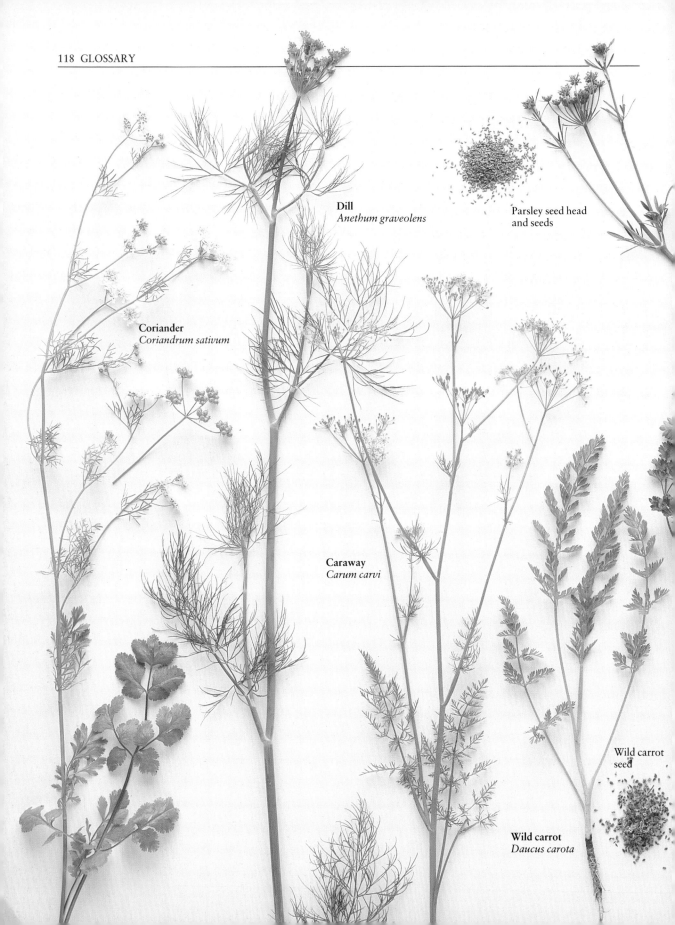

Dill
Anethum graveolens

Parsley seed head
and seeds

Coriander
Coriandrum sativum

Caraway
Carum carvi

Wild carrot
seed

Wild carrot
Daucus carota

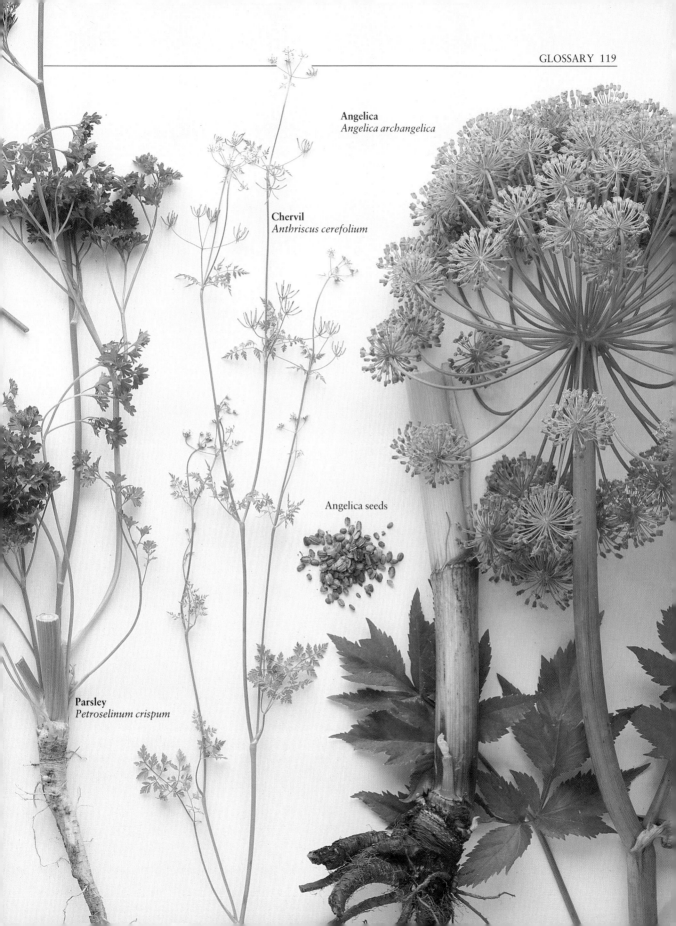

Angelica
Angelica archangelica

Chervil
Anthriscus cerefolium

Angelica seeds

Parsley
Petroselinum crispum

Carum carvi
Caraway

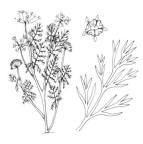

3 ft × 8 ins (90 × 20 cm). See p. 118.

Parts used Seeds.

Constituents Volatile oils (3–7%), fixed oil (8–20%), proteins, calcium oxalate, colouring matter, resin.

Main uses *Culinary* In bread, cakes, and biscuits; with stews and soups.

Fossilized caraway seeds have been discovered at Mesolithic sites, so this herb has been used for at least five thousand years. It was known to Arabian physicians and probably came to be used in Europe by the thirteenth century. Cultivated on a large scale in the Netherlands, the widespread use of caraway is partly due to the seeds' digestive properties. They improve the appetite and prevent flatulence.

Coriandrum sativum
Coriander

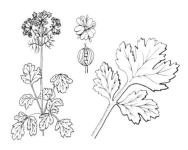

h 1–2 ft (30–60 cm). See p. 118.

Parts used Leaves, dried seeds.

Constituents Volatile oil (containing coriandrol and pinene).

Main uses *Culinary* In salads; leaves as garnish; seeds in garam masala (see p. 69) and in curries.

Coriander, native to the Mediterranean and eastern European regions, is mentioned in the Egyptian Ebers Papyrus, circa 1500 BC. Also known as Chinese parsley, the fresh, pungent flavoured leaves are used in Chinese, Indian, and South East Asian cuisines. Coriander is good for the digestive system, reducing flatulence. It stimulates the appetite, aiding the secretion of gastric juices.

Cuminum cynimum
Cumin

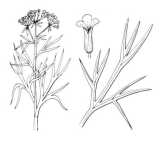

h 8 ins (15 cm). See p. 35.

Parts used Seeds.

Constituents Volatile oil (2.5–4%, comprising 25–35% aldehydes, pinenes, terpenes, cuminic alcohol).

Main uses *Culinary* In Asian cuisine, in curries, and in spice mixtures.

Cumin, indigenous to Egypt, was used by the Romans and was one of the commonest spices in the Middle Ages.

Daucus carota
Queen Anne's lace
Wild carrot

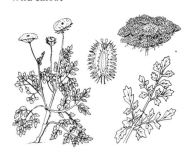

h 1–3 ft (30–90 cm). See p. 118.

Parts used Herb, seeds, and root. (Domestic carrot root may be used.)

Constituents Herb and seeds: volatile oil (that in the seeds contains pinene, carotol, daucol, limonene, geraniol), alkaloid (daucine). Root: Vitamins C, B, B2, carotene (provitamin A), sugars, pectin, minerals.

Main uses *Medical* Urinary disorders.

Queen Anne's lace is the ancestor of our domestic carrot. Its aerial parts are a useful antiseptic diuretic for the treatment of cystitis and prostatitis. The herb also helps prevent or wash out urinary stones and gravel. Because it promotes the excretion of uric acid it is a good remedy for gout. The seeds, rich in volatile oil, are soothing to the digestive system. A tea made from the seeds helps colic and flatulence. The oil has an antispasmodic effect on smooth muscle. Carrot seeds also promote the onset of menstruation.[1]

The root is an excellent source of vitamin A and many minerals. Carrots expel worms and are antacid and so recommended for heartburn and gastritis. In addition, the juice has a reputation for having anti-cancer activity. The pulped root makes an excellent first-aid poultice, particularly for an itchy skin.

CAUTION Queen Anne's lace has several poisonous lookalikes. Avoid seeds in pregnancy.

Foeniculum vulgare
Fennel
See page 123

Hydrocotyle asiatica
Gutu kola
Indian Pennywort

h to 6 ins (15 cm). See p. 82.

Parts used Aerial parts.

Constituents Heteroside, asiaticoside, triterpene acids, glycoside, resin, tannin, volatile oil.

Main uses *Medical* Purgative.

This powerful plant must be used with care. In its native India it is used for TB, bowel complaints, and leprosy.

CAUTION Gutu kola is poisonous. Large doses cause vertigo and coma. RESTRICTED.

Levisticum officinale
Lovage
See page 122

Petroselinum crispum
Parsley

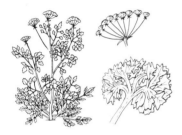

h 12 ins (30 cm). See p. 119.

Parts used Leaves, root, seeds; cultivation see pp. 276–7.

Constituents Essential oil (containing apiol, apiolin, myristicin, pinene), flavonoids, a glycoside, vitamins C and A, iron, manganese, calcium, phosphorus.

Main uses *Culinary* As garnish. *Medical* Urinary infections, gout.

Parsley is a useful medicine as well as a delicious addition to sauces. It is a strong diuretic suitable for treating urinary infections and stones as well as fluid retention. It encourages uric acid elimination and so is good for gout. It also increases mother's milk and tones the uterine muscles. It is a rich source of vitamin C and iron and strengthens the digestion.

Parsley leaves are a well known breath-freshener, being the traditional antidote for the pungent smell of garlic. The seeds or leaves steeped in water can be used as a hair rinse.

Parsley is a widely used culinary herb, valued for its taste as well as for its nutritional content. It is used in bouquet garni and as a garnish.

CAUTION Avoid medicinal use during pregnancy.

Pimpinella anisum
Anise

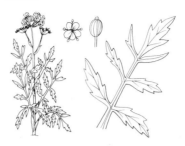

h to 30 ins (75 cm). See p. 35.

Parts used Seeds.

Constituents Volatile oil, coumarins, glycosides, fixed oil.

Main uses *Culinary* In curries; in Chinese and Mediterranean cuisines.

Aniseed tea eases indigestion, flatulence and colic. Its relaxing and expectorant action makes it useful to treat tight coughs. Anethole and other components in the volatile oil are insecticidal[1] and a wash of aniseed clears up lice.

Star anise (*Illicium verum*) comes from a tree indigenous to S.E. Asia having similar properties.

CAUTION Japanese star anise (*I. lanceolatum*) is poisonous.

URTICACEAE

Parietaria diffusa (also known as *P. officinalis*)
Pellitory-of-the-wall

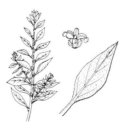

h 8 ins–2½ ft (20–75 cm). See p. 126.

Parts used Aerial parts.

Constituents Bitter glycoside, tannins, sulphur, flavones, potassium, calcium, mucilage.

Main uses *Medical* For urinary infections and stones.

This plant gains its common and Latin names because it grows in old ruins and walls. Herbalists use pellitory as a soothing diuretic to treat retention of urine, cystitis, nephritis, inflammation of the prostate and urinary stones. The fresh plant may be more effective than the dried. In France, a poultice of the fresh plant is applied to the kidney area, or over the bladder, to treat retention of urine and cystitis.

Urtica dioica (and the small nettle *Urtica urens*)
Stinging nettle

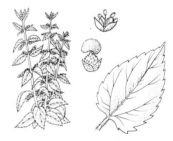

h 3–6 ft (90–180 cm). See p. 127.

Parts used Aerial parts of young plants.

Constituents Formic acid, histamine, acetylcholine, 5–hydroxytryptamine, glucoquinones, chlorophyll, minerals (including iron, silica, potassium, manganese, sulphur), vitamins A and C.

Main uses *General* In hair shampoos and rinses (see p. 146). *Culinary* As vegetable or soup. *Medical* Arthritis, eczema, anaemia.

Nettles grow wherever land is disturbed by human beings. Although we may curse the nettle for its sting, it is invaluable as a food, rich in vitamins and minerals, and as a medicine. In spring, the fresh green leaves may be cooked and eaten like spinach, made into a delicious soup or drunk as a tea. Nettles make a valuable tonic after the long winter months for they provide one of the best sources of minerals. They are an excellent remedy for anaemia – their vitamin C content ensures that the iron they contain is properly absorbed. Net-

Levisticum officinale (also known as *Ligisticum levisticum*)
Lovage
Smallage

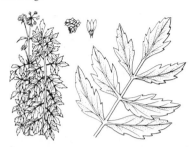

6½×3½ ft (2×1 m)

Parts used Roots and seeds.

Constituents Volatile oil (about 1%, consisting mainly of phthalides, also pinene, phellandrene, terpinene, carvacol, terpineol), isovaleric acid, angelic acid, coumarins (coumarin, umbelliferone, bergapten, etc), gum, resin.

Main uses *Culinary* Leaves in stews and soups, with fish and jam, seeds in breads and savouries.

Lovage is an aromatic stimulant and a warming digestive tonic, similar in action to angelica (see p. 117). Lovage cordial is an old country drink used to settle the stomach and ease the digestion. In hot infusion, lovage is sweatinducing. It also has diuretic properties but should be avoided in kidney disease due to its irritant effect. It also promotes the onset of menstruation. In traditional Chinese medicine, a related species, *Ligisticum chinensis*, is used to relieve painful menstruation. The phthalides in the volatile oil have been reported to be sedative in mice.[1]

The seeds, leaves, and stems of lovage have a strong celery-like flavour, which goes well with many foods, especially vegetarian dishes based on rice or nuts.

CAUTION Lovage should not be used during pregnancy or kidney disease.

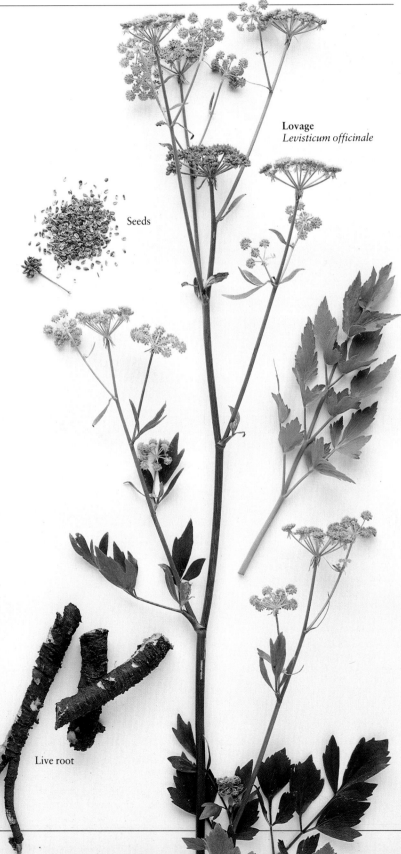

Lovage
Levisticum officinale

Seeds

Dried root

Live root

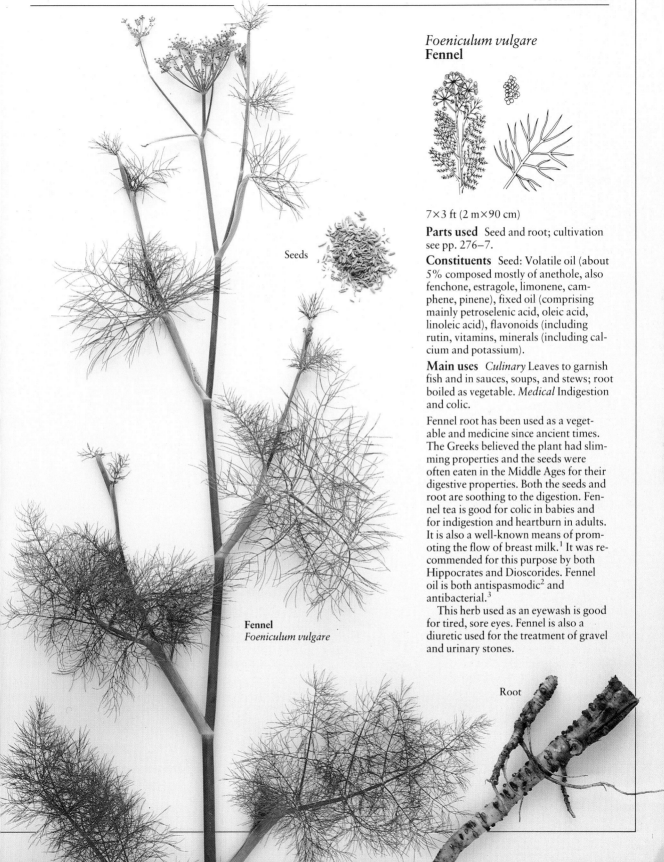

Seeds

Fennel
Foeniculum vulgare

Root

Foeniculum vulgare
Fennel

7×3 ft (2 m×90 cm)

Parts used Seed and root; cultivation see pp. 276–7.

Constituents Seed: Volatile oil (about 5% composed mostly of anethole, also fenchone, estragole, limonene, camphene, pinene), fixed oil (comprising mainly petroselenic acid, oleic acid, linoleic acid), flavonoids (including rutin, vitamins, minerals (including calcium and potassium).

Main uses *Culinary* Leaves to garnish fish and in sauces, soups, and stews; root boiled as vegetable. *Medical* Indigestion and colic.

Fennel root has been used as a vegetable and medicine since ancient times. The Greeks believed the plant had slimming properties and the seeds were often eaten in the Middle Ages for their digestive properties. Both the seeds and root are soothing to the digestion. Fennel tea is good for colic in babies and for indigestion and heartburn in adults. It is also a well-known means of promoting the flow of breast milk.[1] It was recommended for this purpose by both Hippocrates and Dioscorides. Fennel oil is both antispasmodic[2] and antibacterial.[3]

This herb used as an eyewash is good for tired, sore eyes. Fennel is also a diuretic used for the treatment of gravel and urinary stones.

tle tea increases the excretion of uric acid which may explain why nettles are a remedy for arthritis and gout.[1] Nettles have been applied directly to painful arthritis joints used as a counter-irritant. This fairly heroic treatment is often effective. Nettles encourage the flow of breast milk and lower blood-sugar levels. They are also a good astringent, effective in stopping bleeding. Internally they are used for profuse menstruation and externally the powdered leaves used as a snuff will stop minor nose bleeds. A wash is employed for haemorrhoids. The blood-invigorating properties of stinging nettles make them appropriate for girls at puberty and women at menopause. Nettles are useful in treating eczema too. A nettle rinse can eliminate dandruff.

VALERIANACEAE

Valeriana officinalis
Valerian
All-heal, setwall

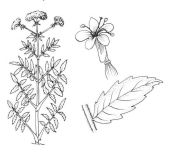

h 8 ins–5 ft (20 cm–1.5 m). See p. 126.

Part used Root.

Constituents Valepotriates (including valtrate and didovaltrate), glycoside (valerosidatum); volatile oil (up to 2%) containing esters of acetic, butyric and isovalerianic acids, which on drying, yield isovalerianic acid, giving valerian's characteristic smell; the oil also contains limonene, a sesquiterpene, valerian camphor, alkaloids, chatinine, valerianine, actinidine and valerine, choline, tannins, resins.

Main uses *Medical* Nervous tension, insomnia, headaches.

The valepotriates in this plant are thought mainly responsible for its seda-

tive effect on the central nervous system.[1,2] One study shows valerian to be sedative for agitated patients, while it stimulates someone who is suffering from fatigue.[3] Valerian is an excellent remedy for anxiety, nervous tension and insomnia. It is good for treating headaches too. Valerian also has a strengthening action on the heart (good for palpitations) and experiments indicate that it lowers blood pressure.[4] The valepotriates are antispasmodic and valerian is a useful remedy for nervous dyspepsia, stomach cramps, and for a spastic or irritable bowel. It is also an effective treatment for menstrual cramps. Tincture of valerian is reported to clear dandruff.

CAUTION Use only as prescribed by a qualified practitioner as valerian may cause headaches, muscular spasm and palpitations. Avoid large doses and prolonged use.

VERBENACEAE

Lippia citriodora
Lemon verbena

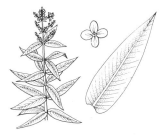

h up to 60 in (150 cm). See p. 127.

Parts used Leaves, flowering tops; cultivation see pp. 276–7.

Constituents Essential oil (comprising mainly citral).

Main uses *Culinary* In refreshing tea; in wines, stuffings, preserves, and desserts.

The name of this herb reflects its strong lemon scent. In its native South America, it was once used in fingerbowls at banquets, and the oil was used to scent soaps and cosmetics. Although today it is used in cooking, it is most familiar as a refreshing tisane. As well as being pleasant to drink, this is good for nausea, flatulence, and dyspepsia.

Verbena officinalis
Vervain

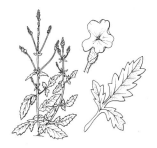

h 1–3 ft (30–90 cm). See p. 126.

Parts used Aerial parts.

Constituents Glycosides (verbenalin and verbenin), alkaloid (unidentified), bitter principle, volatile oil, tannin.

Main uses *Medical* Liver and gall-bladder disease, nervous exhaustion.

Vervain has a wide variety of traditional uses. It strengthens the nervous system, dispelling depression and countering nervous exhaustion. It is effective in treating migraine and headaches of the nervous and bilious kind. Vervain is prescribed for disorders of the liver and for gallstones. Experiments show a scientific basis for the traditional use of vervain to increase the flow of mother's milk and to promote the onset of menstruation (due to its glycosides).[1] The herb makes a good mouthwash for infected gums.

CAUTION Avoid in pregnancy.

Vitex agnus castus
Chaste tree
Chasteberry, monk's pepper

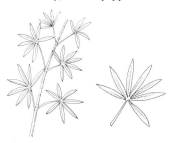

h to 20 ft (6 m)

Parts used Fruit.

Constituents Volatile oil, glycosides, flavonoids, a bitter principle (castine), possible alkaloids.

Main uses *Medical* Menstrual and menopausal disorders.

This plant has a folk use which strongly suggests a hormonal effect. Its Latin (*agnus*, lamb, *castus*, chaste) and common names (monk's pepper and chasteberry) seem to suggest that the plant is an *an*aphrodisiac. In Italy, the flowers are strewn on the ground in front of novices as they enter the monastery or convent. In classical times, the plant was used for disorders of the female reproductive system. Research in Germany now indicates that the plant possesses the ability to increase production of the luteinizing hormone and prolactin.[1,2] Comparitive case studies appear to confirm that it does, indeed, stimulate the flow of milk.[3] It has also been shown that it can regulate periods where there is excessive bleeding, or too frequent menstruation where there is prolonged or excessive bleeding.[4] The plant appears to stimulate synthesis of the hormone progesterone,[5] although it may also have a regulatory effect on oestrogen since herbalists have found it useful for the symptoms of both PMS and the menopause. It has been used to treat fibroids, inflammation of the womb lining, and to reestablish normal ovulation and menstruation after discontinuation of the contraceptive pill. This remedy would repay more research.

VIOLACEAE

Viola odorata
Sweet violet

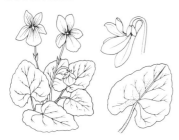

4–6 ins × 4 ins (10–15 cm × 10 cm)

Parts used Leaves and flowers (occasionally root).

Constituents Saponins, methyl salicylate, alkaloid (odoratine), volatile oil, flavonoids.

Main uses *Culinary* In confectionery for flavouring. *Medical* Respiratory disorders and hot swellings.

Due to its saponin and mucilage content violet is an excellent soothing expectorant useful to treat a range of respiratory disorders (a syrup of the flowers is useful for treating children).

Violets have a cooling nature. In France they are used to treat hangover (alcohol is heating) and headaches or migraine where the head feels hot (compresses can be applied directly to the head). Violets are also good to treat feverish colds. The plant makes a good mouthwash or gargle for inflamed gums and throats. The fresh leaves are a soothing and healing poultice for sore, cracked nipples. The leaves also have a reputation for treating tumours.

Violet flowers have a reputation for being slightly sedative, and so helpful for anxiety and insomnia. In Chinese medicine the herb and root together are used to treat hot swellings and mumps.

CAUTION The seeds may cause vomiting. The root in large doses is also emetic and has been used in place of ipecacuanha.

Viola tricolor
Wild pansy
Heartsease, love-lies-bleeding, love in idleness, herb trinity

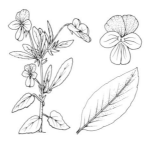

h 4–6 ins (10–15 cm). See p. 127.

Parts used Aerial parts; cultivation see pp. 278–9.

Constituents Salicylic acid and salicylates, saponins, alkaloid (unidentified), flavonoids (rutin is present in high concentrations up to 24%), tannin, mucilage.

Main uses *Medical* Skin disease, arthritis and respiratory disorders.

Wild pansy is a valued remedy for treating skin disease. Used internally and as a compress or ointment applied to affected areas it is good for eczema, psoriasis and acne. It is excellent for curing milkcrust (cradlecap) in babies. The herb is diuretic, employed in treating frequent and painful urination. Both the salicylates and the rutin contained in the plant are anti-inflammatory and herbalists use wild pansy to treat gout and rheumatoid arthritis. The saponins in the plant account for its expectorant action while its mucilage content soothes the chest. Wild pansy is used to treat a range of respiratory disorders such as bronchitis and whooping cough. Due to the high concentration of rutin in the flowers,[1] this herb may be employed to prevent bruising and broken capillaries, to check the build up of fluid in the tissues and to reduce atherosclerosis and in so doing help reduce blood pressure. Wild violet is mildly laxative. An infusion of wild pansy was once reputed to ease a broken heart – hence its common name heartsease.

Vitis vinifera
Grape vine

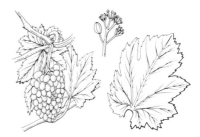

Parts used Fruit, leaves.

Constituents Sugars, tartaric acid, quercetine, quercitrin, tannin, malic acid, gum, potassium bitartrate.

Main uses *Culinary* Fruit in wine; leaves as an accompanient to many foods in Middle Eastern cuisines.

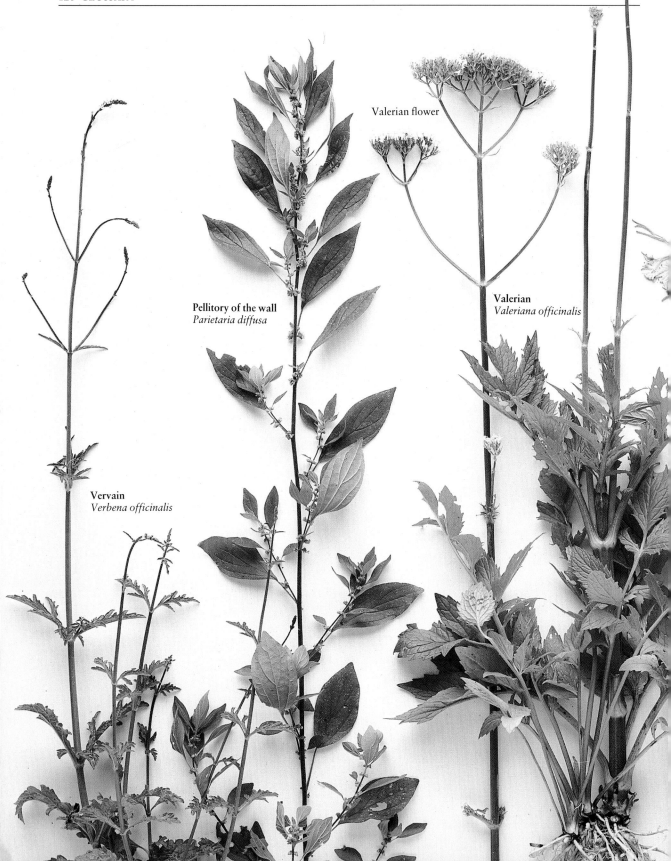

Valerian flower

Pellitory of the wall
Parietaria diffusa

Valerian
Valeriana officinalis

Vervain
Verbena officinalis

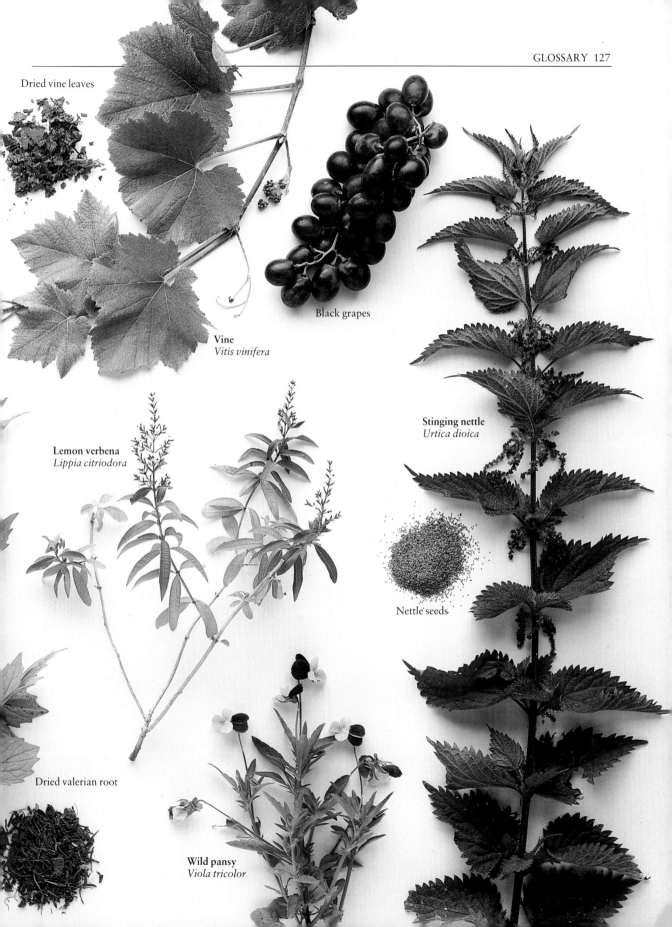

Dried vine leaves

Black grapes

Vine
Vitis vinifera

Stinging nettle
Urtica dioica

Lemon verbena
Lippia citriodora

Nettle seeds

Dried valerian root

Wild pansy
Viola tricolor

ZINGIBERACEAE

Elettaria cardamomum
Cardamom

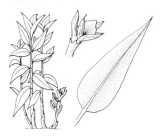

h to 9 ft (3 m). See p. 35.

Parts used Seed.

Constituents Volatile oil (3–6%, containing terpene and terpineol), cineol, starch, gum, yellow colouring.

Main uses *Culinary* In mixtures such as garam masala (see p. 69); in curries; in cakes and Asian sweetmeats. *Medical* Flatulent indigestion.

Cardamom is a common spice used to flavour coffee, cakes, curry and bread in Asia, the Middle East and Latin America. This aromatic spice stimulates the digestion easing bowel spasms and flatulence. Herbalists often combine cardamom with bitter remedies and use it to prevent the griping effect of laxatives.

Curcuma longa
Turmeric

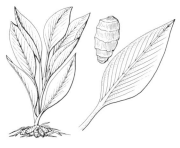

h 3 ft (1 m). See p. 35.

Parts used Root.

Constituents Volatile oil (5–7%), terpene, curcumen, starch (24%), albumen (30%), colouring due chiefly to curcumin, potassium, vitamin C.

Main uses *Culinary* As yellow colouring in curries, with rice and grains, in garam masala, and in lentil dishes.

Turmeric is chiefly cultivated in south east Asia and was used in Thailand to dye the robes of Buddhist monks. It is widely used both as a colouring and flavouring agent in a variety of foods. Turmeric is used in Chinese medicine to treat shoulder pain, menstrual cramping and colic.

Zingiber officinale
Ginger

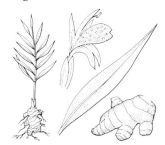

h to 9 ft (2.7m). See pp. 34–5.

Parts used Rhizome.

Constituents Volatile oil (up to 3% comprising mainly zingiberone and bisabolene, also camphene, geranial, linalool and borneol), oleoresin (containing the pungent principles gingerols, shogaols and zingerone), fats, protein, starch, vitamins A and B, minerals, amino acids.

Main uses *Culinary* Roots used widely, especially in far eastern cuisines; stems crystallized in candy. *Medical* Indigestion, flatulence, nausea, poor circulation.

Ginger is warming and stimulating, promoting gastric secretion and aiding the absorption of food. It is excellent for easing indigestion, colic, and flatulence. A piece of ginger chewed (crystallized stem ginger will do as well) is as effective for travel sickness as any drug.[1] A little ginger may also help morning sickness. It also has a stimulating effect on the heart and circulation so it is good for cold hands and feet. Ginger hand and foot baths can help this complaint too.

Ginger has a warming expectorant action on the lungs, dispelling mucus and phlegm. Ginger tea is good for colds and flu; it causes an eliminative sweat. Ginger juice or tea massaged into the scalp is said to stimulate hair growth.

In Chinese herbal medicine a distinction is made between fresh ginger root which is said to be better for treating colds and causing sweating and dried ginger thought to be more suitable for treating respiratory and digestive disorders.

ZYGOPHYLLACEAE

Guaiacum officinale
Guaiacum

Lignum vitae, tree of life, guaiac

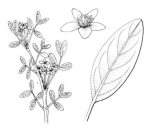

h to 54 ft (18 m). See p. 82.

Parts used Gum or resin or the heartwood.

Constituents Resin acids (guaiaconic acid), saponins, vanillin, polyterpenoid.

Main uses *Medical* Arthritis and gout.

Once reputed to cure syphilis, today guaiacum is used to stimulate the circulation and to reduce inflammation. It is employed in the treatment of arthritis and gout.

PART TWO

Using Herbs

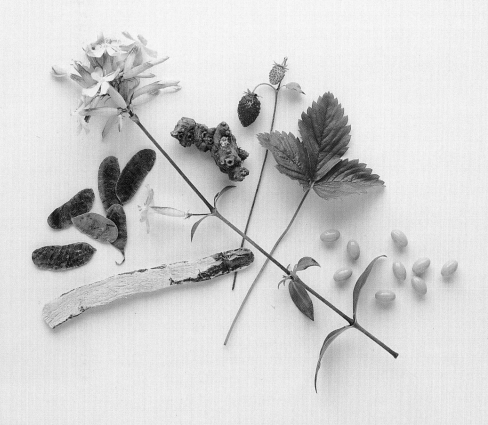

CHAPTER TWO

Practical Herbalism

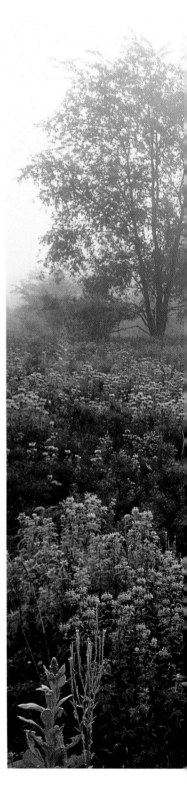

In our everyday lives we take the role of plants almost entirely for granted. If we are fortunate enough to live in the country, the changing seasons may attract our attention; in towns, we may wander to the park. But the cornflakes on the breakfast table are unlikely to remind us of the maize plant, the toast hardly suggests the blowing wheat fields. Still less do our clothes remind us of the cotton plants of the tropics, or our furniture of the hardwood giants of the forest. Least of all do we remember that the air we breathe and the rain that falls are also conditioned by the green world of plants.

Plants are enormously valuable, bought and sold as commodities in markets throughout the world. Food crops such as wheat or soya represent vast sums of money for the traders, and survival for the eventual consumers. We daily use plant products from every corner of the globe – rubber, flax, and hemp; coffee and tea; wine and olive oil from the Mediterranean; morphine and codeine from the Burmese opium poppy; spices from the far east; dyes and gums; timber and fuels and foods; ginseng from Korea; cosmetics from the desert jojoba bush.

In truth, we seldom have direct contact with the plants on which our comfort depends, or any experience of the labour and skill needed to make use of them. We see them more often as ornament or luxury – from the houseplants that grace our homes to the occasional exotic fruit in our diet. We have lost our former close contact with plants, when a herb could represent the difference between nutrition and starvation, or life and death. The true level of our dependence on the plant world escapes our notice in the modern world of plastic packaging and supermarkets.

Learning to use herbs in simple and practical ways can be the first time we truly begin to appreciate the value of plants – the magic of their chemistry, those subtle oils which lend themselves so well to healing the human body, that extraordinary diversity of use and range of properties. Working with herbs, and making simple infusions or decoctions to bring out their actions, also helps bring home the reality of human involvement with plants, over thousands of years of patient trial and error. The basic methods of preparing herbs and extracting

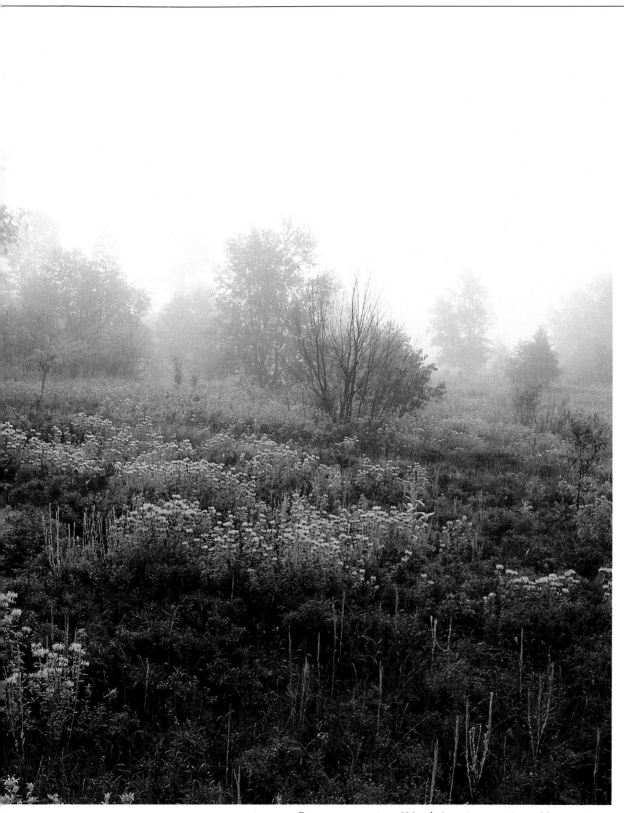

Bergamot, a native of North America, growing wild in Michigan

their active constituents described in these pages have not changed
since Egyptian times, and have been used for generations to build up
our knowledge. They do not require much skill, or any unusual
equipment – you can easily try them out at home. Practical herbalism
is a gentle art, and a pleasurable one, with deep roots in human
experience. It provides a direct and intimate contact with the plant
world – a contact which is often lacking in our urbanized and
consumer-oriented lives.

Herbs and the user

We use herbs in many different ways. But ultimately they all achieve
their effects through one means – by interacting directly with our body
chemistry. Whether herbs are used for food, for medicine, for cosmetics, or for relaxing fragrance, their active constituents must first be
absorbed into the body before they can be of benefit. Once they reach
the bloodstream, they can circulate to influence our whole system. The
essence of the herbalist's skill is to use these effects to balance and
strengthen the body's own responses, not to suppress or disturb them
as many modern products tend to do.

Herbal principles can enter the body in several ways. Food and
medicines are taken in through the mouth into the digestive system –
the most direct route. But there are more indirect routes which herbalists frequently use. We often think of the skin as primarily a protective
covering for our bodies, which keeps out water and protects us from
the elements. So it is, but it is also highly absorbent and, with its
complex network of tiny blood vessels (see p. 140), provides a direct
way into the bloodstream. Herbal cosmetics, as well as medicinal
poultices and compresses, take this route into the body and thus can
have a rapid and often profound effect on our well-being. Like the
skin, the eyes will also readily absorb herbal preparations. Anyone
who has relaxed with slices of cucumber over the eyes knows the
potential of this absorption. Medical herbalists use a range of more
complex lotions and compresses for the eyes. The nose, via aromatherapy, offers another entry for plant-based medicines – essential oils
which are particularly adept at finding a way into the bloodstream (see
pp. 150–1).

Releasing the power within the plant

Many plants yield their therapeutic power very readily, when eaten or
applied to the body whole. Most of our knowledge of herbs must have
begun this way, as our ancestors picked fresh leaves to chew or rub on
a sore or bruise. We still largely use culinary herbs fresh and whole,
and even herbal medicine includes simple remedies involving the
unprepared plant. Herbalists still, for instance, recommend yarrow

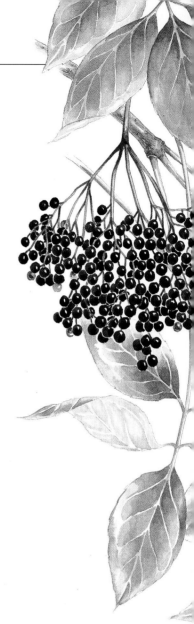

The versatility of plants
*The elder demonstrates well
the many uses of plants.
The twigs were once used in
basket-making and yield a
dye, the berries can be eaten
stewed and in jams and provide a popular wine. The
flowers can be made into a
drink or eaten raw; they are
also used in herbal cosmetics. Medicinally, the plant
is used to treat colds and
throat infections.*

Plants and human use

Plants support and help us at many levels. They condition the natural environment, air, and climate – services we take for granted. They supply shelter, clothing, fuel, furniture, and many other comforts, their products literally surrounding us and protecting us from the elements. But our most intimate and direct contact with plants is through food and herbs. We have to grow or gather the plants and prepare them for use – and we take their products into the body directly as food and indirectly via absorption through the skin, the respiratory system, or the sense organs.

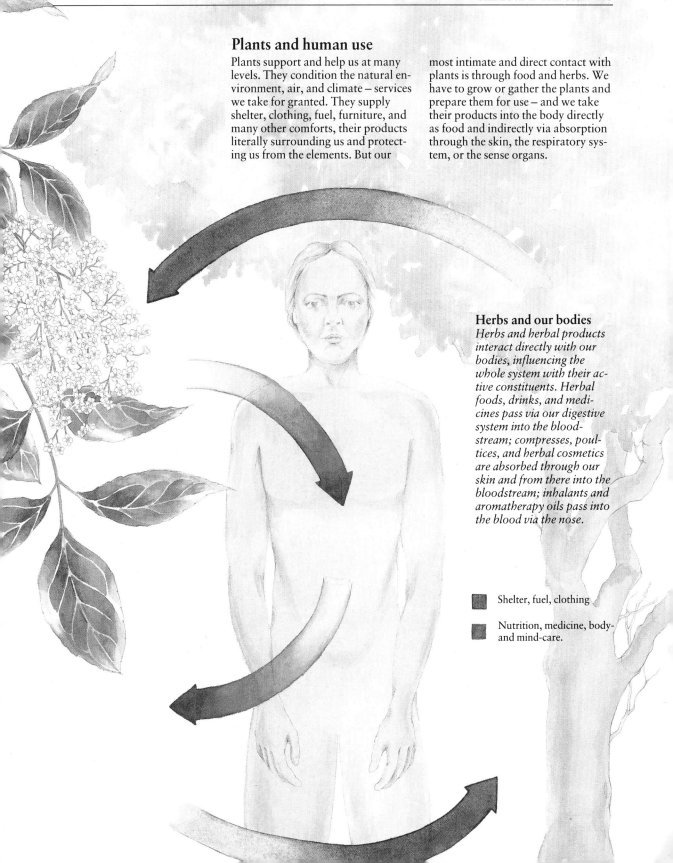

Herbs and our bodies

Herbs and herbal products interact directly with our bodies, influencing the whole system with their active constituents. Herbal foods, drinks, and medicines pass via our digestive system into the bloodstream; compresses, poultices, and herbal cosmetics are absorbed through our skin and from there into the bloodstream; inhalants and aromatherapy oils pass into the blood via the nose.

Shelter, fuel, clothing

Nutrition, medicine, body- and mind-care.

leaf to stop nosebleeds or eating feverfew for migraine, while the country remedy of rubbing dock leaves on nettle stings is widely known.

But people must have learned early on how to increase the power or usefulness of a herb by making some sort of preparation with it – whether to render it easier to absorb or apply, to preserve it beyond its season, or to release its active constituents. Some of the processes involved can easily be carried out at home – making a simple infusion, for instance. Others are more complex; essential oils, for example, are usually extracted commercially.

Numerous herbal cosmetics, cleansers, and medicines, for instance, use concentrated extracts from the plant, either essential oils or tinctures. Essential oils are extracted by maceration (saturating oil or fat with the leaves or flowers) or by distillation (heating the plant in water and filtering the oils out of the steam). Tinctures are made by steeping the herb in alcohol. Both are readily available commercially, but you can make tinctures yourself too (see p. 135). Tinctures and essential oils are very useful to the herbalist, as you can combine them with different bases in many ways. You can use the oils for aromatherapy, combine them with vegetable oils for massage, or heat them in water for inhalation. You can add tinctures to purified water to make perfumed skin tonics such as rosewater or elderflower water, or mix them with a base of fat, lanolin, oil, or beeswax to make creams and balms. Dilute tinctures are also used by homeopaths as the basis for their medicines.

The useful commercial herbal preparations (see right) include lozenges, capsules or perles (such as garlic capsules), liniments, and syrups (such as the nutritious rosehip syrup). You could also make syrups yourself, either by boiling the herb or fruit with sugar like a jam, or by adding a tincture to a sugar.

But the simplest herbal preparations are often the most effective, and four in particular are the standby of home herbal medicine: infusions, decoctions, compresses, and poultices. Infusions are usually made with the aerial parts of a herb or its flowers. They are prepared like a tea, by steeping the herbs in hot water; because the time that the herbs are exposed to heat is quite short, there is a minimal loss of volatile oils. Decoctions are used mainly for the woodier parts of plants and the roots, and involve boiling them in water for about 15 minutes; they are ideal for extracting bitter principles and mineral salts but the longer exposure to heat means that more volatile oils are lost. Compresses are wads of material soaked in herb infusions or decoctions and applied to the skin, while poultices involve wrapping the herbs themselves in material applied to the skin, so that their active constituents can be taken into the system by absorption.

Oils Extracted essential plant oils for use in inhalants and, diluted with a suitable vegetable oil, for massage.

Tinctures Herb essences prepared by steeping herbs in alcohol.

Syrups Tincture added to sugar syrup, for medicinal use.

Lozenges Powdered herb or oil combined with dry sugar and mucilage or gum into pills.

Capsules Gelatine containers filled with finely powdered herbs, extracted juice, or oils.

Ointments Herbs or tinctures combined with a base such as beeswax, white wax, oil, fat, or vaseline, for direct application to the skin.

Liniments Extracts of herbs in an oil or spirit base, designed to be applied to the skin.

Working with herbs

This page contains the basic instructions for making the preparations referred to in the next three chapters. Use these instructions in conjunction with the standard doses on page 193. For culinary uses, chopping and grinding herbs and spices (see p. 169) helps release their flavour and scent. Pounding before use will have a similar effect, and these techniques will also help to bring out the perfume of many herbs for cosmetics. Another method of releasing flavour is to wilt the herbs by heating them in butter, or putting them in hot water or a warm oven. Herbs used in medicine or body care usually require adding to a base such as water or alcohol. Preparations made with a water base, such as infusions and decoctions, do not keep well and should be used immediately. For cosmetic purposes, infusions can be made with bottled spring water for better keeping qualities. You can keep alcohol-based tinctures much longer. Another advantage is that alcohol is a very good solvent for most of the healing constituents in herbs. This is the reason why many herbal medicines are based on tinctures. They can be taken orally with hot water, or combined with syrups, or mixed with fats (to make ointments).

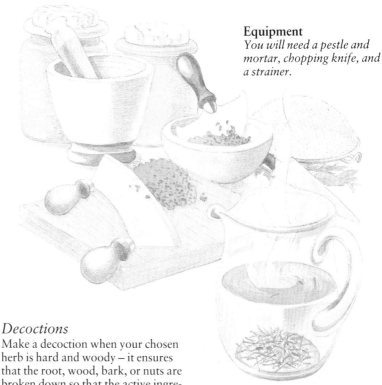

Equipment
You will need a pestle and mortar, chopping knife, and a strainer.

Decoctions

Make a decoction when your chosen herb is hard and woody – it ensures that the root, wood, bark, or nuts are broken down so that the active ingredients enter the water in solution. Cut up the fresh herbs into small pieces or grind dried ingredients. Measure the required amount into an enamelled pan and add water. Bring to the boil, cover, and simmer for 10 to 15 minutes. Strain the decoction while still hot.

hol, try cider vinegar. Tinctures can be taken undiluted or with water, added to compresses or teas, or put into the bath. They can also be used to make ointments by mixing with beeswax or cocoa butter.

Infusions

Infusions are useful when you want to use the active constituents of a plant that is rich in aromatic oils, especially if you are using the leaves or petals. Making an infusion is like making tea. Take a warmed porcelain or glass teapot, measure in the required amount of fresh or dried herbs (one part of dried herb is equivalent to three parts fresh) pour over boiling water, and cover. Leave the infusion to steep for 10 to 15 minutes before straining. If you require large quantities of an infusion, keep your stock in a jar or bottle in the refrigerator.

Tinctures

These preservative mixtures of alcohol, water, and herbs are very concentrated, so the amount needed will be smaller than an infusion or decoction. The ratio of herb to fluid used is 1:5 (e.g. 7 oz (200 g) of herbs to 2 pts (1 l) of fluid). Measure the required amount of your chosen herb into a dark, screw-top jar and cover it with a spirit, such as vodka. Keep the tincture tightly covered in a warm place and shake the bottle well twice daily. After 14 days, strain the residue through a muslin cloth, squeezing well. Keep in tightly stoppered dark bottles. If you prefer not to use alco-

Compresses and poultices

These help the body to absorb herbal compounds through the skin. For a compress, soak a clean piece of linen, gauze, or cotton in a hot decoction or infusion. Apply it as hot as possible to the affected area and change it when it has cooled. To make a poultice, wrap the herbs themselves in thin gauze, or apply them to the skin directly. You should mix dried herbs with water or cider vinegar to make a hot infusion or decoction. Keep the poultice hot and change it when it cools. A hot water bottle placed on the poultice will help keep the heat in longer.

Plants and human technology

Many apparently ingenious human inventions are simply adaptations of basic plant engineering – plants have had millions of years to develop such solutions to living in diverse environments and communities. Sir Joseph Paxton's famous design for London's Crystal Palace in 1850 was based on the natural strutting in the recently discovered giant water-lily, *Victoria amazonica*. Strength from corrugation was copied from the leaves of palm trees. The idea of micro-encapsulation – the enclosing of scents in minute, easily broken "bubbles" – was modelled on the way aromatic herbs store their volatile oils in glands.

Often the structural devices of plants have been turned to human use in ways that echo their function in the plant. The immense capacity of the bog-dwelling sphagnum moss to absorb moisture led to its use in wound dressings. The soft piths that provide lightweight "foam-fillings" for fast-growing plants like elder and rushes have been used as lamp-wicks, cork substitutes, and as oil absorbents by precision engineers and clockmakers. The shrubby leguminous plant dhainca owes its ability to grow in wet and salty soils partly to a water-soluble gum in its seeds which helps them settle in their marshland habitat. This gum can be turned into a smooth elastic film for stabilizing mud around oil drillings – or for sizing paper and textiles. Gums and resins from trees are pressed into economic roles that exactly mimic those in the parent plant, for sticking surfaces together, and coating them with an antiseptic seal into the bargain. Plants sometimes cope with environmental stress – for instance the presence of high levels of metals in the soil – by subtly changing their metabolism, and consequently the colour of their foliage. This means that certain species can be used as indicators of minerals in the soil.

The ability of some species to take maximum advantage of the meagre resources in areas of poor soil has sometimes made them the basis of whole economies. The Paiute Indians in Nevada were dependent on the reedmace for much of the year. They ate its shoots as a green vegetable, wove the leaves into boats, baked the pollen from the flowers into bread and used the downy seedheads as a stuffing for cradles, beds, and clothing. On the impoverished moorlands of Scotland that resulted from forest clearance, heather played a similar role, providing material for roofing, fuel, rough ropes, beer, tea, dyes, and even food for sheep.

Many species are newly being exploited. The water hyacinth, *Eichhornia crasipes*, offers itself as a pasture at our convenience. A free-floating nomad, it can be pushed or pulled around as required to provide a cheap source of cattle fodder or to clear a waterway of many poisonous or polluting substances. Since it is highly prolific, (it is known as the rabbit of the botanical world) the main problem is keeping its abundance within bounds. Today, renewable resources like jojoba and sunflower are being investigated as alternative sources for raw materials once supplied by fossil fuels.

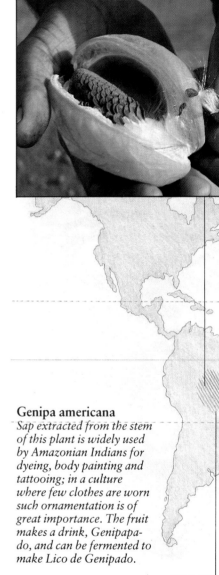

Genipa americana
Sap extracted from the stem of this plant is widely used by Amazonian Indians for dyeing, body painting and tattooing; in a culture where few clothes are worn such ornamentation is of great importance. The fruit makes a drink, Genipapado, and can be fermented to make Lico de Genipado.

Silk cotton
The kapok tree (Ceiba pentandra), *a native of South America, was introduced into Africa and the Far East. Today, 90% of the world's kapok comes from Indonesia. This fibre from the seeds is not suitable for spinning but is water-resistant (good for life-jackets) and used as stuffing for pillows and insulation.*

Sphagnum moss
A plant of water-logged bogs, this moss (Sphagnum cymbilifolium) *can absorb huge quantities of moisture. This makes it useful both for lightening the soil in hanging baskets and for stanching bleeding. Used for this latter purpose since ancient times, and in World War I, its healing properties are thought to be due to the antibiotic action of associated micro-organisms.*

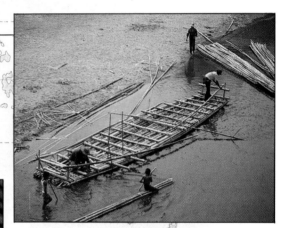

Bamboo
The various bamboo species are of great value to human societies. The illustrated species (Dendrocalamus giganteus), *is used in the Far East for building and making rafts. The many other species furnish vegetables (young buds), paper (fibres in wood), compounds used in growing chemical cultures (shoots), deodorant (leaves), and diesel fuels (culms).*

CHAPTER THREE

Herbs for Natural Living

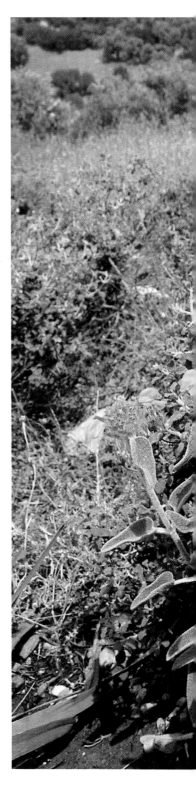

Among the greatest benefits of herbs is the sheer pleasure living in their midst can give us. The variety of their scents and the delicacy of their colours can enhance and enrich our homes, whether we plant them out in the garden or enjoy them as houseplants inside. But even at this simple level, herbs are therapeutic in ways of which we are barely conscious. Most of us find the fragrance of lavender or roses pleasing, to be sure – but few of us realise that the emotional uplift these plants provide is due to more than their scent or their beauty. The essential oils which the plants release affect our nervous system in ways which we are only just beginning to understand. It is this potential that aromatherapists use and that we can exploit as relaxation aids – in the form of massage oils, vaporizers, or simply the living plants.

Growing plants in and around the home reminds us how close and important our relationship with the world of plants can be – and how essential this relationship is to our well-being. Now that scientists are beginning to discover the full extent of the damage to our health that can result from chemical toxins in products as diverse as air fresheners and skin cleansers, the time is ripe for a renaissance of the use of natural products. The gentle, balanced action of herbs is healthier not only for our bodies but also for the environment, and allows us to bypass products that contain harmful chemicals, products that have been tested on animals, and those that have been made or packaged with scant regard to the earth's resources. Making herbal preparations also enables us to adjust each recipe to our own requirements.

The herbs that are used in beauty and skin-care and for home-care products are the ones that are most enjoyable to grow and have around the home. Many of them are fragrant, like lemon balm, rosemary, and the various species of rose. Others, such as soapwort, contain cleansing saponins, chemicals that produce a soap-like lather. And yet others have properties that benefit the skin, nourishing, soothing, and healing blemishes – such as the healing oils in lavender and the soothing mucilages in Irish moss.

The preparations in this chapter should not be taken internally. Store them out of the reach of children.

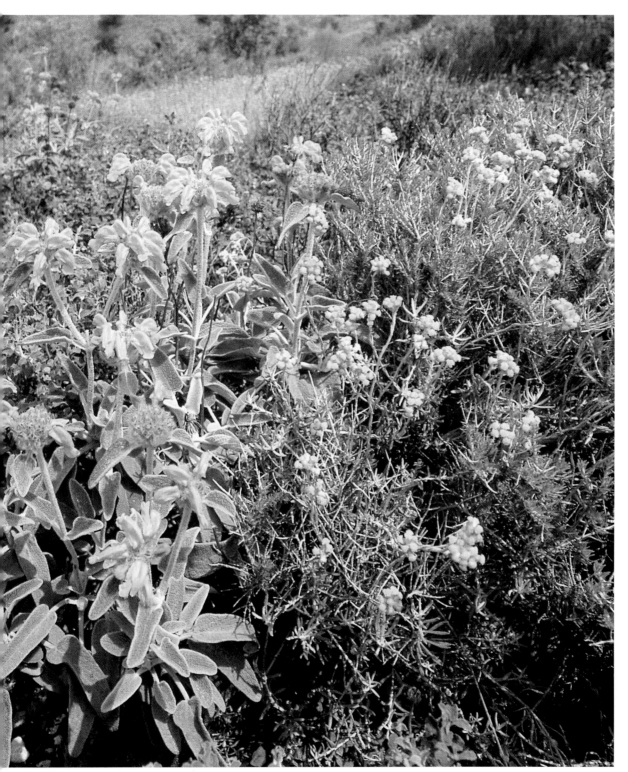

Jerusalem sage, one of the many species of this herb, growing in Crete

Body care

Our bodies serve us throughout our lives, and so deserve our care. Many people now realise the importance of a good diet, and use relaxation to combat stress, both areas in which herbs can help (see pp. 148–51 and 220–3). But we often ignore a simpler means by which herbs can exert an influence over our well-being: the daily care we take of our bodies and the products we use on our hair, in oral hygiene, and especially on our skin.

The skin is our frontier with the world, its elasticity protecting us against shock and damage, its surface layers guarding against infection and pollution. It is a vital organ, involved in functions from temperature control to waste removal. And it is our major sensory contact with the environment, with pleasure and with pain.

Though it guards us, the skin is not impermeable; in fact it has remarkable powers of absorption, taking in both healing and harmful substances, which may pass into the body. Chemicals from cosmetics, for example, have been found in the blood stream; garlic applied to the skin can later be detected on the breath; aromatherapy oils rubbed into the skin can affect the nervous system.

The skin profoundly affects our health and sense of well-being. Yet we use commercial skin-care products without thought for their effects. Some can cause allergic reactions; others upset the skin's natural acid balance (often called its pH level), which protects it from germs and chemical toxins. Hair care, too, has problems: shampoos, especially for dandruff, may damage the hair, while colourants and lighteners can contain chemicals which, if absorbed, will hurt your health as well. Ironically, many products sold specifically to promote personal comfort are potentially harmful. In America, eight common ingredients of deodorants and antiperspirants have been withdrawn over the last ten years, because of health risks. Skin irritation caused by commercial antiperspirants is still common.

Herbs and body care

Herbal products care for the body gently, with low chemical risk – cleavers, for example, is a safe alternative deodorant, sage a good tooth cleaner. They are also both effective and delightful to use, and many have healing properties besides their cleansing actions.

Your skin needs regular care in three ways: cleansing, toning, and nourishing. Fragrant herbal soaps and cosmetics will cleanse the skin deeply, tone it to restore its natural pH level, and nourish it with plant oils. For hair, shampoos with soapwort are mild and cleansing, rinses such as henna are conditioning and nourishing. The following pages will show you how to make a range of herbal preparations to care for your hair, skin, and teeth naturally, and with pleasure.

The structure of the skin

Our skin is a complex organ made up of three layers – the epidermis at the top, the dermis in the middle, and the subcutaneous tissue below. The two lower layers make up the living skin. They are criss-crossed with nerves and blood vessels.

Oil/water layer
This invisible layer is secreted by the sweat and sebaceous glands. It acts as a moisturizer, balancing the skin's pH level.

Epidermis
This outer part consists of dead cells, which are continually being replaced from beneath. Many skin creams affect only this layer.

Dermis
This layer consists entirely of living cells, which give the skin its strength and form. It contains the oil-secreting sebaceous glands.

Subcutaneous tissue
This is a layer of fat, which provides a protective padding. The sweat glands are found in this layer.

Nerve endings
These transmit touch sensations to the brain. Substances that penetrate the skin can sedate or stimulate the nerves, so influencing our level of relaxation.

Capillary endings
The skin has many tiny blood vessels into which chemicals – both beneficial and harmful – can find their way. From here, the bloodstream will distribute them.

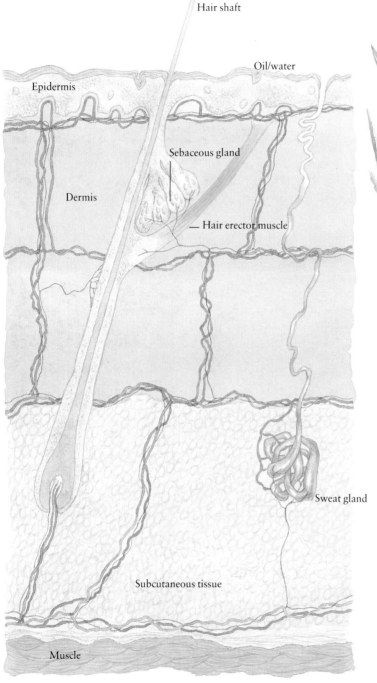

Hair shaft

Oil/water

Epidermis

Sebaceous gland

Dermis

— Hair erector muscle

Sweat gland

Subcutaneous tissue

Muscle

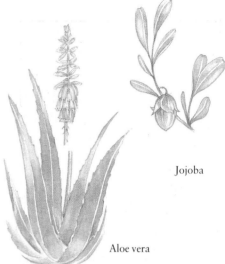

Jojoba

Aloe vera

Cosmetic plants
*Some "wonder plants"
much used in natural
cosmetics actually mimic
the skin's own functions.
Jojoba oil is similar in structure to our natural sebum;
aloe vera's fleshy pulp
assists the healing of blemishes.*

Basic infusions
For the infusions in this section use
these amounts. To each 1 pt (½ l)
boiling bottled spring water:

Dried herbs
*½ oz (14 g) for weak infusion
1 oz (28 g) for normal strength
2 oz (56 g) for strong infusion*

Fresh herbs
*1½ handfuls for weak infusion
3 handfuls for normal strength
6 handfuls for strong infusion*

For more information on making
infusions, see pp. 134–5. Because of
the chemicals added to the domestic
water supply, it is best to use bottled
spring water for cosmetic purposes;
the infusions will also keep longer.

Herbs for the skin

You should match herbal cosmetics to your skin type, as you would any other skin-care products. If you have oily skin, select preparations containing astringent herbs, which tighten the skin, encouraging the closing of pores and the healing of blemishes. For dry skin, use emollient herbs, which soften, soothe, and lubricate, supplementing the skin's own protective oils. You should use such herbal cosmetics for an overall programme of cleansing, toning, and nourishing the skin. But in practice you will find that many herbal preparations combine several properties, so that even a simple infusion for cleansing can be beneficial in other ways. For a simple cleanser, try using a normal strength infusion of chamomile, elder flowers, marigold, violet, or yarrow, choosing the herb for its extra properties listed in the chart. Strain the liquid through a filter paper and store it in the refrigerator. Rinse your face with lukewarm water afterwards.

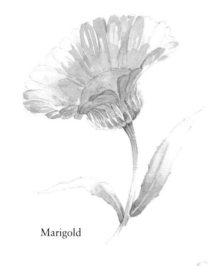

Marigold

Astringents

Marigold and witch hazel, traditionally known as two of the best natural healers, are astringents. This group of plants contains tannins – compounds that react with proteins to produce a contracting and tightening effect on tissues to which they are applied.

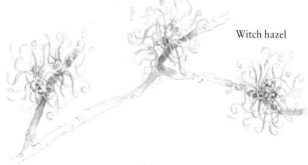

Witch hazel

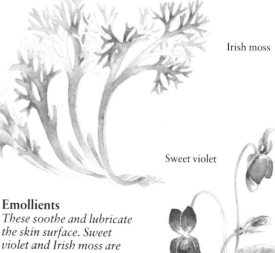

Irish moss

Sweet violet

Herb	Actions
Elder flowers	Cleansing, emollient, lightening, promotes sweating
Irish moss	Emollient
Violet	Cleansing, emollient
Marsh mallow	Emollient
Comfrey	Emollient (no internal consumption)
Marigold	Cleansing, astringent, promotes healing of wounds, toning
Witch hazel	Astringent, promotes healing of wounds
Horsetail	Astringent
Lady's mantle	Astringent
Thyme	Toning, refreshing, disinfectant
Yarrow	Cleansing, toning, promotes sweating
Chamomile	Cleansing, cooling, lightening, anti-inflammatory
Lavender	Antiseptic, stimulating

Emollients

These soothe and lubricate the skin surface. Sweet violet and Irish moss are two of the most effective. Both contain mucilages – compounds that form gels when mixed with water making them easy to use on the skin.

Herbs for the hair

As well as shampooing, your hair needs conditioning to replace lost oils and restore its bounce and shine. Many herbs, such as elder flower and chamomile, combine both cleansing and conditioning qualities – those in the chart work well with cleansing soapwort in herbal shampoos (see p. 146). When choosing these herbs, remember that different hair types respond to herbs in different ways. Dry hair, for example, benefits from emollients such as marsh mallow, while for dull, lifeless hair, herbs like southernwood, which has essential oils that pass to the roots and act as a conditioner, are ideal. Other plants that are rich in oils, such as rosemary and thyme, are all-round conditioners suitable for all hair types. Chamomile and sage, with their colouring properties, are suitable for light and dark hair respectively.

Hair type	Fresh herbs	Dried herbs
Fair	Chamomile, elder flowers, yarrow	Chamomile, lime flowers, yarrow
Dark	Rosemary, thyme, sage	Rosemary, sage, henna (powder)
Red	Marigold flowers	Marigold flowers
Oily	Lavender, peppermint, white dead-nettle	Lavender, peppermint, white dead-nettle
Dry	Marsh mallow	Marsh mallow
Dull, lifeless	Stinging nettle, fennel leaves, southernwood, parsley, rosemary	Southernwood, stinging nettle
All	Rosemary, thyme, stinging nettle, marjoram, horsetail stems and branches	Elderflower, thyme, rosemary
To prevent dandruff	Cleavers, burdock root, southernwood	
To encourage hair growth	Horsetail branches and stems, catnip, southernwood	

Herbs for oral hygiene

Many herbs have cleansing and antiseptic properties that make them suitable for oral hygiene. The most important herbs for oral hygiene are sage (astringent), cloves, peppermint and thyme (antiseptics), parsley, marjoram, bramble and blackcurrant leaves, and juniper berries. Chewing juniper berries, peppermint, or parsley will kill the odours of onion, garlic, or alcohol; rubbing the teeth with sage will clean them and sweeten the breath. Strawberries whiten and clean the teeth, and remove plaque. You can make an effective mouthwash with a normal infusion (see p. 141) of sage, mint, thyme, or marjoram. Another useful herb for the mouth comes from the tree Salvadora persica. Its stems are traditionally used in Africa, India, and the Middle East to clean the teeth and gums. Some of the herbs used for oral hygiene should not be used under certain circumstances. Consult the Glossary for cautions before use.

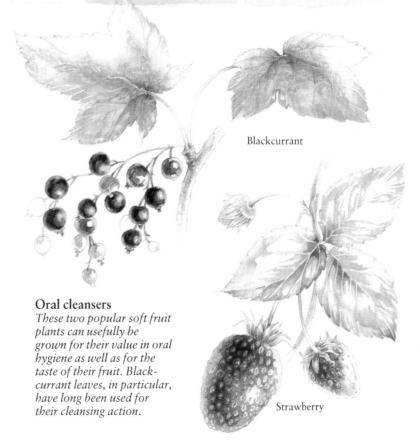

Blackcurrant

Oral cleansers
These two popular soft fruit plants can usefully be grown for their value in oral hygiene as well as for the taste of their fruit. Blackcurrant leaves, in particular, have long been used for their cleansing action.

Strawberry

Skin care

These two pages include recipes for cleansers, toners, and nourishers. Use cleansers night and morning on cotton balls to remove dirt and make-up. Use toners after a bath or facial steam – gently wipe the face and neck with moistened cotton balls. Massage nourishing cream into the skin at night.

Herb soap

For normal and oily skins nothing is more refreshing than a simple soap and water wash, though if your skin is dry you should wash with warm water only. The alkalinity of most soaps can upset the skin's natural acidity, making it feel tight and irritated, so use this gentle herbal soap with warm or cool water – avoid excessive heat or cold.

*5 oz (140 g) simple uncoloured
  unscented soap
3 oz (85 g) whole fresh herbs:
  rosemary or marjoram
10 fl oz (300 ml) water
2 teaspoons oil of rosemary or
  sandalwood*

Coarsely grate the soap into a bowl. Make a normal-strength infusion of your chosen herb (see p. 141), and let stand for 30 minutes. Strain the infusion on to the soap and stand the bowl over a pan of simmering water. Stir as the soap melts and whisk hard until smooth. Remove from heat and beat in the essential oil. Pour quickly into moulds, such as small waxed paper cake cups. When cool, cover with greaseproof paper and leave in a warm, dry place for about eight weeks until hard.

Variation For wash balls, a favourite Elizabethan toiletry, use 5 fl oz (140 ml) rosewater instead of the herb infusion. Rosewater is slightly astringent. Form the soap into small balls and dry in a warm place. To finish, moisten your hands with rosewater and smooth each ball to make the surface shiny.

Cleansing complexion milk

To remove ingrained grease and dirt, deep cleansing is often necessary. Used night and morning, this milk will cool and cleanse your skin. Apply it on cotton balls or soft tissue. It contains several ingredients that are good for the skin. Oil of lemon is acidic and refreshing. Marigold is an astringent that is good for blemished skins (see p. 142). Almond "milk" is also very good for the complexion. It keeps for much longer than cow's milk.

*2 oz (56 g) ground almonds
5 fl oz (150 ml) water
3 tablespoons strong infusion of
  marigold (see p. 141)
1 teaspoon borax
2 tablespoons grape seed oil
5 drops oil of lemon*

Tie the almonds in a muslin bag and soak in the water in a bowl for several hours, pressing occasionally with a spoon. Lift out the bag of almonds and squeeze dry. (You can set this aside for use as a bath bag, see p. 149). Reserve the milky almond liquid. Put the marigold infusion in a cup with the borax and stand in a pan of hot water, stirring until the borax dissolves. Heat the grape seed oil and vigorously whisk in the borax solution. Add 4 tablespoons of almond milk and the oil of lemon. Cool, then pour into a bottle and shake well. Shake the complexion milk again before using.

Quick cleansing milk

This preparation is easy to make with common ingredients. It is good for dry skins. The lemon juice it contains is astringent and quickly restores the pH balance of the skin.

*½ small carton natural yoghurt
1 tablespoon safflower oil
½ tablespoon lemon juice*

Whisk together all the ingredients and use within two days.

Cleansing facial steam

This is a useful cleansing process for blackheads and oily skins; do not use it if you have thread veins, or your face flushes easily. Choose from the herbs listed. Most contain essential oils that aromatherapists use to influence mood (see pp. 150–1). A short, five-minute steam is also a good cleansing method for dry skins, provided that you follow it by massage.

*2 handfuls of fresh herbs or 2
  tablespoons of dried herbs, selected
  from:
Lavender, dried lime flowers
  (calming)
Peppermint (stimulating)
Rosemary, sage (soothing,
  refreshing)*

Cover your hair and lean over a bowl of hot water containing the herbs of your choice. Tent a thick bath towel over your head and shoulders and inhale the reviving aroma for 5–10 minutes. Afterwards you can squeeze out blackheads using a clean face tissue, not fingernails. Apply a dab of witch hazel to the spot.

Toning flower lotion

Many soaps and cosmetics upset the skin's natural level of acidity. A healthy body restores the balance after a while, especially if you use a gentle, natural soap (see left). This toning lotion speeds up the process, closing the pores, and tautening the skin to leave it cool and refreshed. The lemon juice provides acidity, while the witch hazel acts as an astringent.

*4 tablespoons witch hazel
4 tablespoons lemon juice
4 tablespoons flower water (rose,
  elderflower, orange, or lavender)
A few drops of oil of lemon,
  lavender, or rose geranium*

Mix all the ingredients in a jug. Pour into a bottle and shake well.

Toning face packs

You can use a face pack once a week to condition and tone your skin, or to brace it after a facial steam. This type of treatment is especially good for oily skins. First clean your face thoroughly, then cover your hair. Spread the mix fairly thickly over your face, avoiding the area around the eyes and mouth. Lie down for ten minutes, during which time your skin will start to feel tight and stiff. Then rinse the pack away thoroughly with warm water. Choose herbs that suit your skin (see p. 142). Good herbs are elder flowers, fennel leaves, marigold petals, thyme leaves, and yarrow leaves and tips.

*2 tablespoons finely chopped herbs
   or flowers, or 2 tablespoons strong
   infusion dried herb (see p. 141)
2 tablespoons natural yoghurt
Fine oatmeal, or kaolin powder*

Put the herbs and yoghurt into a bowl and stir in enough oatmeal or kaolin to make a soft spreadable paste. You will need a little more oatmeal or kaolin with dried herbs, to absorb the infusion.

Rich, nourishing night cream

This cream is soothing and fragrant. The moisturizing properties of the lanolin, sunflower oil, and almond oil make it especially good for faces dried and roughened by the weather, and for chapped hands. The lavender oil is soothing.

*3 tablespoons lanolin
1 tablespoon sunflower oil
1 tablespoon almond oil
1 teaspoon oil of lavender*

Melt the lanolin in a small bowl over a pan of hot water. Add the first two oils, and beat well to combine. Remove from the heat and cool a little, beat as the mixture thickens, then stir in the oil of lavender. Pour into a small jar and screw on the lid when the cream is cold.

Nourishing hand gel

The mucilage in this seaweed makes it a rich emollient. You can buy Irish moss dried, or pick it from the rocks at low tide, and dry it and bleach it in the sun yourself.

*½ oz (15 g) dried Irish moss
7 fl oz (200 ml) water
2 teaspoons strained lemon juice
2 tablespoons glycerine
½ teaspoon borax
A few drops oil of lemon or orange*

Soak the seaweed for 20 minutes. Put it into an enamel pan with the water. Bring to the boil, cover, and simmer slowly for 20–30 minutes. Remove from the heat and let it cool. Strain into a bowl, pressing the gel through the strainer with a wooden spoon. Stir in the lemon juice. Warm the glycerine and add the borax, stirring until it has dissolved, then beat into the Irish moss mixture. Add a few drops of citrus oil and pour the gel into screw-top jars.

Nourishing hand and body oil

Smooth this light, fragrant oil over your body after bathing. The rosewater gives it a tonic and astringent quality.

*3 fl oz (90 ml) rosewater
1 teaspoon borax
2 tablespoons almond oil
2 tablespoons grape seed oil
1 teaspoon oil of rosewood, or rose
   geranium*

Warm the rosewater in a bowl over a pan of simmering water, add the borax and stir until dissolved, then add the oils and stir briskly until thoroughly combined. Bottle, and shake well before use.

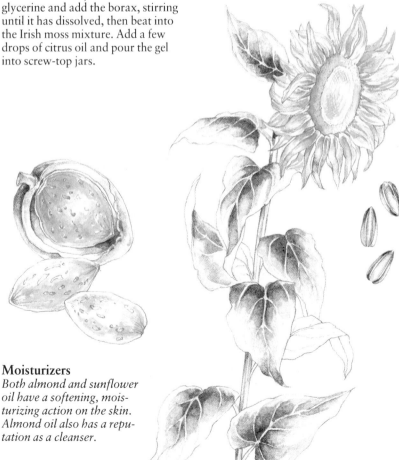

Moisturizers
Both almond and sunflower oil have a softening, moisturizing action on the skin. Almond oil also has a reputation as a cleanser.

Hair care and hygiene

Fresh soapwort shampoo

Soapwort contains saponins, chemicals that foam when added to water. All parts of the plant produce a gentle, cleansing lather that does not sting the eyes or make the hair brittle. You can combine it with other herbs. Do not take soapwort internally.

About 10 leafy soapwort stems, 6–8
ins (15–18 cm) long
1 pt (½ l) water
Herbs (see p. 143)

Cut the stems into short lengths and put them into an enamel saucepan, bruise lightly with a wooden spoon, and add the water. Bring to the boil, cover, and simmer for 15 minutes, stirring two or three times. Remove from the heat. Allow the liquid to cool, then strain and bottle for future use. Before you use the shampoo, add 3 tablespoons of strong herb or flower infusion (see pp. 141, 143). For immediate use, and while the pan of liquid is still hot, add a few sprigs each of several mixed fresh herbs, or two large handfuls of any one herb. Cover the shampoo, allow it to cool, and then strain. Use all the liquid for one hair wash.

Dried soapwort root shampoo

Herbal suppliers sell dried soapwort root. You should prepare the root in advance; before you add the herbs, boil, and simmer the mixture. Avoid internal consumption.

1 oz (30 g) dried soapwort root
1¼ pt (generous ½ l) boiling water
1 oz (30 g) dried herbs and flowers
(see p. 143)

Pour the boiling water on the broken up roots, cover, and leave to soak for 12 hours, or overnight. Tip the root and liquid into an enamel pan, bring to the boil, cover and simmer for 15 minutes. Remove from the heat, add the dried herbs or flowers, stir, cover, and leave to cool. Strain into a jug, and use for one hair wash.

Stinging nettle
Nettles have a long-standing reputation for preventing hair loss and making the hair soft and shiny.

Nettle rinse and conditioner

Nettle is an excellent hair conditioner. It is an acidic plant and promotes a healthy gloss. It also has a reputation for arresting hair loss. Use it as a final rinse after washing your hair, or massage it into the scalp and comb through the hair every other day. Keep it in small bottles in the refrigerator.

A big handful of nettles
Water (see recipe)

Wear rubber gloves to cut the nettles. Wash thoroughly and put the bunch into an enamel saucepan with enough cold water to cover. Bring to the boil, cover, and simmer for 15 minutes. Strain the liquid into a jug and allow it to cool.

Lotion for unruly hair

Rub a little lotion into the scalp and comb through your hair. You can use any suitable herbs (see p. 143).

8 tablespoons herb or flower
infusion, normal strength (see page
141)
1 tablespoon eau-de-cologne
1 tablespoon glycerine

Pour the first two ingredients into a bottle. Add the glycerine one drop at a time and shake well.

Horsetail hair rinse and tonic

Herbal hair tonics and conditioners help restore the scalp's natural acidity and strengthen the circulation, giving a healthy shine to the hair. Horsetail provides a good all-round conditioner. Its contains saponins, which create a lather, flavone-glycosides, which act on the scalp's tiny blood vessels to stimulate the circulation, and silica, which gives the hair body. Other conditioning herbs that you can use instead of horsetail are rosemary, southernwood, and stinging nettle.

About eight horsetail stems, 6–8 ins
(15–18 cm) long (or other
conditioning herbs)
1 pt (½ l) boiling water

Pound the horsetail stems with a spoon before adding the boiling water to make an infusion. Cover and leave until lukewarm, then strain off the liquid. After shampooing and rinsing, pour the infusion over your hair and massage it into the scalp. Blot up excess moisture with a towel, and comb through the hair. Cover your head with a warm towel and wait for 10 minutes before drying your hair in the usual way.

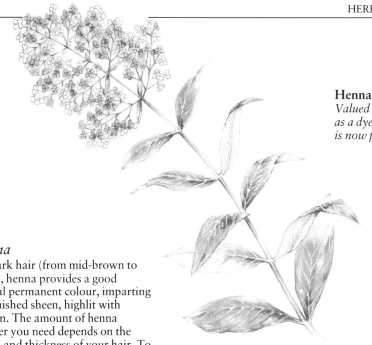

Henna
Valued in eastern countries as a dye for the hair, henna is now popular in the West.

Henna

For dark hair (from mid-brown to black), henna provides a good natural permanent colour, imparting a burnished sheen, highlit with auburn. The amount of henna powder you need depends on the length and thickness of your hair. To deepen and enrich the colour, mix the powder with strong real coffee instead of water. For a redder shade, add red wine to the water; add a tablespoon of lemon juice or cider vinegar to "fix" the colour. Wear rubber gloves, use an old towel, and take care to protect your clothes from stains when using henna.

Henna powder (see recipe)
Hot water or coffee (see recipe)
1 egg yolk, beaten

Put about a cupful of henna powder in a bowl, stir in enough hot water to make a thick paste, stir in the egg yolk and mix thoroughly. Aim for a medium thick paste, gradually adding more liquid or powder. Too thick a mixture will be crumbly, too thin will trickle down your face and neck. Shampoo and rinse your hair once. Towel dry. Paint the henna paste on to your hair with a square-tipped paintbrush, working down to the hair roots. Cover the hair with a plastic bag and test after 30 minutes by rubbing a strand of hair with a damp cloth. If it has reached the desired colour, rinse out right away; shampoo, and rinse again. If you want a deeper shade, leave the henna to work longer until you have the desired effect.

Leaf mouthwash

Pick the leaves when they are young and fresh, taking the bramble leaves from the tops of the stems.

One large handful blackcurrant or
*   bramble leaves*
1 pt (½ l) water
2 teaspoons lemon juice

Put the leaves and water into an open saucepan and boil until the liquid is reduced by half. Add the lemon juice, strain, and use immediately.

Toothpaste with peppermint

This mixture cleans the teeth and freshens the mouth. Use it with a damp toothbrush.

1 tablespoon arrowroot
1 teaspoon milled sea-salt
½ teaspoon bicarbonate of soda
15–20 drops oil of peppermint

Mix the ingredients with a spoon, then pound to a dry paste with a pestle and mortar. Keep in a screw-topped jar.

Variation Substitute 1 teaspoon ground cinnamon and 15 drops oil of cloves for the last two items.

Toothpowder with sage

Use fresh sage for this powder – it tastes good and its volatile oil has antiseptic properties. Rinse your mouth well after use.

1 small handful fresh sage leaves
Sea-salt – see recipe

Wash the sage. Pick off the tips and the freshest leaves and chop finely or put through a parsley mill. To each spoonful of chopped sage, add ½ spoonful milled sea-salt. Measure on to a flat ovenproof dish and bake in pre-heated oven (150 °C, 300 °F, Gas 2) for 20 minutes, until the sage is dry. Remove from the oven and pound the mixture to a fine powder with a pestle and mortar. Return to the oven for a further 15 minutes, until powdery. Cool and store in a screw-topped jar.

Cleavers deodorant

When you wash after using a deodorant you will usually notice the skin has a slight resistance to soap. Cleavers has the same effect on the skin, which is entirely harmless. If you prefer to use dried herbs as a deodorant powder, try a mixture of dried powdered orange peel, lemon peel, and orris root.

1 large handful of fresh, green
*   cleavers stems and leaves*
2 pt (1 l) water

Put the cleavers and water in a saucepan. Bring to the boil and simmer in the open pan for 15 minutes. Allow to cool, then strain and bottle. The deodorant keeps for 4–5 days in the refrigerator, so make fresh batches regularly.

Mind care and relaxation

Today the pace of life is faster than ever before. The pressures that it exerts on us are often overwhelming. The increasing tempo and demands of change leave us little time in which to relax. A wholesome diet, quiet meditation and healthy exercise that releases tension can help. But centuries of experiment and use by medical herbalists and aromatherapists have shown that herbs in various forms can have a powerful effect on the mind, both by encouraging feelings of calm relaxation and by stimulating and invigorating the system.

One of the simplest ways of relaxing with herbs is to add them to a bath. Soaking in a warm bath is in itself enjoyable and by adding herbs to the water in various ways you can make a bath even more relaxing – the essential oils in the herbs are released by the heat and absorbed directly through the skin into the blood stream. There are several different methods of introducing herbs into a bath in this way – and a number of herbs are suitable (see opposite).

Herbs for the nervous system

You can use most of the techniques on the following pages regularly, or resort to them at times when you have a particular problem such as stress at work or an inablility to sleep. But if you have had a long period of stress, anxiety, or nervous exhaustion, you should also take regular infusions of one of the plants that herbalists use to feed the nervous system. There are three that are particularly good for this – oats, skullcap, and vervain. A regular infusion of a teaspoon of one of these dried herbs in a cup of boiling water will revivify the whole system while easing tension and helping you to relax. A milder relaxant that is particularly good for children is lemon balm, which you can also use as an infusion. It soothes the nerves and can help with stomach problems that are often linked with anxiety and stress. **Note:** Check with your doctor before attempting these treatments for stress, especially if you are pregnant.

Many of the relaxing herbs have a dual effect that is also stimulating and invigorating. This is because being relaxed is itself a renewing state, in which you are far better able to rise to life's challenges and problems. But there are some herbal preparations (see opposite), and certain essential oils, that are particularly stimulating and refreshing. As with the relaxing herbs, the ones that work best will depend partly on the individual – so if one is not effective, experiment with different herbs or oils. A variety of herbs are used in aromatherapy. Some, such as lavender, rose, and chamomile, are familiar for their uses in herbal medicine, or for their perfume or other properties. But some more exotic herbs are also used, including oil extracted from the "perfume tree" and from frankincense (see p. 151).

Herbs to relax the eyes
There are several effective herbal remedies for eye strain and inflammation, which can be caused by artificial light, a smoky atmosphere, or lack of sleep. For quick relief, relax for 10 minutes with slices of cucumber placed over your closed eyelids. Cucumber is well known for its gentle cooling and soothing action; you can achieve a similar effect with slices of washed and peeled raw potato.

Eye baths and compresses
A number of herbs have a soothing and anti-inflammatory action. You can make an infusion of one of these plants and use it as an eye bath or a compress to soothe tired or inflamed eyes. To make a compress, dip cotton balls or squares of sterilized gauze in the cool liquid and place on the eyelids for 10–15 minutes.

1 teaspoon dried herbs (choose from borage, chamomile, coltsfoot, elder flower, eyebright, fennel seeds, lady's mantle, marigold)
1 cup bottled spring water

Infuse the dried herbs in the boiling spring water. Cover and stand for 10 minutes. Strain through a small funnel, lined with filter paper, and use when cool.

Relaxing herbal baths

One of the most effective ways to use herbs for relaxation is to add them to the bath water and soak for a while. Muslin bags of herbs, bulked out with bran or oatmeal, make a very pleasant bath. Soak the bag in the bath and smooth it gently over your face and body after soaping, to release the fragrance.

1 cupful fine oatmeal or bran
3 cupfuls dried lime flowers
  or chamomile flowers (or 2 cupfuls
  of dried flowers)
1 piece of muslin approx 15 ins (38
  cm) square

Put the oatmeal and herbs into a bowl and stir to mix. You can also add almonds reserved from making complexion milk (see p. 144). Tip on to a square of doubled muslin; gather up and tie tightly with string or thread.

Variation For a similar effect, make a very strong infusion of the dried herb (2 oz/56 g to 1 ½ pt/ 0.8 l water) strain it, and pour into the bath.

Invigorating bath vinegars

Slightly disinfectant, herb vinegars have a distinctive clean fragrance. In hot weather, add a cupful of herb vinegar to a tepid bath. It will leave you feeling invigorated, with your skin tingling fresh.

10 fl oz (280 ml) cider vinegar
10 fl oz (280 ml) water
2 handfuls chopped fresh herbs, or 3
  tablespoons mixed dried herbs and
  flowers (lime flowers, chamomile,
  lavender, or thyme)

Measure the vinegar and water into an enamel saucepan, bring slowly to the boil, then remove from the heat. Put the herbs into a bowl and pour over the hot liquid. Cover and leave for several hours. Strain and bottle.

Bath and shower gel

This gel, produced by the mucilage in Irish moss, is very invigorating. It also softens the skin. Rub handfuls of the gel over the body before rinsing your skin in the bath or shower.

2½ pts (1¼ l) fresh Irish moss
3 pts (1½ l) water
4 tablespoons orange flower or
  elderflower water
A few drops green food colouring
  (optional)

Wash the seaweed in plenty of fresh water to rid it of sand and small stones. Put the prepared seaweed into a large pan with the water, bring to the boil, cover, and simmer for 30 minutes. Rub the mixture through a food mill or strainer, stir in the flower water and add the colouring if required. When cold, pour into jars or wide-necked bottles.

Variation Instead of fresh Irish moss, use 2 oz (55 g) of the dried seaweed. Soak it in water to soften it before boiling.

Relaxing foot baths

For tired feet and aching leg muscles, particularly after vigorous exercise or jogging, soak your feet for 10 minutes in a herbal footbath before rinsing them in cold water. Adding sea salt or Epsom salts to the water is also helpful.

10 fl oz (280 ml) strong infusion
  (see p. 141) of one of the following:
  lavender, lime flowers, rosemary,
  peppermint (avoid prolonged use),
  thyme, yarrow, mugwort
2 tablespoons sea salt (or 1
  tablespoon Epsom salts)

Fill a large bowl with very hot water to which you have added the herbal infusion and the sea salt or Epsom salts. After soaking your feet, finish with a foot rub (see above right); alternatively, end with a massage with a relaxing oil (see pp. 150–1).

Soothing foot rub

As a final restorative for tired feet, massage with this lotion after soaking in a foot bath. Alum hardens the skin, helping to prevent blisters; the oils feed dry patches that tend to crack; and the lavender soothes aching muscles. Dip a piece of rough towelling into the lotion and rub into the feet, giving special attention to the insteps, arches, and ankles.

3 tablespoons sunflower oil
½ tablespoon cider vinegar
½ teaspoon oil of lavender
½ teaspoon alum powder

Put all the ingredients into a jam jar and stand the jar in a pan of hot water. Heat gently and stir. Allow it to cool, then screw on the lid and shake thoroughly. Remove the lid until completely cold. Shake again before use.

Hop pillows

Hops are well known for their sleep-inducing properties, which come from a substance called lupulin. A good way to utilize this is to make a hop pillow. You can add other relaxing herbs to the hops.

2 or 3 handfuls of dried hop flowers
Additional herbs (see recipe)
Muslin (see recipe)

Make a muslin bag to fit inside a small pillowcase and fill it loosely, so that it lies flat beside your ordinary pillow. With the hops you can include dried lime flowers, mignonette, dried, crumbled marjoram, and lemon balm.

Aromatherapy

For thousands of years, people have used aromatherapy as an aid to physical and emotional well-being. We can trace its use back at least as far as the ancient Egyptians, who recognized the therapeutic powers of essential oils, and there is also a long tradition of aromatherapy in the Far East, particularly in China. The oils, which are volatile compounds that occur naturally in plants, are important to the plant because they contribute to its characteristic scent (thus helping to attract pollinating insects) and because they help in water retention (see p. 23). Oils are extracted (either by distillation or maceration) from the flowers of some plants and the leaves of others. Their use in aromatherapy is effective because it links two potent forces – the healing ability of the oils themselves and the receptivity of the human skin and sense of smell.

There are many accounts of the physical healing powers of essential oils, one of the most famous being that of Gattefossé, the early French aromatherapist, who burned his hand, immediately thrust it into a bowl of essence of lavender, and found it healing very rapidly. There has been little scientific testing of the way aromatherapy works on the mind, although research at Milan University has shown that the oils are effective in treating anxiety and depression. They stimulate the nerves in the olfactory organs, which are linked directly to the parts of the brain that control the emotions. They also stimulate the nerve endings on the skin surface, and aromatherapists believe that their effect passes back along the nerves until it eventually reaches the pituitary gland. This master gland controls all the body's other glands, including the adrenals, which in turn regulate our stress or relaxation response (see pp. 220–1).

Using aromatherapy

Essential oils must never be taken internally. But there are several other ways we can use the oils, to make aromatherapy part of our everyday lives. In so doing, we will not only be able to relax more easily, we will also regain touch with our sense of smell – a sense that suffers badly as a result of pollution from many products in common use around the home (see p. 152). One of the most effective ways to use the oils is in massage. This activates the nerve endings and stimulates the blood circulation near the skin's surface, speeding the entry of the oils into the body (see p. 140). Another good method is to put two drops of oil in a hot bath and soak in the water for at least ten minutes. Close the doors and windows to retain the vapours, which will be absorbed through the pores in the skin and nose. Alternatively, you can inhale the vapour from a few drops of oil placed in a bowl of very hot water. Another method is to use a commercial vapourizer but do be careful to observe the manufacturer's instructions that accompany the unit.

Choosing essential oils
Amongst the wide range of essential oils on the market, there are a number that you can use for their soothing and relaxing properties. The chart opposite includes a selection of the most useful. You can use all of them as bath oils (adding two drops to a hot bath, unless otherwise specified), while some of them, diluted in a carrier such as soya oil or grape seed oil, also make good massage oils.

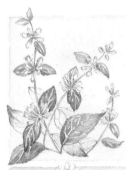

Melissa

The essential oil from the lemon balm plant is generally known to aromatherapists as melissa. They use its soothing properties to disperse depression and black thoughts. Add five or six drops of melissa to a hot bath.

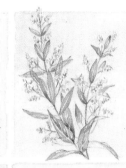

Sandalwood

This heavy, luxurious oil is useful for tension and anxiety. It also has a folk reputation as a sexual stimulant.

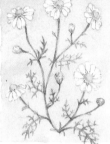

Chamomile

This oil is frequently used in aromatherapy to calm overwrought nerves. You can use it in a bath (adding five or six drops), or make a massage oil by adding two drops of chamomile oil to five teaspoons of soya oil.

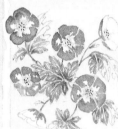

Geranium

You may find this oil sold as Geranium Bourbon-la-Reunion, after the island where the plant originates. Relaxing in small quantities, geranium makes a good massage oil. Dilute two drops in two teaspoons of soya oil.

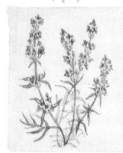

Bergamot

Aromatherapists have found that this oil is particularly good for depression, as well as being effective in helping the body to fight infections.

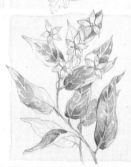

Ylang ylang

Far eastern "perfume trees" provide this strongly scented oil which you can use in the bath. A sedative and antidepressant, it is good for shock and pain. As it has a heavy scent, you should use it sparingly.

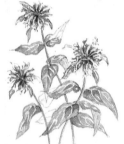

Lavender

As well as being known for its ability to heal burns and wounds (see opposite), lavender is an excellent relaxant. Dilute a drop and add it to a baby's bath to help it to sleep.

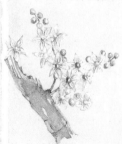

Frankincense

Extracted from the gum resin of the tree *Boswellia Thurifera*, this oil is calming and deepens the breathing. Use it on a vapourizer to produce a contemplative state during meditation. Add five drops of frankincense to a bath.

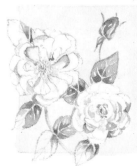

Rose

This oil comes from the damascena, centifolia, and gallica varieties of rose. Aromatherapists value it for tension in women, particularly for post-natal depression and the stress that follows the break-up of a relationship.

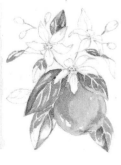

Neroli

This oil comes from the bitter orange tree. In cases of nervous tension and anxiety it will induce calm; it is also used to encourage sleep. You can make a massage oil by mixing five drops with two teaspoons of soya oil.

Home care

Plants are highly versatile. Just as plant preparations can benefit your physical and emotional health, so they can also be used widely in the care of your home environment. On the simplest level, this means no more than bringing plants into your home and enjoying their appearance and scent, growing them in pots and decorating your house with vases of cut herbs. Using herbs in this way is not only enjoyable and convenient, it also brings you still closer to the natural world, providing ample proof that the indoor environment is just as much a part of the living world as your garden. What is more, you can make natural herbal home-care products – ranging from pot-pourris to cleaners and polishes – that are highly effective, pleasant to use, and safe. Research at several American centres for environmental health and human ecology has shown that fears about the toxicity of many commercial products – air fresheners, detergents, fly killers – are justified. Natural alternatives to all these products are much healthier for everyone in your home.

On the pages that follow, you will find recipes for a variety of products used in the home. Soaps, polishes, and scented sachets for closets, pot-pourris, natural dyes, and herbal insect repellents are all covered.

Housekeeping

Herbs can play a number of practical roles around the home. You can use their fragrance in sweet bags to scent closets. Other herbs can be used to make household cleaners and furniture polishes. All of these are safe, "natural" products, made from simple ingredients without synthetic chemicals. They have the added advantage of spreading the subtle aromas of herbs further around the house.

There are many other ways of using herbs and plants in the home. Wood sorrel, for example, contains a large amount of oxalic acid, and an extract of the plant makes a natural bleach. The juice from its leaves will remove rust spots from white cotton or linen and reduce ink stains. Many plants can be used in the home with little or no preparation. Brazil nut, walnut, and hazelnut kernels make excellent polishes. Brazil nuts are especially effective for darkening white marks on polished furniture. You simply rub the kernel's cut surface in a circular movement before going over the surface in the direction of the grain. After the oil has dried a little, you can polish with a clean, dry cloth. Another valuable fruit is the sloe, which you can use as a permanent ink. You stab a pen into a raw sloe and write with the juice on handkerchiefs or linen. Horsetail makes a good metal polish. A bunch of the stems will clean and shine metal pans and pewter objects. Wash pans before cooking in them.

Keep all the preparations in this section out of the reach of children.

Soapwort
With its lather-producing saponins, this is one of the most useful household cleansing herbs.

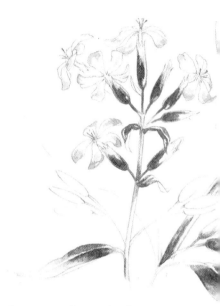

Closets and wardrobes

A pleasant, healthy way of scenting clothes and linen, sweet herb bags can contain any mixture of aromatic leaves or flower petals that combine well together. You can use one of the pot-pourri mixtures (see p. 155), or any suitable blend of dried, crumbled aromatic herbs with added oil of rosemary or oregano. For lavender bags, intensify the fragrance of the dried lavender flowers with a few drops of oil of lavender. Another successful mixture is a selection of wild flowers – dried, crumbled meadowsweet, woodruff, elder flowers, and ground ivy leaves combine well; you can sharpen the fragrance with a little oil of citronella. Use small rectangular cotton bags for closets, loosely filled sachets for drawers, and tiny bags tied with cord for hanging from coat hangers.

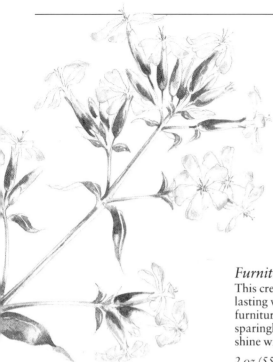

Liquid cleaner-polisher

This polish is easy to apply and thoroughly cleans any dirty, dry wood. Its liquid consistency makes it ideal for carved furniture and its oils feed and give a gentle shine to pine and beech furniture without darkening the wood. Apply it with a soft rag and polish off with a clean duster.

5 fl oz (140 ml) pure turpentine
5 fl oz (140 ml) raw linseed oil
2.5 fl oz (70 ml) wood spirit
2.5 fl oz (70 ml) cider vinegar
3 teaspoons lemon oil

Measure all the ingredients into a bottle and shake well. Shake again before applying.

Soapwort fabric shampoo

The gentle cleansing power of the saponins in soapwort makes this shampoo ideal for upholstery and delicate fabrics. The plant is used in parts of the Middle East for washing wool and has recently found favour for cleaning old tapestries and hangings. For upholstery, dampen a sponge with the solution and squeeze out the surplus, or use a very soft brush. Rub the material lightly and allow it to dry before applying again if necessary and rinsing. For delicate fabrics, soak in cool water, wash gently in cool soapwort shampoo, and rinse in cool water. Test on a hidden piece of fabric first.

½ oz (15 g) dried soapwort root, or
2 large handfuls of the fresh stems
1½ pts (¾ l) water

Crush the root with a rolling pin, or chop the fresh stems into shorter lengths. If using dried soapwort, prepare it by soaking overnight. Put the soapwort into an enamel pan with the water. Bring to the boil, cover, and simmer for 20 minutes, stirring occasionally. Allow to stand until cool. Strain through a fine strainer.

Furniture cream

This cream gives a beautiful, long-lasting wax finish to antique polished furniture. You should apply it very sparingly and polish to a brilliant shine with a soft, clean cloth.

2 oz (55 g) beeswax
10 fl oz (300 ml) pure turpentine
2 oz (55 g) soap flakes
7 fl oz (200 ml) normal strength
  rosemary infusion (see p. 141)

Measure the beeswax and turpentine into a bowl and melt together over a pan of simmering water. Dissolve the soapflakes in the hot herbal infusion. Cool both mixtures a little, then stir together to make a thick cream. Pour into a screw-topped glass jar.

Floor polish

Useful for wood-block and oak floors, this durable and protective wax polish gives a beautiful shine. Rub it well into the floor with a pad of soft cloth and leave for an hour or two before polishing to a shine.

2 oz (55 g) beeswax
5 fl oz (140 ml) pure turpentine
2 tablespoons raw linseed oil
2 teaspoons cedar oil

Melt the first three ingredients together in a bowl over a pan of barely simmering water. Remove from the heat and stir to a soft cream. Add the cedar oil and stir again. Pour into a screw-topped jar.

Household soap

You can use this richly lathering soap for all types of household cleaning. The antiseptic power of the oil of cloves and the emollient quality of the honey make it gentle and pleasant to the skin.

½ lb (225 g) soap flakes
2 tablespoons corn oil
2 oz (55 g) honey
2 teaspoons oil of cloves

Measure the first three ingredients into a bowl and soften over a pan of simmering water for about 15 minutes. Work the mixture with a wooden spoon, then transfer it into a dry pan and add the oil of cloves. Heat gently and stir constantly until the mixture becomes like marzipan, or a stiff dough. Turn out into oiled moulds (such as miniature loaf tins, or individual pie dishes). When cool enough, press down firmly with your fingers, and smooth the surfaces with oil. Store the blocks of soap in a warm, dry place for a week or two, until they are hard.

Fragrance

Scents are among the most immediate and evocative sensations, and plants provide some of the most delightful scents of all. Although there is something mysterious about the sense of smell (we cannot measure levels of smell, as we can sound and light) it is a simple process, in which the highly sensitive nerves in the membranes lining the nostrils sense volatile compounds in the air. The volatile compounds from plants can be healing (see Aromatherapy, pp. 150–1) or simply enjoyable in themselves, a combination that accounts for the long history of human use of fragrant plants. The ancient Egyptians were the first to record this – they put aromatic herbs in their homes and their tombs, and since then every civilization has used sweet-smelling herbs in its own way. The spice trade, bringing sweet-smelling spices from the Far East to the Middle East and later to Rome, is one of the most ancient links between East and West. The Romans used exotic spices, together with the aromatic herbs that grew naturally on the hillsides of the Mediterranean, for perfumes, cosmetics, and medicines, and to banish insects. Beads made of ambergris and scented gums, and pomanders are other methods that have been used to spread and preserve the fragrance of herbs, and the tradition of using natural perfumes in a variety of ways continued until comparatively recently. By the 19th century it was not unusual to find scented books, writing-paper and even ink.

Many uses of fragrant herbs have passed out of currency because we now have artificially produced substitutes. Disinfectants and air fresheners have replaced the habit of strewing herbs and rushes. But these products often come in aerosols (potentially harmful to the environment) and their perfumes are less pleasant and less wholesome than those from the plants in their natural state. Growing aromatic herbs in and near the house is one of the best ways of spreading fragrance around your home. Roses, lavender, wallflowers, pinks and carnations, violets, heliotropes, lilies, and mignonettes all have beautiful scents (see also pp. 254–5). Hanging up bunches of herbs can provide an additional fragrance. Woodruff, with its scent of hay, makes rooms smell sweet and fresh when used in this way.

Two of the most enduring ways of using fragrant herbs are in pot-pourris, which enable you to combine and preserve perfumes from a wide range of plants, and pomanders, citrus fruit studded with whole cloves and rolled in sweet-smelling powdered spices such as cinnamon, ground cloves, or grated nutmeg. Both are delightfully fragrant, and you can combine them by garnishing a pot-pourri with miniature pomanders made from kumquats. People react differently to these delicate fragrances, so exercise your personal taste when preparing perfumed items for the home, and use your nose when combining the scents of herbs. The lists of ingredients for pot-pourris opposite are intended as starting points – you can vary the mixtures as you wish.

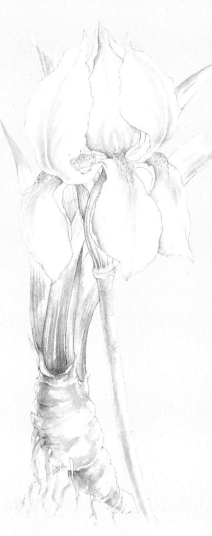

Orris root
The root of the Florentine iris is the principal source of orris root, made by grinding the dried root-stock. Orris root has been used in perfumery since the ancient Egyptians. It is valued for its violet scent and its ability to act as a perfume fixative.

Preparing the herbs

This book suggests the dry method of pot-pourri-making. It is simpler than the traditional moist method, and produces good results. Suggestions for combinations of ingredients are given on this page. You can also add: citrus peel (dried in a low oven for 10 minutes), spices (cinnamon, cloves, mace, juniper berries, fennel seeds), wood raspings (cedar and sandalwood), frankincense, and myrrh. You start by drying the leaves and flowers in single layers on a piece of muslin stretched over a frame. Keep each batch to one type of flower or leaf, as drying times vary. Keep the frames in a warm, dry place out of the sun. When they are dry and crisp, put the ingredients in jars with tight-fitting lids. Over each layer (1 in/2.5 cm deep) of plant material sprinkle ½ teaspoon coarse salt and ½ teaspoon orris root powder. Screw on the lids, label, and store in the dark for three weeks.

Making a pot-pourri

Choose a covered bowl if you want to scent the room occasionally, an open one for delicious wafts of perfume. Assemble all the jars of dried plant material, and any spices you intend to use. Select one or two (rarely more) essential oils that will compliment your choice of plants. Tip out the jars into the bowl, add the spices, and stir all together gently. Shake a few drops of perfumed oil over the material, stir, and test the perfume.

Flower garden pot-pourri

Most gardens contain a number of scented flowers that combine well.

6 tablespoons lavender flowers
4 tablespoons scented rose petals
4 tablespoons carnation, or dianthus petals
2 tablespoons chamomile flowers
2 tablespoons heliotrope flowers
2 tablespoons salt
2 tablespoons orris root powder
About 1 teaspoon oil of lavender

Herb garden pot-pourri

This pot-pourri includes a range of popular culinary herbs.

6 tablespoons peppermint, or spearmint leaves
4 tablespoons rosemary leaves
4 tablespoons lemon balm leaves
2 tablespoons marjoram leaves
1 tablespoon sage leaves
1 tablespoon broken up bay leaves
½ tablespoon thyme leaves and sprigs
2 tablespoons salt
2 tablespoons orris root powder
About 1 teaspoon oil of rosemary
About ½ teaspoon oil of oregano

Forest pot-pourri

For a perfume reminiscent of woods, try this mixture.

2 handfuls cedar twigs and raspings
2 tablespoons sandalwood raspings
4 tablespoons larch or alder cones
2 tablespoons myrtle leaves
2 handfuls pine needles
2 tablespoons crumbled southernwood
Some dried lichen
2 tablespoons salt
2 tablespoons orris root powder
About a teaspoon sandalwood or cedar oil

Herbs for pot-pourris

Material from woodland, spice shop, or flower garden can be used in pot-pourris.

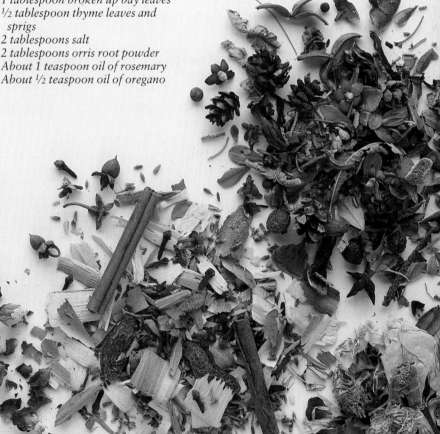

Dyeing with plants

Since prehistoric times humans have embellished their skins and fabrics with colour. The first dyes were probably no more than stains obtained from fruit juices, flowers, and decoctions of leaves and roots. Experiments with earth that contained iron and other minerals would have rendered the stains more permanent. In ancient China, India, and the Middle East, skills in dyeing developed very early. Much of this knowledge spread to Egypt, Greece, and Rome, survived into the dark ages in Europe and was widely used in thirteenth century Italy. Until the nineteenth century, all dyes were "natural", obtained from animal, vegetable, and mineral material. Today we can use herbs to recapture the muted colours and soft lustre of these dyes, which have a beauty and subtlety often lacking in the combinations of synthetic fabrics and crude colours produced today.

The easiest material to dye is wool – silk, linen, and cotton are much more difficult to prepare. It is best to start with skeins of white or pale-coloured wool. You can re-dye (or "over-dye") skeins of wool if they are too pale, but you cannot do this with knitted or woven garments, as they would shrink in the hot dye-bath.

Using herbal dyes

Dyeing is not difficult, but you will need several items of special equipment (see opposite). The best place to work is in a utility room or outhouse with electricity, but if you are careful to avoid splashing you can carry out dyeing in the kitchen. Some of the materials (particularly the mordants) are poisonous, so you should keep them away from children and pets and wear rubber gloves when using them.

Many plants can be used for dyeing but some colours are easier to obtain than others. The most common shades are yellows, browns, and greys; a few plants also yield purples and blues (see pp. 158–9). When you are gathering herbs for dyeing, you will need quite large amounts of plant material, so you should always be careful not to overpick, and limit yourself to common species. If you are not taking plants from your own garden, make sure before you begin that you have the permission of the landowner and that you will only need to take a small proportion of the material growing on the site.

If you are in doubt, limit yourself to plants you have grown yourself, and to commercially grown herbs. Before dyeing, you should prepare the wool by tying the skeins loosely in several places. Then wash the wool in a hot solution of well dissolved soap flakes to remove the grease. Rinse it several times in water of the same temperature until the water is clear. This process is called "scouring". The next process is applying a mordant to help the wool absorb the colour and to make the dye permanent. Most mordants are based on metallic compounds, which should be treated with care. Some natural dyers advocate omitting mordants, but this will produce a result that runs very quickly.

Many of these preparations are toxic. Keep them out of the reach of children.

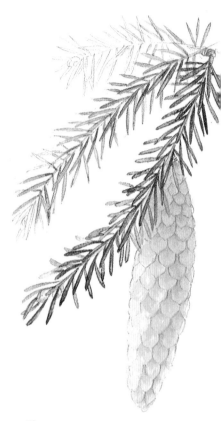

Pine cones
Cones from pine trees like these of the Norway spruce, yield a number of different colours – orange-yellows with an alum mordant and browns with an iron mordant.

Alum mordant

The most useful mordant is potassium aluminium sulphate, known to dyers as alum. Sometimes potassium hydrogen tartrate (usually called "cream of tartar", but different from the substance used in baking) is added to the alum to help the dye to penetrate evenly and brighten the colour.

4 oz (120 g) aluminium sulphate
1 oz (30 g) cream of tartar
1 lb (450 g) wool in skeins
Water

Put the alum and cream of tartar into a dye bath full of cold water. Stir well, and when dissolved, add the wool. Gradually bring the water to the boil, turn down the heat, and simmer gently for 1 hour. If the wool is very fine and soft use 3 oz (90 g) of alum and simmer for ¾ hour. Lift out the wool, drain, and squeeze gently. It is now ready for dyeing.

Tin mordant

Tin is sold as crystals of stannous chloride. It brightens reds and yellows and is usually added towards the end of the dyeing process.

Materials for alum mordant (above)
½ oz (15 g) stannous chloride
2 oz (60 g) cream of tartar
1 lb (450 g) dyed wool in skeins
Water

Mordant the wool with alum (see above) and simmer in the dye bath for 45 mins. Lift out the wool. Add the cream of tartar to the dye bath, stir to dissolve, then stir in the tin crystals. When these have dissolved add the wool and simmer for a further 15 mins. Drain and squeeze out the wool as before.

Onion
Onion skins give golden browns with an alum mordant.

Iron mordant

Available as ferrous sulphate, iron is used in conjunction with cream of tartar. Iron darkens colour and dyers generally use this mordant at the end of the dyeing process.

½ oz (15 g) ferrous sulphate
1 oz (30 g) cream of tartar
1 lb dyed wool in skeins
Water

Simmer the wool in the dye bath for 30 mins, then remove it from the water. Add the iron and cream of tartar to the water and stir until they are dissolved. Then return the wool to the dye bath and simmer until you achieve the required depth of colour.

Chrome mordant

Bichromate of potash (chrome) is light-sensitive and should be kept in the dark. It makes colours fast and gives a soft, silky feel to wool.

CAUTION Chrome is poisonous.

½ oz (15 g) bichromate of potash
1 lb wool in skeins
Water

Put the chrome in a bath of cold water, heat, and stir well. When it has dissolved, add the wool. Slowly bring to the boil; turn down the heat and simmer for 1 hour. Lift out the wool, drain, and squeeze out gently.

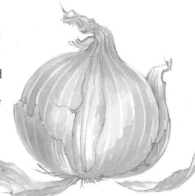

Equipment
A large stainless steel vessel, such as a preserving pan, is required for the dye-bath, together with a stainless steel or enamel bucket and bowl. You will also need: tongs (stainless steel or wooden) for lifting; stirring rods (wood or glass); a graduated quart or litre measure; scales; and rubber gloves.

The dyeing process

You can use dried plant material, which you can buy or dry yourself, or use fresh plants. Pick the latter when the leaves and shoots are young and green. If you are using flowers, pick them just as they are coming into bloom. Roots for dyeing should be dug up in the autumn. Smash up twiggy material, roots, and bark, and put all the material you are going to use into a muslin or nylon bag.

1 lb (450 g) mordanted wool in
* skeins*
1 lb (450 g) plant material
Water

Put the dye bath on the stove and fill three-quarters full with cold water. If you are using dried, powdered material, dissolve this in the water. For fresh plants, put them into a mesh bag, tie it securely, and lower it into the water. Add the skeins of wool, bring the water slowly to the boil, stirring occasionally; then turn down the heat, and simmer for 1 hour. Remove from the heat, and leave the wool and plant material in the dye bath until cold, or until you think the colour is right. After lifting out the wool with the tongs, gently squeeze it out and rinse in water of the same temperature until no colour runs out. Reds and yellows are improved by a hot soap and water wash before rinsing. Dry skeins over a rod or cord, with a light weight tied at the bottom to stop kinking.

Dye plants

Certain plants are particularly valuable to dyers because they yield rare colours. One of the best examples is woad (*Isatis tinctoria*), an ancient dye plant which gives blue. It also illustrates another principle of dyeing – that the colours produced can vary greatly according to the mordant used and the timings of the dyeing and mordanting processes. The range of blues and beiges on this page were all dyed with woad. Madder, famous for its reds, and sorrel can also produce a variety of results.

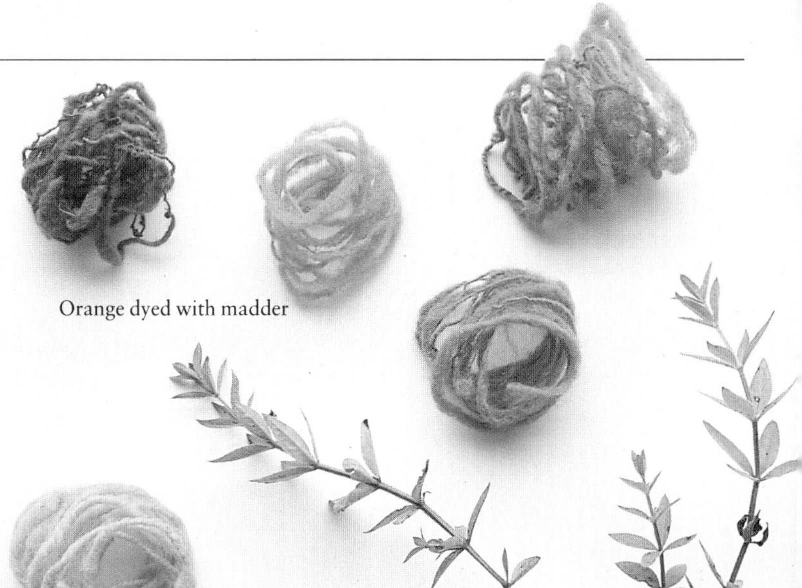

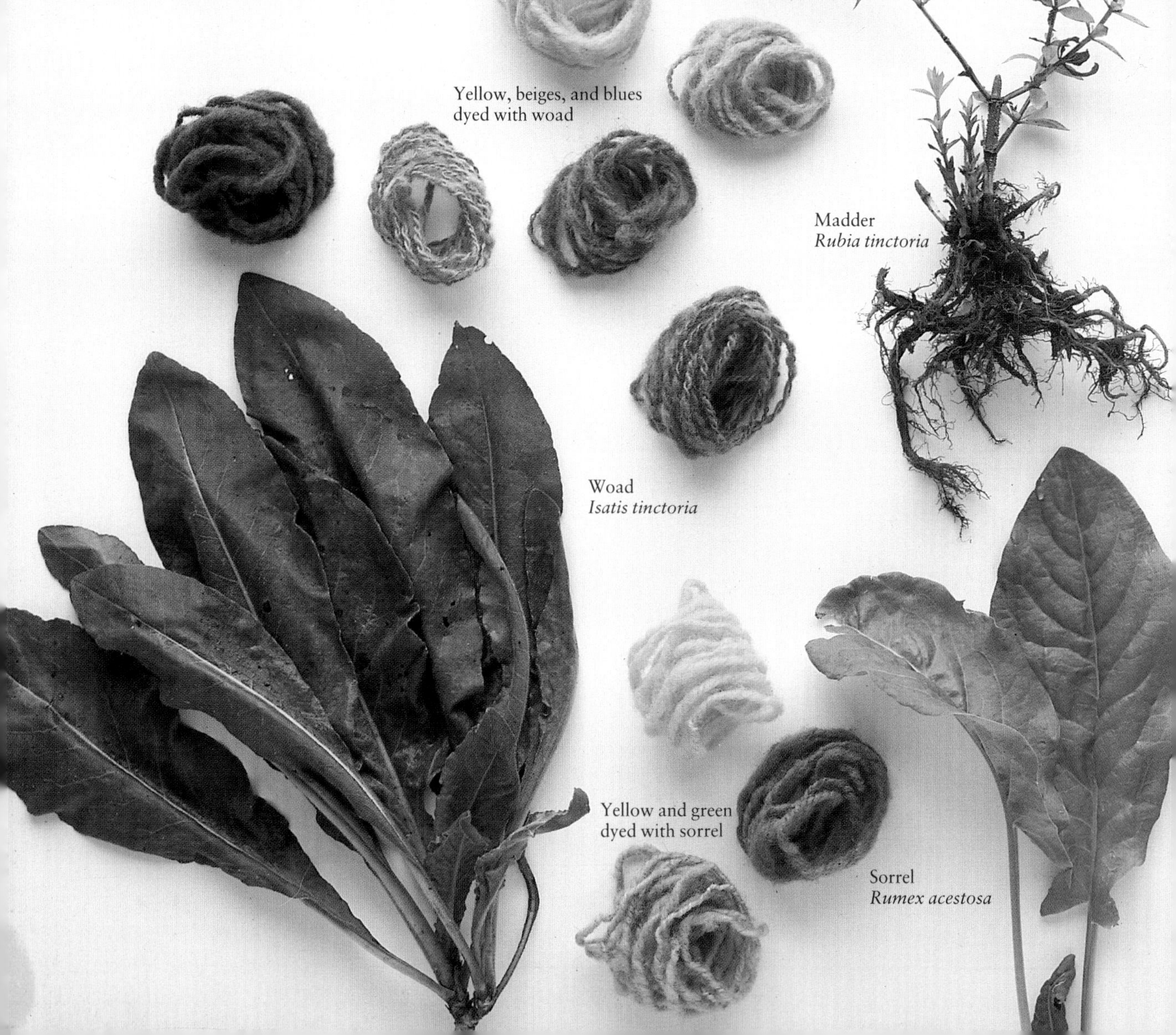

Orange dyed with madder

Yellow, beiges, and blues dyed with woad

Madder
Rubia tinctoria

Woad
Isatis tinctoria

Yellow and green dyed with sorrel

Sorrel
Rumex acestosa

Plants to gather

The selection of plants (right) produces a good range of colours with the mordants shown in parentheses. They are all common enough to gather from the wild, provided that you collect them responsibly. Pick your dye material where there are plentiful supplies – you should always leave far more material behind you than the amount you take away. You will probably obtain the best results with fresh plants, particularly if you are using leaves, although roots and onion skins can give good results when dried. Fruits are best when they are fresh, ripe, or even overripe.

Plants to buy

If you cannot obtain the plants you want from the wild, you can buy many different dried dye plants from craft stores and herb suppliers. These will provide a range of colours similar to the native plants you can gather, but there are certain plants that are useful because they yield the rarer colours. Bearberry and woad give blues, horsetail can produce a range of shades from fawn to pink, madder yields reds and browns, and logwood chips (available from dye suppliers) give tones from slate grey to black.

Bramble *Rubus fruticosus*
Shoots (Iron) Blacks/greys

Bramble *Rubus fruticosus*
Berries (Alum) Blues/greys

Bilberry *Vaccinium myrtillus*
Fruits (Alum) Blues/purples

Elder *Sambucus nigra*
Berries (Alum) Violets/purples

Privet *Ligustrum ovalifolium*
Fruits (Alum) Blues/greens

Elder *Sambucus nigra*
Leaves (Alum) Greens

Bracken *Pteris aquilina*
Young shoots (Alum) Yellows/greens

Heather *Calluna vulgaris*
Shoots (Alum) Olives/yellows

Fig *Ficus carica*
Leaves (Alum) Lemon yellows

Birch *Betula pendula*
Leaves (Alum) Yellows

Privet *Ligustrum ovalifolium*
Leaves (Alum) Yellows

Ragwort *Senecio jacobaea*
Whole plant (Alum) Yellows

Tansy *Tanacetum vulgare*
Flowers (Alum) Yellows

Golden rod *Solidago canadensis*
Whole plant (Chrome) Golden yellows

Pine *Pinus spp*
Cones (Alum) Orange yellows

Bracken *Pteris aquilina*
Roots (Alum) Oranges/yellows

Onion *Allium cepa*
Skins (Alum) Golden browns

Walnut *Juglans regia*
Shells (no mordant) Pinkish browns

Pine *Pinus spp*
Cones (Iron) Browns

Insect repellents

We are so used to "knock-out" pesticides in our chemically dominated lives that we often overlook the way the natural world deals with the problem. The plant world offers a perfectly effective range of natural insect repellents and yet the chemical companies continue to produce products whose effects on animal and bird life are lethal and on human health uncalculated. Stores still display products with poison warnings and the public goes on buying them. Very often the pesticide is more harmful than the pest. But we should not under-estimate the power of plants. There are wild plants that can kill a man, so the belief that plants can both kill and repel insects is not unreasonable. Pyrethrum and derris (see p. 267) are potent pesticides derived from plants, requiring common sense in handling, but harmless to humans and pets, except reptiles and fish. Another example is elecampane. Spanish country people use the sticky roots of this herb as a natural fly-paper. They hang the roots by their windows to attract and trap flying insects. This section concentrates on ways of keeping different types of insects away.

Some of the herbs used are toxic if ingested, so you should keep them away from children and pets.

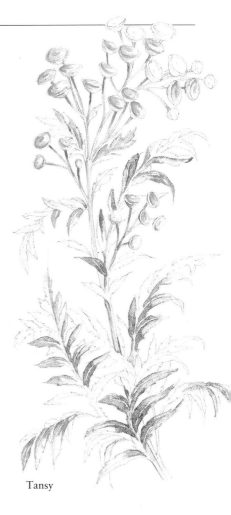

Tansy

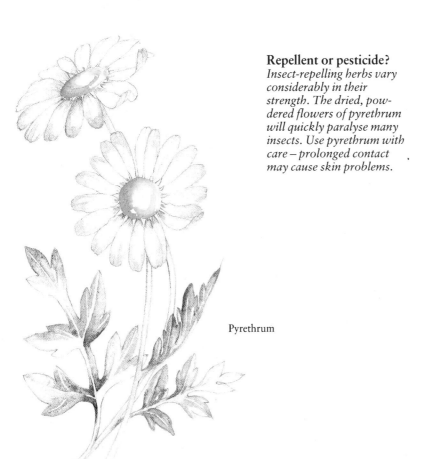

Pyrethrum

Repellent or pesticide?
Insect-repelling herbs vary considerably in their strength. The dried, pow-dered flowers of pyrethrum will quickly paralyse many insects. Use pyrethrum with care – prolonged contact may cause skin problems.

Fly repellents

One way of deterring at least some flies is to hang up bunches of insect-repelling herbs in the house, or to put vases filled with aromatic and pungent-scented fresh herbs on the windowsills. In summer, collect eau-de-cologne mint, pennyroyal, rosemary, rue, southernwood, thyme, or tansy to hang up or stand in a jug or vase. Many of these were strewn on the floors of houses in the Middle Ages to help repel flies. Tansy, one of the old strewing herbs, has a good reputation as an insect repellent. Its clean pungency when crushed underfoot helped keep flies away. An old method of keeping flies off meat was to rub it with tansy, but the use of this potentially highly toxic herb is not recommended today.

Ant and mite repellents

For ants in the house, a strong decoction of walnut leaves (6 handfuls of leaves boiled in 1 pt/½ l water for 20–30 minutes) can be painted round floors or on work surfaces. And if you are a home-baker with a large amount of flour to store, keep 2 or 3 nutmegs or a few peeled elder shoots in the bag or bin to prevent mites.

Walnut

The leaves of the walnut tree have a distinctive aroma. A decoction repels ants.

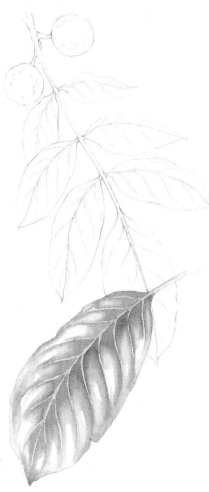

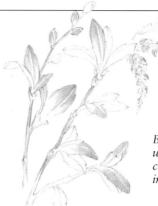

Bog myrtle (left) is rare; wormwood (right) is more common but toxic if taken internally.

Moth repellents

To deter moths, lay whole sprays of dried herbs among blankets or woollens. Put southernwood (its French name of *garderobe* confirms its usefulness), santolina, rosemary, and lavender among clothes between sheets of tissue paper. The rarer bog myrtle, or sweet gale (*Myrica gale*), has the old country name of flea-wood and was used to scent linen and to drive out fleas.

Moth-repellent sachets

Sachets or bags filled with a mixture of pungent herbs and spices, and placed in closets and drawers, are a good protection against moths.

3 tablespoons southernwood
2 tablespoons mugwort (handle
  with care)
1 tablespoon rosemary leaves
1 tablespoon chamomile flowers
1 tablespoon thyme
1 teaspoon cinnamon
1 teaspoon ground cloves
½ teaspoon grated nutmeg
1 teaspoon salt
1 teaspoon orris root powder
Oil of cloves, or lavender, or lemon
  oil (see recipe)

Crumble the dried herbs into a bowl. Add the spices, the salt and orris root. Store in a screw-topped jar, away from the light, for 2 weeks. Have the bags ready for filling, and shake enough oil on to the herbs to scent them quite strongly. Fill the bags and stitch or tie the opening.

Outdoor insect repellents

To prevent the evening onslaught of mosquitos in summer, rub a handful of fresh elder leaves on your arms, legs and neck. This is effective for about 20 minutes, but must then be renewed. Alternatively, strong infusions of chamomile or elder leaves are useful to dab on the skin to prevent insect bites; carry a small bottle of the infusion in your pocket for frequent applications. You can even wear elder leaves or lavender in your hair to repel insects. Oil of lavender and citronella (the oil of the stone root, *Collinsonia canadensis*) are both lovely scents to wear outdoors on the hair or skin, and effectively keep off mosquitos.

CHAPTER FOUR

Herbs for
Nutrition and Health

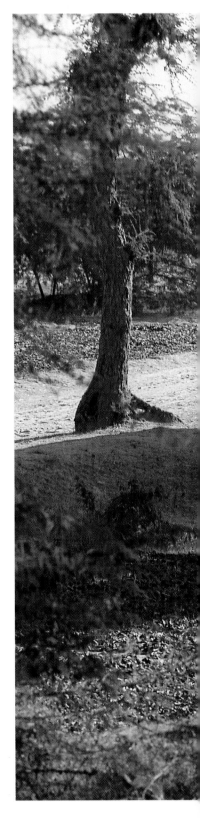

We are what we eat. Systems of medicine from East to West recognize the importance of diet for our health. Some complementary medicine practitioners, especially naturopaths and medical herbalists, regard food as a therapy in itself, prescribing special diets for particular ailments, as well as recommending a basic regime for general well-being. And the dietary principles of both yoga and macrobiotics are intended to balance the body and promote natural energy flow. But simply eating the right foods is not always enough to ensure that we are getting the best out of our diet. We must be able to digest and assimilate the right nutritents to stay in optimum health.

Herbs have a vital role to play here, and it is one that is recognized in every ancient culinary tradition. For herbs were originally used in cooking less for their flavour than for their digestive and preservative properties. For the viewpoint of digestion, the volatile oils are the most important constituents of culinary herbs – and they are found especially in plants of the mint family, Labiatae, such as marjoram, peppermint, and rosemary, and the carrot family, Umbelliferae, such as caraway and parsley. These herbs have what herbalists describe as a carminative action, soothing the walls of the digestive tract, stimulating peristalsis, and reducing flatulence. But culinary herbs also contain tannins, bitter principles, and other pharmacologically active constituents. And many have an antiseptic action too – a vital property in hot climates, where contaminated food is a hazard to health.

The range of herbs that may be employed in cooking is vast, and used with imagination and flair, herbs will not only add zest and variety to your diet, they can also open up new horizons in your eating and drinking habits. "Tea" need no longer be limited to a drink made from the leaves of a single plant, it can mean refreshing herbal infusions of anything from mint to lemon verbena; flavouring can come from a whole range of plant-based alternatives to sugar and salt; and the most unlikely-looking plants – from stinging nettles to burdock roots – can provide meals at once delicious and nutritious.

Some herbs are unsafe in certain circumstances. Consult the Glossary for cautions before use.

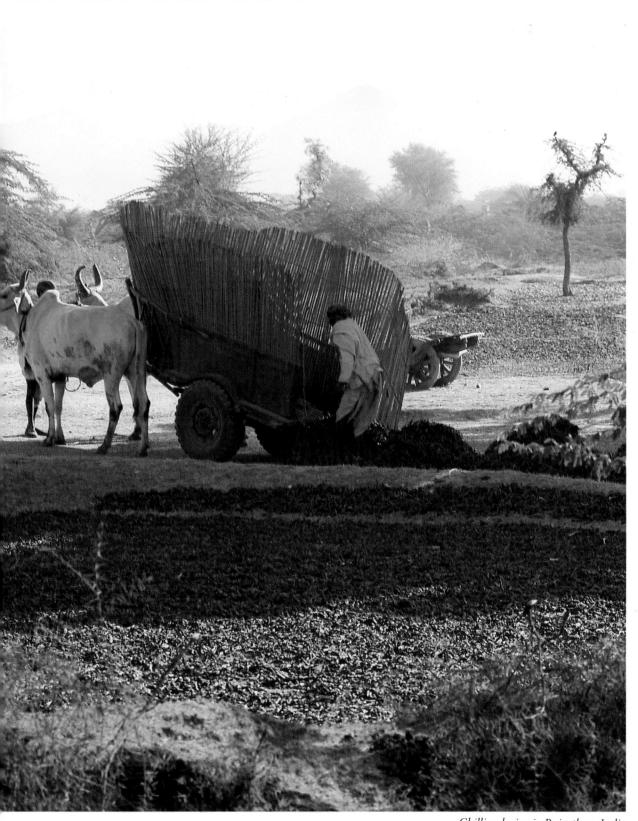

Chillies drying in Rajasthan, India

Properties of culinary herbs

In modern western cuisine, herbs tend to be used as "extras" to please the palate and enliven our menus. But their value is more profound: they stimulate our appetite, enhance our digestion, and preserve our food. In many places they remain guardians of health in the diet – as they were everywhere in the days before chemical preservatives and refrigerators were available.

The principal active constituents of digestive herbs are their volatile oils. These stimulate our secretion of digestive juices, prevent fermentation (which causes flatulence) and decomposition of food, and soothe the digestive system. Angelica or savory, for instance, eaten after a meal, will help prevent flatulence; fennel or cardamom will sweeten the breath. Some herbs also contain tonic and astringent bitter principles which rouse the appetite, and so are helpful for invalids – two with a long history are marjoram and rosemary. Others may contain tannins which help prevent dyspepsia, secretins which aid the pancreas (found in nettles for example), or organic acids which help us to digest fats. All these properties are at their best in freshly picked herbs, but are still effective in properly dried ones (see p. 272). The anti-bacterial and preservative properties make culinary herbs and spices valuable for use in vinegars, oils, pickles, wines, and all stored foods, where they slowly release their essential oils. And herbs regularly added to our diet in reasonable quantities – in fresh salads and liberal garnishes especially – can enrich its nutritional content with a whole range of vitamins, minerals and trace elements. Rose hips, for example, contain twenty times as much vitamin C as oranges; dandelion leaves are rich in vitamin A; parsley and kelp are good sources of calcium as well as containing many vitamins.

Nutritional constituents
The chart gives a breakdown of the active nutritional constituents of a range of common culinary herbs. Dandelion and mustard greens, for example, are sources of vitamin A, which promotes, amongst other things, good vision and strong bones and teeth. Chicory and garlic are both useful potassium sources. Kelp, watercress and parsley leaves contain good supplies of calcium, a must for healthy bones and teeth, for blood-clotting, and for healthy muscle function. The vitamin C in rosehips is the valuable element of rosehip syrup for infants.

Healing through food
Many culinary herbs are also healers with wider actions on the body systems. Garlic has a range of health benefits (p. 80) and is a good addition to any diet. Not only does it act as an internal purifier and help to keep cholesterol down, but it can also keep colds and flu at bay. Some culinary herbs are good for the mouth – cinnamon strengthens the gums, sage with its astringent and antiseptic actions helps heal mouth ulcers. In fact many herbs, from mint to cloves, have antiseptic or antibiotic actions. Not only culinary herbs but many food plants too are potential healing agents. Oats, for example, calm the nervous system; carrots aid the function of the liver; rice water is rich in vitamin B and commonly used to treat vomiting with diarrhoea. Dietary healing is a major part of the herbalist's practice, with special diets being recommended for many illnesses – from colds to arthritis.

Herb (leaves)	Constituent	Amount per 100 g
Chicory	Potassium	180 mg
	Folic acid	50 mg
Comfrey (avoid over-consumption, see p. 33)	Protein	35%
	Vitamin A	Quantities unknown
	Vitamin B12	Quantities unknown
Dandelion	Vitamin A	14,000 IU
Kelp	Calcium	1 g
	Iron	Quantities unknown
	Iodine	
	Vitamin B1	
	Vitamin B2	
	Vitamin B12	
Mustard Greens	Vitamin A	7000 IU
	Vitamin B2	0.22 mg
	Vitamin C	95 mg
Nettle	Calcium	Quantities
	Iron	unknown
	Vitamin A	
	Vitamin C	
Parsley	Calcium	330 mg
	Copper	0.5 mg
	Iron	8 mg
	Potassium	1080 mg
	Vitamin A	1165 IU
	Vitamin C	150 mg
Watercress (use only commercially grown plants, see p. 53)	Calcium	220 mg
	Folic acid	200 mg
	Vitamin A	4900 IU
	Vitamin B2	0.16 mg
	Vitamin C	80 mg

Chicory

Comfrey

Dandelion

Kelp

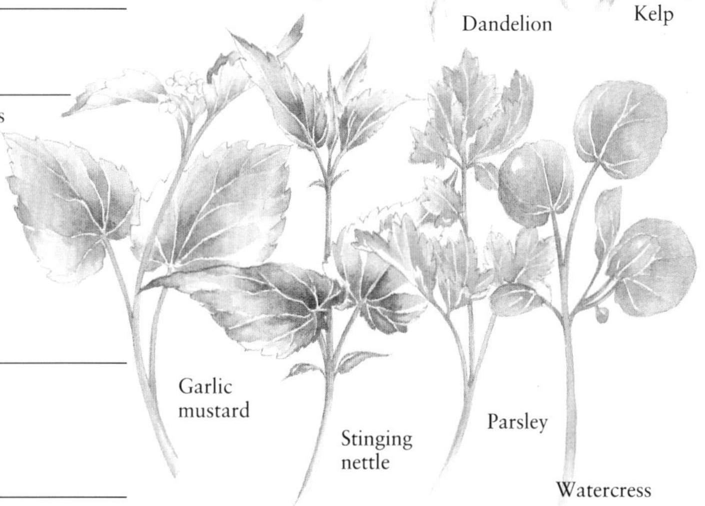

Garlic mustard

Stinging nettle

Parsley

Watercress

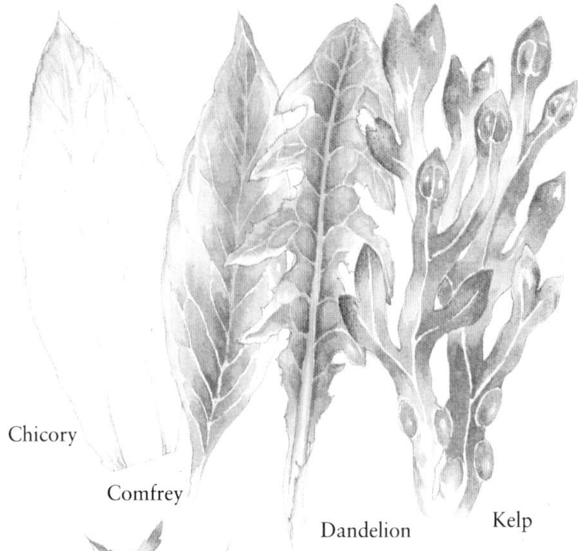

Herb (fruit)	Constituent	Amount per 100 g
Elderberries	Vitamin A	600 IU
	Vitamin C	35 mg
Peppers (capsicum)	Vitamin C	130 mg
	Folic acid	10 mg
Raspberries	Calcium	41 mg
	Vitamin C	25 mg
Rosehips	Vitamin C	295 mg
Sunflower seeds	Vitamin B1	2 mg
	Vitamin B3	5.5 mg
	Vitamin B6	1 mg

Elderberries

Sunflower seeds

Green pepper

Rose hips

Herb (root)	Constituent	Amount per 100 g
Garlic	Potassium	530 mg
	Vitamin C	15 mg

Garlic

Ginger root

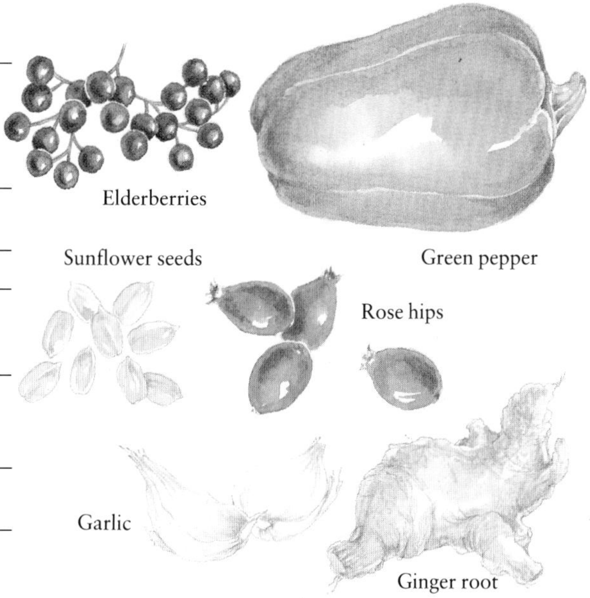

Which diet?

The diverse cultural regions of the world have evolved a huge range of cuisines, each with its own philosophy and its own claim to be the healthiest. From China to Italy, however, common basic principles apply: they are based on a staple carbohydrate food such as rice or wheat, with the judicious addition of green vegetables and fruits and oils; many make a fairly low use of meat, fish, or eggs, as elements of recipes or feast menus; and they rely on the expert use of herbs and spices to please the palate, aid digestion, and balance and vary the diet. In affluent western society, by contrast, meat, fish, and eggs dominate the diet, not wholefoods and carbohydrates – we eat too much, and in the wrong proportions. And even though there is a bewildering range of health diets put forward, the knowledge of herbs and spices that makes these healthier regimes palatable and digestible is often sadly lacking. Some of these diets are discussed opposite, with the appropriate herbs and spices.

Natural diets

Many people now believe that, in view of the diversity of plant foods, and since meat is not necessary for nutrition while its saturated fats are harmful in excess, we would do better to eat a vegetarian diet. And the implications of vegetarianism go far beyond personal health. Producing plant proteins for human consumption, rather than feeding them to animals that are subsequently fed to us, is a more efficient use of the earth's already overstretched resources. There are obvious humanitarian reasons too for boycotting foods from the abattoir or the factory farm. As well as true vegetarians there are also many who restrict their meat intake considerably. Herbs are a delight to largely vegetarian eaters – eaten fresh in salads, used to flavour stocks and the blander rice or legume dishes, or lavishly and creatively combined in "green cuisine".

Meat is a vexed question, but whatever diet you choose there are basic guidelines for health. First and foremost, eat foods as near to their natural state as possible – whole, fresh, raw or lightly cooked, and free from additives. Such foods have higher nutritional value, greater energy or *chi*, and retain the fibre which helps keep the digestive system healthy. The exquisite flavour of freshly picked, naturally grown herbs can help to counteract the bulkiness of wholefood diets and aid digestion.

The second basic rule of a good diet is not to eat too much of foods which stress your system – saturated fats in meat, eggs, butter, cream and cheese, and coffee, tea, sugar and salt. The olive, corn, sunflower, and many other plants provide oils which can replace saturated fats; herbs can happily flavour dishes in place of salt, and provide refreshing tisanes in place of tea or coffee; fruit is nicer and healthier than sugar. Finally, don't eat too much, and never eat when you are full.

High-fibre diet

Unrefined foods such as whole grains, vegetables, and fruit, make up the bulk of the high-fibre diet. Cutting out processed foods means a reduced intake of sugar and saturated fats. Use herbs and spices liberally to flavour high-fibre legume dishes, and avoid flatulence! Mix fresh herbs such as dandelions, coriander, and nasturtium leaves with raw vegetables to make unusual salads. You can also include lean meat and fish, using herbs to bring out their full flavour. Your health will benefit from the low fat, high vitamin and mineral content of this diet.

Typical daily diet

Breakfast
Home-made, sugar-free granola with dried fruit

Lunch
Baked potato with low fat cottage cheese and chives and parsley
Crunchy coleslaw

Dinner
Chilli con carne with garlic and peppers, brown rice, green salad with fresh herbs
Fresh fruit

Drinks
Vegetable juices (such as carrot juice)
Whole fruit juices

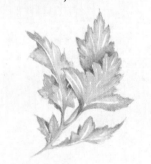

Coriander leaves

Naturopathic health diet

This diet is safe for anyone wishing to improve their general health. It focuses on fresh fruit, vegetables, and raw salads. You should eat food as near as possible to its natural state, using fresh herbs for flavour, extra vitamin content and digestive benefits. Intake of animal fats, salt, and sugar is low, but fish is permitted. The diet builds energy, cleanses the system, and eases constipation. Nuts, seeds, and yoghurt make healthy garnishes for salads. Herbal teas such as peppermint and chamomile are natural alternatives to coffee, strong tea, and alcohol.

Typical daily diet

Breakfast
Fresh fruit salad with
   wheatgerm and yoghurt

Lunch
Peppers stuffed with walnuts,
   breadcrumbs, and mushrooms
Tomato and basil salad

Dinner
Poached salmon with sorrel
   sauce and lightly steamed
   vegetables
Tofu desert

Drinks
Fruit juices
Herbal teas
Cereal coffee substitute

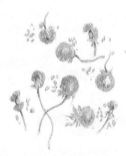

Dried chamomile flowers

South Indian diet

Spices such as turmeric, cloves, cinnamon, pepper, ginger, and coriander have been used for centuries in India to preserve food. This has always been necessary in a climate of baking summer temperatures and intense humidity. Seasonings of fresh and dried herbs also enrich simple vegetable dishes in a country where many people cannot afford meat, or avoid it for religious reasons. Fennel and cardamoms aid digestion while fresh coriander is rich in vitamin A. Paans, made of mixed herbs, such as cardamoms, cloves, fennel, aniseed, and betel, round off a meal.

Typical daily diet

Breakfast
Fresh mango, rice cakes with
   mustard seed, yoghurt

Lunch
Chapatis and spiced dahl
Samosas
Gujerati carrot salad

Dinner
Tandoori chicken with rice
Spiced spinach with ginger and
   coriander
Creamed almonds with saffron
   and cardamom

Drinks
Lassi (yoghurt drink)
Fresh lime soda with mint

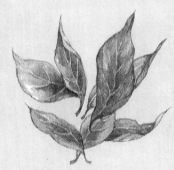

Curry plant leaves

Macrobiotic diet

The philosophy behind macrobiotics is the balancing of yin and yang foods, which are opposite in nature but complementary. Yin foods, generally cooling, tend to grow above ground in spring and summer, and be aromatic; yang foods, generally warming, tend to ripen later, often below ground, and be less aromatic. Brown rice is the purest, most balanced food and whole cereal grains usually make up a large proportion of the diet. Herbs are usually yin foods, and chives, parsley, ginger and mustard are used liberally. Strong, salty flavours are yang.

Typical daily diet

Breakfast
Scrambled tofu, or rolled oat
   porridge

Lunch
Poached white fish with shoyu
   and ginger
Brown rice
Cucumber and seaweed salad
Stewed fresh apple

Dinner
Miso soup
Sourdough bread
Rice with roasted pumpkin seeds
   and steamed green vegetables

Drinks
Twig or stem tea; mu tea
Apple or vegetable juices

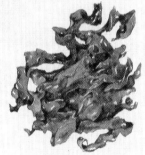

Dulse

Ways to use herbs and spices

If you are a beginner you should use herbs and spices with care. Each has its own subtle and individual flavour, its own favourite companion food, and you should add only one kind at a time to a dish until you discover how they can enhance, rather than overwhelm, the natural flavour of the food. Another convenient way to begin is to use a well known culinary mixture such as bouquet garni (see below), fines herbes, or herbes de Provence. Bouquet garni uses whole herb sprigs while the others combine the leaves only. Such mixtures release a rounded flavour into a dish. Spice mixtures often reflect the flavour of a region – garam masala, for instance, is unmistakeably Indian in flavour (see opposite). Chilli powder, with its pungent blend of hot spices, is distinctly Mexican. You create a characteristic Chinese aroma when you combine certain ground spices to make five-spice powder (see opposite page). Spices are also useful to help combine flavours: sweet and savoury combinations, such as meat and fruit, marry more successfully through the introduction of spices.

Once you are familiar with the particular properties of each, you can combine two or three herbs or spices together yourself in harmonious variations. There are a huge number of ways to use culinary herbs and spices, fresh or dried, whole or ground, and a surprising range of foods you can try them in if you are enterprising. Some of these ways are explored here and on the following pages, providing an aromatic and varied cuisine.

Using fresh herbs

Certain herbs have classic associations with particular foods – basil, for instance, is well known as "the tomato herb"; fennel is paired with fish; rosemary goes with lamb. There are also special combinations of herbs that go well together. The classic mixture of fresh herbs, fines herbes, contains parsley, chives, chervil and tarragon, and goes particulary well with eggs. Another well known combination is bouquet garni (see below). You can adapt it to suit the food you are preparing, for example adding a sprig of fennel if you are cooking fish. But herbs are versatile, and there are many combinations with which you can experiment.

There are also innumerable ways to bring out the flavour of herbs. Use them in marinades for meat, poultry, and fish – this both flavours and preserves the food, and you can use the

Bouquet garni
There are many variations of this classic seasoning mixture. Here is the basic recipe:

2 sprigs thyme
2 sprigs marjoram
1 bunch parsley stalks
1 bay leaf

Tie the herbs together with some string or thread.

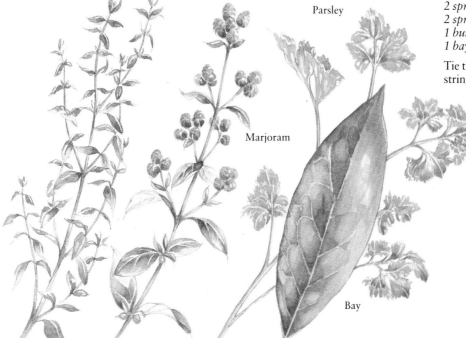

Thyme

Parsley

Marjoram

Bay

Fines herbes
Combine 4 tablespoons of fresh parsley, 2 tablespoons each of chives and chervil, and 2 teaspoons of tarragon. Use immediately.

marinade to make delicious sauces once you have removed the meat or fish. For eggs, try adding herbs to the water in which they are boiled – the eggs will absorb the flavour through the shells. Steeping herbs in vinegar is a highly effective way to bring out their flavour too. Try, also, adding flowers such as rose petals, violets, or elderflowers to vinegars, for a lighter, delicate flavour. Use herb vinegars in salad dressings, soups, and marinades (see p. 180–1). Another useful way to make use of herb flavours is to add fresh herbs to mayonnaise (see p. 178–9). Add garlic and you've made aioli, a classic French mayonnaise which is delicious with fish soup, spread on croutons with cheese. Other classic accompaniments are herb butters, cheeses, and stuffings.

You can use fresh herbs widely as garnishes. Sprinkle them over steamed vegetables – try mint with peas, or ginger with spinach. Best of all, add freshly picked herbs to green salads or fruit salads and fruit cups, lavishly mixing the flavourings – or serve fresh herbs such as mint, coriander, or nasturtium on side dishes with meat or fish. They will help to freshen the palate and aid the digestion.

You can use many herbs in delicious desserts, sorbets, and ice creams, and even make herbal milkshakes by whisking elderflower, lemon balm, or sweet cicely into milk which has already been flavoured with raspberry, strawberry, or honey. You can use some herbs, like lady's bedstraw, instead of rennet to curdle milk when making cheese. This is of particular use to vegetarians.

Preparing fresh herbs
Chop your fresh herbs on a wooden board with a heavy, sharp, kitchen knife. The most popular types designed specially for cutting herbs are the hachoir (with a small blade and central handle), and the mezzaluna (with two handles).

Using whole spices
Spices, defined in culinary terms as the dried seeds of certain plants, have been used for centuries in many cuisines. Indispensable in hot, humid climates for their preservative properties, spices add welcome flavour and colour to many foods.

You can use large, whole spices, such as cinnamon, vanilla, and allspice berries, in stocks, soups, and vinegars. Strain the liquid after cooking for a clear result. Leave smaller whole spices, such as dill, cumin, caraway, and fennel, in the dish when it is cooked.

Many recipes call for ground or grated spices. The process of grinding helps to release the flavour and also allows you to mix the spices thoroughly into the food you are preparing. It is worth buying whole such spices as cardamom, coriander, allspice, juniper, nutmeg, and pepper, so that you can grind or grate them as necessary. Cinnamon, mace, chillies, cloves, cumin, ginger, mustard, and turmeric can be difficult to grind at home so keep them ground in dark, airtight jars. Choose peppermills to grind round, hard spices like peppercorns, allspice, and mustard seeds or, for a coarser texture, a pestle and mortar. The latter is useful for softer-textured spices such as juniper berries. You can grate nutmegs on the fine section of a kitchen grater.

Add ground spices to casseroles, stews, sauces, chutneys, cakes, and biscuits. Make use of mild, not hot, paprika and cayenne to garnish dishes such as humus and dips. Commercially packaged spice mixtures like curry powder are convenient, but it is well worth your while to assemble and grind your own mixtures at home – you will taste the difference. A good curry powder consists of equal quantites of coriander, turmeric, ginger, pepper, black mustard, cloves, and fennel, ground together finely with one or two dried chillies (to taste). For Chinese dishes, grind together a five-spice mixture of aniseed, szechuan pepper, fennel seeds, cloves, and cinnamon.

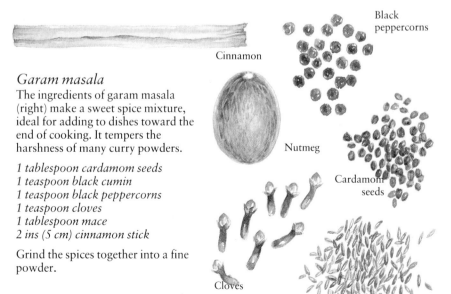

Garam masala
The ingredients of garam masala (right) make a sweet spice mixture, ideal for adding to dishes toward the end of cooking. It tempers the harshness of many curry powders.

1 tablespoon cardamom seeds
1 teaspoon black cumin
1 teaspoon black peppercorns
1 teaspoon cloves
1 tablespoon mace
2 ins (5 cm) cinnamon stick

Grind the spices together into a fine powder.

Cinnamon

Black peppercorns

Nutmeg

Cardamom seeds

Cloves

Cumin

Herb salads

Spring salads have always been an important source of nutrition, and herbs can give your salads extra goodness as well as flavour. Many large-leaved plants, such as dandelions and nasturtiums, make excellent salad vegetables, while many other herbs can provide variety. You can also use flowers in salads, to add different colours, textures, and flavours from soft, velvety pansies to strong-flavoured lavender.

Greens and garnishes

Some familiar salad vegetables, such as watercress and fennel (*Foeniculum vulgare*), are also known as herbs because of their healing properties. These plants are valuable nutritionally too: fennel is good for the digestion, while watercress is a rich source of vitamins and minerals. Amongst the other traditional salad vegetables, spinach is a good source of iron and vitamin A.

Your herb garden can offer a variety of nutritious salad greens. Dandelion leaves are an excellent source of vitamins, iron, and other minerals. They taste slightly bitter, but if you blanch the leaves some of this bitterness will be removed. Many herbs taste similar to other ingredients used in salads or dressings: use them as substitutes or to reinforce a particular flavour. For a refreshing lemon taste, use lemon verbena or lemon balm leaves; summer and winter savory have a peppery flavour; salad burnet leaves (*Pimpinella saxifraga*) have a taste reminiscent of cucumber; the stems and leaves of lovage are similar to celery (avoid lovage in pregnancy or if you have kidney disease).

Try using stronger tasting herbs in smaller quantities as a garnish for salads, especially if you are limited to using traditional salad greens such as lettuce and watercress. Rosemary has a particularly powerful taste, so use it sparingly; parsley provides a nutritious garnish; mint is used in many Mediterranean and Middle Eastern salad recipes; fresh coriander leaf is often served with Indian foods. A garnish of chives provides a gentler alternative to onions.

Flowers

One way to increase the visual appeal of your salads is to include flower petals. Few of these have much direct nutritional value, but they will make any food in which they are included look more appetizing. Marigold petals have a subtle but peppery flavour, much less strong than that of nasturtiums. Of the scented flowers, you can add rose, lavender, and violet petals to salads. Rose petals have a gentle, sweet flavour, violets are also sweet but slightly spicey, and lavender is very strong – you should use it in moderation. Pansies are valued mainly for their texture, while borage flowers have a delicious cucumber-like taste similar to the leaves of the plant. Woodruff flower sprigs are pretty, and if lightly warmed, give off their refreshing vanilla-like scent.

Dandelion salad

This is a healthy, spring-time salad. Watercress and dandelions can either be called vegetables or herbs. Either way, they are rich in vitamins and iron, and have been eaten for many centuries as spring-time blood cleansers.

1 small lettuce
3 oz (90 g) watercress
4 oz (120 g) radishes
2 oz (60 g) young dandelion leaves
4 spring onions
4 tablespoons chopped parsley
Freshly ground black pepper
4 oz (120 g) seaweed (optional)
2 tablespoons olive oil
2 tablespoons cider vinegar

Shred the lettuce, chop the watercress, slice the radishes and chop the dandelion leaves and spring onions. Mix them together in a salad bowl, seasoning with the pepper.

Chop the seaweed. Heat the oil in a frying pan on a medium heat. Put in the seaweed and cook it, stirring frequently until it browns. Take the pan from the heat and swirl in the vinegar.

Spoon the contents of the pan over the salad. Toss them into the vegetables and serve immediately.

Chinese cabbage salad

All sprouted beans and seeds have a high vitamin and mineral content. The smaller types can be sprinkled into soups and casseroles as garnishes, the larger ones stir-fried or added to salads as a vegetable.

1/2 large Chinese cabbage
4 oz (125 g) bean sprouts
1 tablespoon tahini (sesame paste)
3 tablespoons sesame oil
2 tablespoons cider vinegar
1 tablespoon tamari sauce
1 tablespoon tomato purée
2 tablespoons sesame seeds

Shred the cabbage and put it into a bowl with the bean sprouts.

Put the tahini into a small bowl and gradually beat in the sesame oil and then the vinegar, tamari sauce, and tomato purée. Fold the resulting dressing into the salad.

Put the sesame seeds into a heavy frying pan with no fat. Set them on a medium heat and stir until they brown. Turn them on to a plate to cool before sprinkling them over the salad.

Rice salad with marigolds

Marigold petals add a delicate flavour and attractive appearance to many different types of summer salads. Serve this rice salad with cold vegetarian dishes.

8 oz (225 g) long grain brown rice
1 pt (575 ml) water
1/2 teaspoon sea salt
1/2 teaspoon ground turmeric
2 lb (900 g) fresh green peas
   (unshelled weight)
1 mint sprig
4 fl oz (125 ml) buttermilk
4 tablespoons olive oil
2 tablespoons chopped mint
Petals from 4 marigold heads

Put the rice into a saucepan with the water, salt, and turmeric. Bring it gently to the boil. Cover and simmer for 40 mins, or until the rice is tender and all the water has been absorbed. Drain the rice, run cold water through it and drain it again.

Shell the peas. Steam them, with the mint sprig, for 15 mins, turning them once during cooking. Mix the peas with the rice.

Beat together the buttermilk and olive oil to make the dressing. Fold it into the rice and peas while they are still warm.

Leave the salad until it is completely cold. Just before serving, fold in the chopped mint and the marigold petals, reserving a few petals to scatter on top.

Persian wheat salad

This is an old recipe made by travellers on the silk route. Most of the ingredients could have been gathered on the way and made up so that the dish would have been ready to eat. At the end of the day, the salad was eaten on fresh grape vine leaves.

3 oz (90 g) bulgar wheat
2 spring onions, finely chopped
3 oz (90 g) chopped fresh parsley
1 1/2 oz (45 g) chopped fresh mint
5 tablespoons olive oil
Juice of 1 1/2 lemons
6 dried apricots
12 young fresh grape vine leaves

Chop the apricots and soak them in the lemon juice. Soak the bulgar wheat in enough cold water to cover it and leave for 15 mins. Drain the wheat well using a sieve and turn it into a salad bowl. Add the lemon juice and apricots, plus the onions, parsley, mint, oil, and seasoning to taste and leave the salad to stand for 2 hours. Serve by spooning the salad on to the vine leaves. Roll up the vine leaves to eat.

Warm chick-pea salad

You can eat this salad while it is warm, adding black olives or chopped hard-boiled eggs. Alternatively, leave it to cool, when the chick peas will have absorbed all the flavours.

8 oz (225 g) chick peas
3 fl oz (90 ml) olive oil
3 cloves of garlic, crushed
2 bay leaves
1 sprig rosemary
1 teaspoon oregano
Juice of 1 lemon
1 small red onion, finely sliced

Soak the chick peas in boiling water for 2 hours and then drain. Place them in a pan with half the olive oil and top up with water so that the peas are just covered. Add the garlic, bay leaves, and rosemary and fast

boil for 10 mins. Then simmer for 2 hours or until the chick peas are tender. Drain away the water while the chick peas are still hot and add the rest of the ingredients. Season to taste and serve on a bed of lettuce.

Spicy eggplant salad

This salad has a delicious blend of hot and spicy and sweet and sour tastes. The yoghurt helps to mellow the spices. Sprinkling with salt stops the eggplants absorbing too much oil.

1 lb (550 g) eggplant
Juice of 1/2 lemon
Salt
3 tablespoons oil
1 teaspoon sesame oil
1 oz (30 g) ginger root, finely grated
1 clove of garlic, finely chopped
1/4 teaspoon five-spice powder
2 spring onions, finely chopped
2 chillies (optional)
1/2 teaspoon sugar
4 fl oz (120 ml) water
1 tablespoon rice vinegar
2 tablespoons Chinese rice wine
5 fl oz (155 ml) thick Greek yoghurt
1 tablespoon chopped chives
1 pinch of cayenne pepper

Cut the eggplant into 3/4 in (2 cm) cubes and mix with the lemon juice. Put the cubes into a colander, sprinkle with salt, and leave for 30 mins. Then rinse the eggplant cubes in cold water and drain them. Heat the two oils and sauté the eggplant for 3 to 4 mins, stirring once or twice; remove from the pan and drain off the oil using a sieve. Put the drained oil back into the pan and fry the ginger, garlic, five-spice powder, spring onions, and chillies for 2 mins on a medium heat. Stir in the sugar, water, vinegar, and rice wine and add the eggplants. Remove from the heat when the eggplants are cooked and the liquid is absorbed. Leave to cool. Stir in the yoghurt. Garnish with the chives and cayenne pepper.

Main meals with herbs

The recipes on the following pages show the diverse ways in which you can use herbs to flavour and enhance your soups and starters, main dishes, and desserts. Many use herbs as the main ingredient, so that you can make full use of their nutritional properties as well as their flavour. A number also contain suggestions for varying the recipe so that you can include other herbs. If you want to sweeten a dish or bring out its flavour try using a herb or spice rather than sugar or salt. Sweet cicely and cinnamon are particularly useful herbal sweeteners. To cut down the fat content of recipes containing butter or cream, try substituting low-fat margarine or natural low-fat yoghurt.

As well as the many individual herbs that you can use to flavour your food, there are numerous plant-based preparations that are invaluable in the kitchen. You can buy most of these ready-prepared. Many of them are based on soya beans, which have a very high protein content as well as containing vitamins (particularly vitamin A and the B complex) and numerous trace elements. Herbs such as sesame, vanilla, and mustard yield further useful flavourings. Most of these preparations are based on health-giving ingredients and you can use them freely. But some, particularly miso and soya sauce, contain a high proportion of salt, and you should therefore use them sparingly on your food.

Note: servings
The recipes in this section are designed to serve four people, except for drinks and preserves, which are made in larger quantities for storage.

Plant-based flavourings
The chart shows a selection of common plant-based preparations used to flavour food, along with their constituents and common uses. Some, like soya sauce, tamari, miso, and yeast extract are particulary strong-flavoured. Use Dijon mustard if you want a gentler flavour than the hot English varieties.

Flavouring	Ingredients	Uses
Miso	Fermented soya bean paste; the lighter coloured varieties contain less salt	Sauces, soups, stews; as a savoury spread
Soya sauce	Fermented soya beans; rice, barley or wheat; salt; check labels for additives	Oriental dishes; instead of salt
Tamari	Wheat-free soya sauce	As soya sauce; suitable for those on a gluten-free diet
Gomasio	Ground, toasted sesame seeds mixed into powder with salt	Salt substitute; low sodium
Tahini	Ground sesame seeds made into paste; dark or light varieties available; salt added	Middle Eastern dishes; added to hummus; sauces, salad dressings; as a savoury spread
Yeast extract	Yeast; high in B vitamins and salt	As a savoury spread; soups, stews; use sparingly
Mustards	Mustard seeds; French varieties often contain vinegar, spices, and herbs such as tarragon	Sauces, marinades, dressings, mayonnaise, with meats
Vanilla essence	Distilled from vanilla pods	Sweet dishes, custards, fruits, ice-cream, and confectionery
Pesto	Fresh basil, olive oil, garlic, pine nuts, parmesan cheese, lemon — pounded to a paste	Classic ingredient of Mediterranean cuisine; sauce for pasta; soups, dressing for vegetables and salads

Lovage soup

Lovage gives this soup a clean, slightly sharp taste, not unlike celery and coriander. Avoid lovage if you are pregnant or have kidney disease.

1 tablespoon olive oil
4 slices wholemeal bread
1 bunch of fresh lovage leaves,
    chopped
1 clove garlic, chopped
½ small bunch of parsley, chopped
A little butter or low-fat margarine
2 pt (1200 ml) good chicken stock
2 whole eggs and 1 yolk

Pour the olive oil over the bread and grill until brown. Sauté the lovage, garlic, and parsley in butter until wilted. Pour on the stock and simmer for 2 mins. Beat the eggs with the salt and pepper. Place one slice of bread in each warmed bowl. Bring the soup to the boil and slowly pour in the egg, stirring gently with a wooden spoon, so that it separates into strands. Pour the soup over the bread and serve.

Variation As an alternative, try replacing lovage with basil, adding 2 oz (60 g) parmesan cheese to the beaten eggs. Or try using spinach, sorrel, or nettle, simmered for an extra 3 mins.

Sorrel soup

Garden sorrel (*Rumex scutatus*) gives this soup a pleasant, lemony taste. It makes a good, substantial winter starter.

1 small onion, chopped
2 cloves of garlic, chopped and
    crushed
2 bunches of finely shredded fresh
    sorrel, stems removed
A little butter or low-fat margarine
Nutmeg, to taste
2 medium potatoes, chopped
2 pt (1200 ml) good light stock
Salt and pepper to taste
½ small 5 oz (150 g) tub low-fat
    yoghurt

Parboil the sorrel and then sauté it lightly with the onion, garlic, and nutmeg. Add the potatoes, stock, and seasoning. When the potatoes are cooked, put the mixture into a blender and purée until smooth. Return the soup to the pan and heat it through. Pour into a hot tureen, add the yoghurt, and serve.

Lemon mushrooms

Lemon juice helps to enhance the sharp flavour of the lemon balm, fennel, and dill. This makes a good starter, served with lemon wedges and french bread.

½ oz (15 g) each fresh parsley and
    lemon balm, chopped
¼ oz (7.5 g) each dill, fennel, and
    lemon thyme, chopped
2 spring onions, finely chopped
Salt and plenty of black pepper
1 teaspoon lemon juice
2 oz (60 g) butter
16 large flat or cap mushrooms
2 oz (60 g) white bread crumbs
2 oz (60 g) parmesan cheese

Heat the oven to 350 °F (180 °C or gas mark 4) or pre-heat the grill. Mix the herbs, spring onions, seasoning and lemon juice, with the butter. De-stalk the mushrooms and spread herb butter on each. Sprinkle some breadcrumbs and parmesan on each and bake or grill for 10–15 mins.

Curry spiced mushrooms

Serve with bread and lemon wedges.

1 clove of garlic, finely chopped
2 tablespoons chopped coriander
½ teaspoon each ground coriander,
    cumin, fenugreek, paprika
A little each ground chilli, mixed
    spice, black pepper, turmeric
2 oz (60 g) butter
16 large flat or cap mushrooms

Mix all the ingredients together and follow the method above.

Six-herb soufflé

This makes an excellent lunch or supper dish, or you can serve it as a starter. Never open the oven door during cooking.

5 eggs, separated
5 yolks
8 oz (225 g) grated cheddar cheese
1oz (30 g) grated parmesan
2 oz (60 g) butter
2 oz (60 g) plain flour
½ pt (300 ml) milk
½ oz (15 g) each of fresh dill, mint,
    basil, french parsley, chives
2 sage leaves, finely chopped

Pre-heat the oven to 350 °F (180 °C or gas mark 4). Lightly butter a 2 ½ pint (50 fl oz) soufflé dish. Melt the butter in a pan, stir in the flour to form a ball, and beat for 1 min. Lower the heat. Slowly stir in the milk with a wooden spoon, beating out any lumps. Remove from the heat. Stir in the cheeses. Cool for a few minutes, then beat in the egg yolks until the sauce is smooth and glossy. Add the herbs and season. Whip the egg whites until very stiff, fold one-third into the mixture with a metal spoon, then fold in the rest. Pour into the greased soufflé dish, making sure the dish is only two-thirds full. Bake for 15 mins until puffed and golden. Take to the table and serve immediately.

Variation To make an individual soufflé dish, use an onion. Peel one large onion per person and cut the base so that it will not fall over. Cut ⅓ off the top and use a small knife to cut away the inner layers. Part cook the onion shell in boiling water for 3 mins, drain, and leave to dry. Butter the inside, fill with the soufflé mixture, and bake.

Wild plants as food

Among the seductive shelves of a modern supermarket's fruit and vegetable section, it is easy to forget that many of these clean, bright, bountiful and sometimes exotic varieties are, somewhere, somebody's naturally occurring weeds. Every vegetable food we know was once a wild plant, even if most of them have been "improved" out of all recognition: the most gothic marrows all derive from a modest American pumpkin; modern strawberries have ancestors in three different continents; and as for garlic, it has been cultivated and modified for so long it is impossible to disentangle which wild species was its true forbear. In the developing countries of the Third World wild green plants are still valuable in supplying trace elements, variety, and extra vitamins in the diet. Palms (for seeds, edible oils, and sago) and seaweeds (for salads, cooked vegetables, and soups) are two important groups still harvested from the wild.

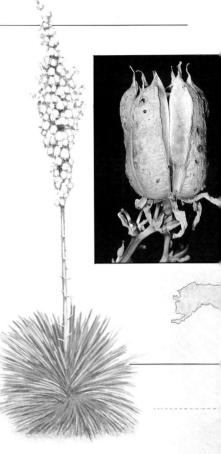

In temperate zones, too, unimproved wild plants and species that have never been cultivated are harvested in their season: fungi in Russia and eastern Europe, wild fruit in central France, spring green herbs in Italy. And in the last 20 years foraging for wild foods has become popular in industrialized areas of America and Europe. This may in part be a fashionable fad for primitivism but, in part too, it is a deep-rooted inquisitiveness about what wild food was like before being adapted, adulterated, and tailored to modern expectations.

Foraging has yielded some surprising results, both in the unexpected flavours revealed and in the nutritional constituents which wild vegetables have proved to have retained. At 14,000 IU per 100 mg, dandelion leaves have nearly twice as much Vitamin A as spinach (8,100 IU per 100 mg), the prime source among conventional vegetables. Blackberries are rich in dietary fibre, rosehips in Vitamin C.

Wild vegetables usually have subtle genetic qualities that tend to be bred out during cultivation: in general they are more resistant to disease and resilient to climate; they often have longer flowering and cropping seasons; they are always more varied in almost all characteristics. As cultivars become more specialized and pampered, plant breeders increasingly need to go back to wild sources for new genetic stock. Small yellow tomatoes from South America have recently been brought back into the breeding line to restore taste and nutritional quality while resistance to wilt is obtained from the wild Peruvian tomato. Wild artichokes from the Middle East have been brought in to provide varieties of a height which will facilitate mechanical harvesting. Work is underway on wild cabbages to exploit their resistance to pests.

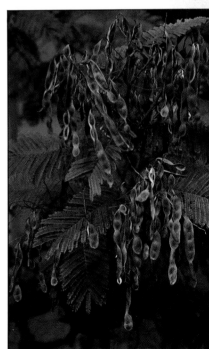

The potential value of wild plants to humans, whether eaten direct, or as animal fodder, or used in the strengthening of cultivated crops, may best be appreciated when it is realized that 95 per cent of our global nutritional requirements are presently derived from only 30 basic plant kinds and a full three-quarters of our diet is based on only eight crops.

Yucca

Yuccas (Yucca spp.) like other desert plants, dispense with seasonal regularity: when rainfall creates the right conditions they flower and leaves sprout. When the rain stops the leaves fall – maybe to wait a decade to reappear. The petals of the white flowers and the ripe pulp of the oblong fruits are edible raw or cooked.

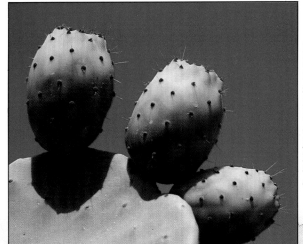

Prickly pear

Prickly pears (Opuntia spp) have been introduced to many arid areas. In Australia they took over 24 million hectares and had to be eradicated. The peeled fruits are edible raw; the young leaves are cooked; seeds are roasted for flour; and stems contain water.

Date palm

The date palm (Phoenix dactylifera), has the most illustrious history of all the palms. Over 800 uses have been recorded. The young leaves are edible cooked and the fruits raw, and sap from the trunk is rich in sugar when boiled down.

Acacia

Acacias (Acacia spp.) occur abundantly from Africa to northern Australia. Their tolerance of arid conditions makes them useful in savannahs and desert scrub where they restore fertility to the soil. Their young leaves and shoots may be boiled, their seeds roasted, and their roots tapped for water.

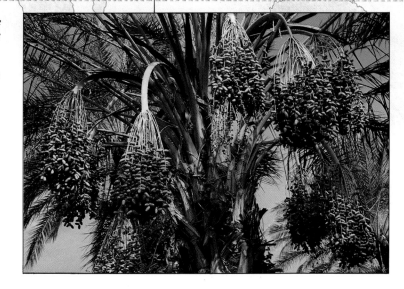

Mackerel with fennel

Both the fennel and the orange juice in this dish help to counteract the oiliness of the fish, while the mint adds a clean, sharp taste.

8 fillets of mackerel
2 heads fennel
Juice and rind of 1 orange
1 orange peeled and sliced
1 tablespoon fresh oregano
1 glass white wine or lime juice
Salt and pepper
1 tablespoon chopped fresh mint

Halve the fennel lengthways and simmer in salted water for 10 mins. Slice ½ in (1 cm) thick. Grate the rind of the orange. Remove any bones from the fish. Arrange alternate layers of mackerel, fennel, and orange in an oven-proof dish. Add the white wine and orange juice. Sprinkle on the orange rind, oregano, salt, and pepper, and bake in a hot oven 350 °F (180 °C or gas mark 4) for 15–20 mins. Remove the fish to a hot dish and reduce the remaining sauce in a pan. Correct the seasoning, pour over the fish and garnish with chopped mint.

Salmon baked in salt and blackcurrant leaves

The salt crystallizes and seals in the flavour of the fish. This dish is particularly good with a tossed green salad.

1 small salmon
large blackcurrant leaves to wrap fish
1 kg (2 lb) coarse sea salt
3 oz (90 g) butter
1 bunch watercress
1 bunch chives
1 bunch parsley
1 Romaine lettuce
1 bunch stinging nettles, young leaves
  only
10 leaves sorrel
½ glass dry white wine
8 strands saffron
1 oz (25 g) plain flour

Scale and clean the fish. Remove the main bone but leave on the head. Roughly chop half the herbs and heat for a few minutes in half the butter. Stuff the fish with herbs. Wrap up the fish with the blackcurrant leaves, tucking in any edges that might flap out. Spread ⅓ of the salt on the bottom of a cast iron oven dish, placing the wrapped fish on top. Cover with the remaining salt. Bake at 425 °F (220 °C or gas mark 7) for 15–20 mins.

For the sauce, melt a little butter and lightly toss the rest of the chopped herbs in it. Add ½ glass of dry white wine and 8 strands of saffron. Bring to the boil and thicken with 1 oz (30 g) of plain flour mixed with 1 oz (30 g) butter. Whisk it in a little at a time until thick.

When the fish is cooked, break the salt crust and remove leaves. Serve fish and sauce separately.

Chicken parcels with wild herbs and raspberries

The sharpness of the raspberry stuffing helps to counteract the richness of the sauce.

½ oz (15 g) each fresh
  wild thyme, marjoram, water mint
4 oz (125 g) fresh young raspberry
  leaves, very finely chopped
1 oz (30 g) white bread crumbs
6 oz (175 g) natural low-fat yoghurt
8 oz (225 g) raspberries
Rind and juice of ½ lemon
Pinch nutmeg
1 egg
4 boned chicken breasts
Oil
Butter
1 glass dry white wine
¼ pt (150 ml) chicken stock
Salt and pepper
1 small onion, 1 carrot, and 1 stick
  celery, all roughly chopped
1 bayleaf

Sauté the herbs and raspberry leaves lightly in butter until they wilt, then remove them from the heat. Add the breadcrumbs, 2 oz (50 g) yoghurt, half of the raspberries, and the lemon rind and juice, nutmeg and egg. Bind well to make the stuffing. With a meat hammer, flatten out the breasts. Put them between two sheets of plastic, to avoid making a hole in the flesh. Place a spoonful of the stuffing at one end, roll up the meat, and secure with string or cocktail sticks.

Gently brown the chicken parcels in oil and butter, with the onion, carrot, and celery for about 5 mins. Add the white wine and reduce a little. Add the stock, salt and pepper and simmer for 10–15 mins or until cooked. Be careful not to overcook or the chicken will dry out. Take out the chicken, arrange on a warm serving dish, lift out the vegetables, and if they are firm enough, serve on the side. Reduce the stock. Add the raspberries to the liquid and remove from the heat. Gradually stir in enough low-fat yoghurt to make a smooth sauce. Adjust seasoning.

Variation If you prefer, use 1 large turkey breast: prepare as for chicken, cook for longer and serve sliced.

Elderflower honeycomb mould

This colourful sweet separates naturally into three layers. The concentrated jelly at the bottom of the mould is topped by two lighter layers, like a honeycomb.

Fresh flowers from 2 heads of elder
5 fl oz (¼ pt) elderflower wine
Juice and rind of ½ lemon
¾ pt (450 ml) milk
3 large eggs separated
¾ oz (18 g) gelatine
2 oz (60 g) fine granulated sugar
¼ pt (150 ml) double cream

Warm the milk with the flowers until hot. Strain. Whisk the milk into the egg yolks, gelatine, sugar and cream in a large bowl. Cook in a double boiler, or in a bowl over simmering water, until the mixture thickens slightly to the consistency of thin cream. Add the wine, rind and juice of lemon and cool. Whisk the egg whites until stiff and fold in the custard mixture with a metal spoon. Pour into a slightly wet 1–1½ pt (575–875ml) mould and set in the refrigerator.

Variation For an elderberry mould use the berries from 2 heads of elder instead of elderflowers. Gently simmer in 5 fl oz (¼ pt) orange or lemon juice, strain, sweeten to taste, and add with the rind and juice of lemon as above.

Rose geranium cheesecake
Herbs can make a welcome addition to an uncooked cheesecake. In this example, rose geranium or lemon geranium leaves give a delicious, fresh-tasting flavour, making an ideal summer dessert.

8 oz (225 g) plain, sweet biscuits
3 oz (90 g) butter
8 oz (225 g) cottage cheese
8 oz (225 g) cream cheese
Juice and grated rind of ½ lemon
8 medium rose geranium leaves, chopped
¾ oz (18 g) powdered gelatine
2 tablespoons hot water
1 egg
¼ pt (150 ml) stirred thick yoghurt
3 dessert spoons fine granulated sugar

Put the biscuits in a plastic bag and crush with a rolling pin. Melt the butter in a saucepan, add the crushed biscuits and stir until all the biscuits are coated in butter. Place in the bottom of an 8-ins (23-cm) loose-bottomed cake tin. Pass the cottage cheese through a sieve, then beat the cream cheese and cottage cheese together with the lemon juice and rind, egg yolk, and stirred yoghurt. Add the chopped geranium leaves. Dissolve the gelatine in the water, fold into the mixture and pour over the base. Chill until set.

Variation As an alternative, try flavouring with elderberry juice. Stew 2 heads of berries in 3 tablespoons of water and sugar to taste. Use half the liquid in the cheesecake mixture and set the rest with 1 teaspoon of gelatine to pour over the cheesecake as a topping.

Cooked golden marigold cheesecake
The marigolds give this cooked cheesecake a rich, smooth, delicate flavour. If there are not many petals on each flower head, you may need to add extra petals.

Petals from 4 heads of fresh or 6 tablespoons of dried marigold petals

Base:
2 oz (60 g) margarine
2 oz (60 g) self rising flour
½ teaspoon baking powder
2 oz (60 g) fine granulated sugar
1 egg, beaten
8 strands saffron infused in 2 tablespoons of hot water

Cheesecake:
3 oz (90 g) butter
2 oz (60 g) castor sugar
pinch of cinnamon
zest and juice of ½ lemon
2 eggs, separated
2 oz (60 g) plain flour
12 oz (350 g) cream cheese, softened with ½ pt (300 ml) double cream

Heat the oven to 375 °F (190 °C or gas mark 5). Simmer a small amount of water. Add the petals, leave for a few seconds, and drain. For the base, cream the margarine, mix in the sieved flour and baking powder, then add the sugar, beaten egg, saffron, and liquid. Bake in a greased loose-bottom 8-ins (23-cm) cake tin for ¼ of an hour. Leave to cool in the tin. Meanwhile, for the cheesecake, separate the eggs, cream the butter and sugar, and beat in the egg yolks and infused marigold petals until light and fluffy. Fold in the flour, then the cream cheese mixture, lemon juice, and zest. Whip the egg whites until stiff and fold them in. Pour over the cooled cake in its tin. Bake at 325 °F (170 °C or gas mark 3) for 1 hour 25 mins. When cool remove from the tin and dust with confectioner's sugar.

Elderflower fritters
These unusual sweet fritters make a delicious snack or starter. Try experimenting with the flower heads of other herbs, such as marjoram.

20 fresh elderflower sprigs
1 egg, separated
1 tablespoon water
1 tablespoon oil
Pinch salt
Rind of 1 lemon
3 oz (100 g) flour, sifted
Rind of ½ orange
Castor sugar
Oil for deep frying

Beat the egg yolk with the water, oil, salt, and lemon and orange rind until well blended. Add the sifted flour, and stir. Leave to stand for 1½ hours. Beat the egg whites until they form stiff peaks and with a metal spoon fold them gently into the batter; dip the flower heads into the batter and fry in hot oil until golden brown. Drain on absorbent paper, sprinkle with fine granulated sugar, and serve with lemon wedges.

Variation To make a savoury version, take out the orange rind, add 1 tablespoon of parmesan cheese to the sifted flour, and do not cover with sugar.

Herbs in bases

You can introduce herbs into many dishes by using a base such as butter, cheese, mayonnaise, or flour. You can use less butter and improve its taste by adding herbs. Use a little herb butter with boiled or steamed vegetables, grilled or baked fish and grilled meats. In its softened state, you can use it to top canapés or to make herb bread.

Herbs and cheese have been closely associated for many centuries. Plants such as stinging nettle and lady's bedstraw were used in the Middle Ages as curdling agents when rennet was not available. And when animal products were used in cheesemaking, herbs were often employed to preserve them. Today, herbs are most often used in cheeses for their taste. They are especially good in cream and cottage cheeses, which are often rather bland. There are several ways in which you can flavour cheese with herbs. The simplest is to beat a mixture of finely chopped fresh herbs (to which you can add crushed garlic) into any soft cheese, thinning with a little natural yoghurt.

Using herbs wisely in salad dressings can make a world of difference – adding flavour and nutrition, and making a plain salad more appetizing. You can use a variety of bases for your herb dressing – oil, mayonnaise, or yoghurt. If you purée the mixture, the dressing becomes a smooth, attractive green. By adding herbs to flour you can flavour a variety of dishes.

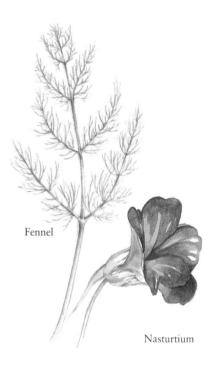

Fennel

Nasturtium

Herb butters

It is very easy to make herb butter by beating chopped, fresh herbs into softened, unsalted butter. You can also add other ingredients, such as crushed garlic, grated lemon or orange rind, a few drops of lemon or orange juice, mustard powder, pepper, or cayenne. And you can vary the taste still further by using one particular herb or a combination. The classic herb butter is the Maître d'Hôtel type, which is flavoured simply with parsley, lemon juice, pepper, and occasionally garlic.

This variation on Maître d'Hôtel butter is excellent with oily fish such as trout or mackerel.

4 oz (125 g) unsalted butter
2 tablespoons chopped parsley
1 tablespoon chopped chives
1/2 tablespoon chopped mint
1/2 teaspoon mustard powder
1 tablespoon lemon juice

Beat the butter to a cream. Beat in the herbs and mustard powder. Add the lemon juice drop by drop, beating well. Place the butter on greaseproof paper and form it into a roll using a flat-bladed knife or small palette knife. Roll the butter up in the paper. Put it into the refrigerator for at least two hours to harden.

To serve, cut the butter into round pats with a sharp knife. If you wish to neaten the edges, stamp the pats into neat rounds using a cookie cutter slightly smaller in diameter than the butter.

Variation You can also use the sweet spices, such as ground cinnamon or nutmeg, to make a spiced butter. Use 4 teaspoons of ground spice per 4 oz (125 g) butter. A little honey or unrefined sugar may also be added. Spread spiced butters on hot toast, scones, tea cakes, fruit loaves and tea breads.

Herb cheeses and dips

One of the classic English cheeses, sage Derby, includes the leaves of sage, and you can improve the taste of many other cheeses by adding herbs. Potted cheeses, made with a grated hard cheese plus a little alcohol, also benefit from the addition of chopped fresh herbs. You can use herbs with a range of other cheeses. Try packing small goats' cheeses, called Crottin, into a jar with oil, herb sprigs, and black peppercorns. Seal and leave them for 2–3 weeks to allow the herb flavour to permeate the cheese.

In the Middle East, a soft cheese made of strained yoghurt is divided into small portions and treated in the same way after first having been rolled in paprika. This is known as labna or labneh. Chopped fresh herbs can also be added to the curds during the cheese-making process itself.

To make herb dips, thin a soft herb cheese with natural yoghurt. A small quantity of lemon juice may be added to taste.

Summer herb cheese

Serve this cheese on tomato or cucumber rings, with toast or crispbreads, or as a sandwich filling.

4 oz (125 g) cottage cheese
2 tablespoons soured cream
1 tablespoon chopped fennel
1 tablespoon chopped lemon balm
2 tablespoons chopped parsley
1 garlic clove, crushed (optional)

Beat the cheese and the cream together. Beat in the herbs.

Serve the cheese as a first course, spooned on tomato or cucumber rings and garnished with nasturtium flowers. The cheese can also be served in small ramekins, again garnished with nasturtium flowers or small fennel leaves, and served with thin, brown toast or crispbreads.

Variation To make a herb cheese dip, add 4 extra tablespoons of soured cream or low-fat yoghurt and serve with small sticks of crisp raw vegetables, as a first course or as part of a buffet.

Herb mayonnaise with tuna

This recipe includes tuna, but you can omit the fish and use the mayonnaise as a dressing for many different foods. It is particularly good with freshly poached or baked fish and also as a coating for a salad of white beans.

Serve as a first course or light lunch or supper.

1 egg yolk
½ teaspoon mustard powder
freshly ground white pepper
4 fl oz (125 ml) sunflower oil
juice of ½ lemon
4 sorrel leaves
2 tablespoons chopped chives
2 tablespoons chopped chervil
2 eggs, hard boiled
one 7 oz (200 g) tin tuna
4 capers

Put the egg yolk into a bowl with the mustard and pepper. Beat them together. Drop by drop, beat in 2 tablespoons of the sunflower oil and then the lemon juice, 1 teaspoon at a time. Gradually beat in the remainder of the oil.

Remove the mid-rib from the sorrel leaves. Put the mayonnaise into a blender or food processor with the sorrel, chives, and chervil. Work them to a smooth, green purée.

Cut each egg in half lengthways. Put each half, cut side down, in the centre of a small plate. Drain and flake the tuna. Surround each egg with a ring of tuna.

Spoon the herb mayonnaise over the eggs only. Top each egg half with a caper.

Herb coating for Cornish hens

A flour coating seasoned with ground dried herbs plus more herbs inside, will gently flavour roasting poultry besides giving a delicious crisp skin.

4 Cornish hens
2 oz (60 g) wholewheat flour
1 teaspoon ground dried thyme
1 teaspoon ground dried marjoram
1 lemon
Freshly ground black pepper
2 teaspoons dried thyme
2 teaspoons dried marjoram
1 egg, beaten
2 oz (60 g) butter

Heat the oven to 400 °F (200 °C or gas mark 6). Put the flour into a bowl. Add the ground herbs and the grated rind of half the lemon and season with the pepper. Toss the mixture.

Truss the chickens, putting ½ teaspoon of each of the dried herbs plus a slice of lemon inside each one. Brush them with the beaten egg and coat them with about three quarters of the flour.

Put the butter into a roasting tin and put it into the oven to melt. Put the chickens into the tin and baste them with the butter. Put them into the oven for 30 mins. Baste again with the butter in the tin and sprinkle a little more flour over them. Return them to the oven for 15 mins, or until they are golden brown with a crisp skin. Baked potatoes and a salad are the best accompaniment.

Berbere

Berbere originated in Ethiopia. It is a fiery spice paste, used for dipping meat and vegetables and for flavouring curries.

1 teaspoon ground ginger
½ teaspon ground cardamom
½ teaspoon ground coriander
½ teaspoon fenugreek seeds
½ nutmeg, freshly grated
¼ teaspoon ground cloves
¼ teaspoon ground cinnamon
¼ teaspoon ground allspice
2 tablespoons finely chopped onions
6 garlic cloves, finely chopped
2 tablespoons fine sea salt
3 tablespoons dry red wine
8 oz (225 g) paprika
2 tablespoons chilli powder
½ teaspoon freshly ground black pepper
12 fl oz (350 ml) water
2 tablespoons peanut oil

Put the ginger, cardamom, coriander, fenugreek, nutmeg, cloves, cinnamon, and allspice into a large, heavy frying pan. Stir them over low heat for 2 mins to heat through. Take them from the heat and cool them for 10 mins. Put them into a blender with the onions, garlic, salt, and wine and work to make a smooth paste.

Mix together the paprika, chilli powder, pepper, and remaining salt. Put them into a frying pan and toast them, stirring, for 2 mins over low heat. Gradually stir in the water and then add the blended mixture. Cook, stirring all the time, over a very low heat, for 15 mins.

Pack the paste into a jar and cool it to room temperature. Pour in the oil to cover the top. Seal tightly.

The berbere can be stored in the refrigerator for up to 6 months.

Herb vinegars and preserves

Herbs or spices suspended in vinegar are eye-catching as well as delicious, and an excellent way of preserving herb flavours. For the best combination of flavour and a preserve that is visually attractive, use both herbs and spices whole.

Flavoured vinegars are the good cook's standby. Mixed with an equal volume of olive or sunflower oil, they make excellent salad dressings. You can also add them to sauces and gravies and use them for pickling and making mustards. Two tablespoons added to a light stock for poaching fish or to the water used for boiling meat will lighten and improve the flavour. You can use almost any herb to make a herb vinegar, but the most popular are garlic, mint, tarragon, thyme, basil, fennel, dill, and rosemary. Spices most frequently used include whole dried chillies, bruised, whole coriander seeds, and dill, fennel, and caraway seeds. You can also use pickling spice, which is based on mustard seeds and includes pepper, cloves, and chillies.

Herbs and spices added to preserves are essential to their keeping qualities and their flavour, whether you are making chutneys, pickles, jellies, or bottled vegetables.

Spice vinegar

Whole spices will keep this vinegar clear and attractive.

One 17.5 fl oz (500 ml) bottle white wine vinegar
6 dried chillies or, 2 tablespoons bruised whole spice, such as coriander

The method is the same as for herb vinegar (below left), but after steeping on the windowsill, strain the vinegar and add no further spices.

Variation For a fast spice vinegar, put the spices and vinegar into a covered heat-proof bowl over a pan of cold water. Bring the water to the boil and take out the bowl. Leave it to cool for about 2 hours, before using the vinegar.

Herb vinegar

Make this vinegar with one of the herbs listed above.

17.5 fl oz (500 ml) bottle white wine vinegar
4 large sprigs of your chosen herb, or, 4 peeled garlic cloves

Pour off a little vinegar from the bottle. Push in two herb sprigs. Top up with the reserved vinegar if necessary. Reseal the bottle. Leave on a sunny windowsill for 2 weeks. Change the herb sprigs for fresh ones.

The vinegar is now ready for use. It is possible to keep herb vinegar in a sealed bottle for up to 2 years.

Variation *Lemon vinegar* Use half a lemon, finely chopped, including the rind and pith.

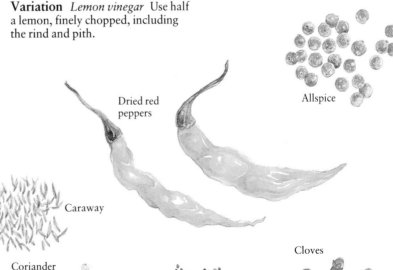

Dried red peppers

Allspice

Caraway

Fennel

Cloves

Dill

Coriander

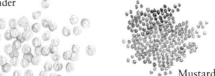

Mustard

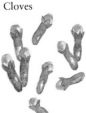

Herb and spice oils

These are ideal for salad dressings, although you can also use them for sautéing and stir-frying. The best herbs to use are basil, dill, fennel, garlic, marjoram, rosemary, and thyme. The most suitable spices are dried chillies, coriander, dill and fennel seed, and mustard seed. Use a good quality mild oil.

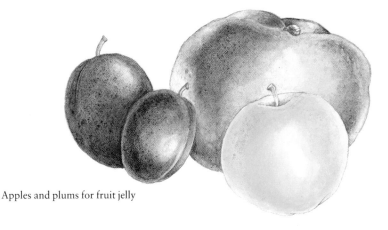

Apples and plums for fruit jelly

Flavoured oil

You can use any of the herbs or spices listed above for this oil.

One 17.5 fl oz (500 ml) bottle olive or sunflower oil
4 herb sprigs
or, 4 garlic cloves
or, 6 whole dried chillies
or, 2 tablespoons whole spices

Pour a little oil from the bottle. Put in two herb sprigs or all the garlic or whole spices. Top up with the reserved oil if necessary. Leave the bottle on a sunny windowsill for 2 weeks. Change the herb sprigs. The spice oil can be strained if wished or the spices may be left in. The oil is now ready for use and should be consumed within three months.

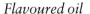

Dill

Sugar-free chutney

Most chutneys and bottled sauces are thick and opaque, with ground spices added in quite large quantities to preserve and flavour them. The long cooking time mellows their flavour further. The following chutney is thick and dark.

1 lb (450 g) cooking apples
1 lb (450 g) pressed dates
8 oz (250 g) onions
3 oz (90 g) raisins
2 oz (60 g) apple butter
1/2 teaspoon sea salt
1/2 teaspoon cayenne pepper
A pinch ground cloves
A pinch ground nutmeg
A pinch ground cinnamon
1/2 pt (290 ml) cider vinegar

Peel, core, and chop the apples. Finely chop the onions and dates. Mix all the ingredients together in a large saucepan or preserving pan.

Bring them slowly to the boil and simmer, uncovered, for about 45 minutes or until the mixture is thick, stirring frequently.

While still warm, put the chutney into warm jars and seal. Leave for 1 month before opening . Fills approximately three 1 lb (450 g) jars.

Mixed fruit and mint jelly

Adding herbs such as mint or thyme to fruit jellies will produce a sweet relish that is good with foods such as cold meats.

2 lb (900 g) dark purple cooking plums
4 lb (1.8 kg) dessert apples
1 lb (450 g) cooking apples
4 lb (1.8 kg) Italian plums
2 pt (1.15 l) water
1 lb (450 g) brown sugar per 1 pt (575 ml) strained liquid
1 1/2 oz (40 g) mint leaves

Halve and stone the plums. Wipe and chop the apples, including the cores. Cut slits round the Italian plums.

Put the fruits into a large saucepan or preserving pan with the water. Bring them to the boil and simmer gently until they are soft, about 1 1/2–2 hours. Skim off as many Italian plum stones as possible during cooking.

Strain everything through a jelly bag and measure the liquid. Return it to the cleaned pan. Weigh out the sugar and warm it in a low oven for 5 mins.

Bring the liquid to the boil. Stir in the sugar and keep stirring until it has dissolved. Boil until setting point is reached. Take the pan from the heat and cool the jelly until it is lukewarm. Stir in the mint, making sure that it is evenly distributed.

Pour the jelly into pots. Cover it with waxed paper circles. Cool it completely and cover it with cellophane circles or lids. Fills approximately three 1 lb (450 g) jars.

Herb drinks

Herbal teas were being drunk long before conventional Indian and China teas came on the scene. They are as simple to prepare as regular teas and have the added benefit of being health-giving. Their main health advantage is that, unlike conventional tea, they do not contain caffeine. Even in the mid eighteenth century, Jonas Hanway claimed that over-indulgence in tea "hurts the nerves and causes various distempers, as tremors, palsies, vapours, fits, etc.", while country doctors recommended the use of balm, sage, and blackberry leaves. Few people followed this advice, but today we are much more aware of the dangers of caffeine in tea and coffee. Herbal teas are widely available from health stores and supermarkets, and you can easily make your own with loose herbs. Chamomile tea is widely drunk for its soothing, calming, and relaxing properties. Other relaxing teas include infusions of bergamot, dill, fennel, marigold, lemon balm, marjoram, or rosemary. Peppermint tea not only acts as a reviving pick-me-up, it is also a refreshing treatment for indigestion. Borage, marjoram, thyme, and sage make excellent tonic teas.

Making herbal wines and beers is a more involved process, but the new combinations of flavours make it worthwhile. You can use herbs either as a basic ingredient in wine-making or as an additive to a ready-made wine or beer, in which case the herbs will improve its flavour, and add health-giving properties. Originally, herbs were added to grape wines during fermentation and vermouth is still made in this way. Spirits can be spiced too; one of the most unusual is ginseng vodka from Korean cuisine. But adding herbs just before drinking, to make a punch or mulled wine, is a much simpler process.

Herb and spice wines

Most of the recipes on the opposite page entail adding herbs to ready-made alcoholic beverages, so no special equipment is required. However, for the lemon balm wine, and beer, you will need buckets with lids, large capacity bottles called demijohns, together with airlocks, straining cloths, a plastic tube for syphoning, and bottles and corks. You can buy everything from a specialist supplier of wine-making equipment. Avoid using iron, copper, zinc, brass, or aluminium utensils to make the drinks, as they will contaminate the wine or beer. Use glass, stainless steel, or enamel instead.

Herbs for wine cups
Herbs such as woodruff and borage make pleasant additions to summer drinks. Wilting the herbs (see right) will enhance the flavour.

Herb teas

Generally you need 2 teaspoons of dried herbs per cup of boiling water. Put them into a teapot. Pour on the boiling water and cover. Covering is important especially if the teas are also to have a medicinal use. It stops valuable properties being carried away by the steam. Leave to brew for 2–3 mins. Strain into a cup. Herb teas may be sweetened with honey to taste.

Early morning herb tea
1 oz (30 g) dried powdered rosehips
1 oz (30 g) dried hibiscus
½ oz (15 g) dried lemon balm
½ oz (15 g) dried peppermint
¼ oz (7 g) dried meadowsweet

Mix and store in a dark, air-tight tin. Make into tea as described, left.

Soothing tea
1 oz (30 g) dried chamomile
½ oz (15 g) dried lime flowers
¼ oz (7 g) dried lemon verbena
¼ oz (7 g) dried rose petals

Mix, store, and infuse as above.

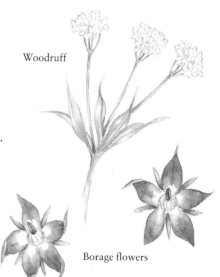

Woodruff

Borage flowers

Hot honey wine punch

Although red wine is most popular for punches, honey wine blends well with sweet spices resulting in an unusual, medium sweet, full-flavoured drink.

1 bottle honey wine
1 pt (575 ml) dry cider
1 pt (575 ml) apple juice
2 oranges
12 cloves
5 ins (12.5 cm) cinnamon stick
2 oz (60 g) honey, or to taste

Put the honey wine, cider and apple juice into a saucepan. Thickly slice the oranges and stick the cloves into the slices. Put them into the saucepan with the cinnamon stick. Stir in the honey. Bring the punch to just below simmering point and hold it there for 20 mins. Serve hot, in warmed mugs or thick glasses.

Summer wine cup

Woodruff gives a gentle, vanilla-like flavour to a wine cup. The fruit tinges it pink and the ginger ale gives a fresh, sparkling appearance. Both woodruff and borage are said to "cheer the heart".

6 fresh woodruff sprigs
1 bottle dry white wine (not too cheap)
½ pt (275 ml) orange juice
4 oz (120 g) strawberries or raspberries
7 fl oz (200 ml) ginger ale
3 fl oz (90 ml) brandy
20 borage flowers

Leave the woodruff sprigs for 1 hour to wilt slightly. This will bring out their vanilla-like flavour. Put them into a bowl and pour on the wine and orange juice. Leave for 1 hour and strain. Quarter the strawberries if they are large. Leave the raspberries whole if using. Put the fruit into a punch bowl. Pour on the strained liquid. Cover with plastic wrap and chill for 30 mins. Chill the ginger ale separately. Pour the brandy and the

ginger ale into the bowl. Float the borage flowers on top. Serve as soon as possible in tall glasses so as not to lose the slightly sparkling effect of the ginger ale.

Lemon balm wine

This is a sweet dessert wine, fragrant and golden.

1 pt (575 ml) lemon balm leaves
2 lb (900 g) raisins
2 ½ lb (1.25 kg) sugar
1 gal (4.5 l) water
Wine yeast (see manufacturer's instructions for amount needed)
Yeast nutrient
1 Sulphite tablet

Finely chop the lemon balm leaves. Chop or mince the raisins. Put the leaves and raisins into a bucket with a lid. Pour on the boiling water. Cover and leave for ten days, stirring every day. Put all the sugar into a second bucket, strain the liquid and pour it over. Add the yeast and yeast nutrient. Cover and leave in a warm place for 2 weeks. Strain the wine, put it into a demijohn, and fit an airlock. Leave until fermentation is complete. Pour into another demijohn, leaving the sediment behind. Add one crushed Sulphite tablet. Leave for one week and then bottle. Leave for at least three months before opening.

Herb beers

Before hops were generally used as the main ingredient in beer, ale was flavoured during its making with locally growing herbs. The same herbs as well as spices were also included in the barrel with the newly made ale to preserve and flavour it and to impart health-giving properties. Costmary, ground-ivy, meadowsweet, agrimony, sage, burdock, and dandelion were some of the many herbs that were used. Most

herb ales were originally thought to carry the health-giving and restorative properties of their flavouring herbs. Burdock ale was thought to cleanse and purify the blood and nettle beer was drunk to ease the pains of gout and rheumatism. In fact, many of the healing constituents are removed during brewing today.

Dandelion and burdock beer

Herb beers and ales like this nettle, dandelion, and burdock bitter are easy to make. They generally have a lighter, more fragrant flavour than ordinary hopped beers and so make ideal summer drinks. They are also more wholesome than ordinary beers, containing only natural ingredients.

1 lb (450 g) young nettles
4 oz (120 g) dandelion leaves
4 oz (120 g) fresh, sliced or 2 oz (60 g) dried burdock root
½ oz (15 g) root ginger, bruised
2 lemons
1 gal (4.6 l) water
1 lb (450 g) plus 4 teaspoons soft brown sugar
1 oz (30 g) cream of tartar
Brewing yeast (see manufacturer's instructions for amount)

Put the nettles, dandelion leaves, burdock, ginger and thinly pared rinds of the lemons into a large pan. Add the water. Bring to the boil and simmer for 30 mins.
  Put the lemon juice, 1 lb (450 g) sugar and the cream of tartar into a large container and pour in the liquid through a strainer, pressing down well on the nettles and other ingredients. Stir to dissolve the sugar. Cool to room temperature.
  Sprinkle in the yeast. Cover the beer and leave it to ferment in a warm place for 3 days. Pour off the beer and bottle it, adding ½ teaspoon brown sugar per pint.
  Leave the bottles undisturbed until the beer is clear – about 1 week.

Herbs in the kitchen

The following charts contain a summary of information about 54 of the most useful and popular culinary herbs and spices. They indicate which parts of the plant are used, whether you should use the herbs fresh or dried and whether the spices are recommended for whole use or ground. They also summarize the types of foods in which you can include each herb or spice. As well as showing the classic combinations (mint with lamb and basil with tomatoes) a variety of other suggestions are shown, including herbs for use with cheeses, sweet sauces and custards, wine cups, pickles, and preserves.

Spice	Uses	Spice	Uses
Allspice Whole or ground	Pickles and preserves; salt meats, fish; sweet cakes; pumpkin pie; hot punches	Ginger Fresh, whole; dried whole or ground	Grated in curries; dried, whole in pickles, mulled drinks; with fruits; in baking; in Oriental dishes
Caraway Whole	Bread, cakes, biscuits; soups, casseroles; cabbage, beetroot; sugar coated to make candy	Juniper Whole, crushed before use	Rich meats, game, and pâtés; with cabbage; avoid if you are pregnant or have kidney disease
Cardamom Whole or ground	Garam masala; legumes; chicken; cakes, biscuits, waffles; coffee or chocolate drinks	Lovage Whole or ground	Ground seed as aromatic substitute for pepper; avoid in pregnancy or kidney disease
Cayenne Ground	Fish, seafood; Middle Eastern and Creole food; eggs; cheeses	Mace Ground	As condiment; flavour can be used widely in sweet and savoury foods (see Nutmeg)
Chillies Whole or ground	Fresh for curries, S American foods; whole dried for pickles; ground in chilli powder, curries	Mustard Whole or ground White or black	Pickling spice; marinades, sautés; baking; seasoned flour; sauces, soups, dressings
Cinnamon Whole quills of bark or ground	Mulled drinks; puddings; sweet baked foods; poached fruit; savoury rice dishes	Nutmeg Freshly ground White or black	Sweet desserts, fruit dishes, sauces; green vegetables; meat loaves; eggs
Cloves Whole or ground	Stocks and poached meats; pot roasts; baked ham; apples; mulled drinks; garam masala	Paprika Ground	Goulashes, soups, legumes; fish and shellfish; curries and Middle Eastern dishes; dressings
Coriander Whole or ground	Garam masala, curries; pickling spice; with olives in oil; ratatouille; rice dishes	Pepper Whole or freshly ground	Whole in pickles, stocks, poached meats and fish; ground in all savoury foods
Cumin Whole	Garam masala; curries; rice and other grains; cheeses; bread, cakes, pastries	Poppy Whole White or "blue"	In curries and sprinkled on the surface of bread and cakes
Dill Whole	Fish; bread; in apple pies and cakes; casseroles and soups; pickles	Saffron Whole	As yellow culinary dye, particularly in rice dishes, cakes, and also in some liqueurs
Fennel Whole or ground	As condiment; in baking; with oily fish; with lentils; seeds as breath freshener	Turmeric Ground	Garam masala, curries; rice, grains; fish; pickles; colouring Indian sweet dishes and drinks

Herb	Uses
Angelica Leaves, stems, roots Fresh	Leaves chopped to flavour fruit desserts and fish, stems and roots candied
Basil Leaves Fresh or dried	In pesto, with tomatoes raw or cooked, widely used in Mediterranean cuisines
Bay Leaves Fresh or dried	In bouquet garni; in soups, stocks, casseroles
Borage Leaves, flowers Fresh	Leaves in wine cups and soups, whole as fritters; flowers in wine cups, salads
Chamomile Flower heads Dried	As tea; in the manufacture of certain beers
Chervil Leaves Fresh	Soups, cassseroles; salads; egg dishes, particularly omelettes
Chicory Leaves, root Fresh or dried	Leaves in salads; root roasted as coffee substitute; root baked as vegetable
Chives Leaves, flowers Fresh	Salads, soups, savoury butters, soft cheeses, egg dishes, grilled meats
Comfrey Leaves Fresh or dried	Fresh leaves as fritters or vegetable; chopped in white sauce; use sparingly, see p. 33
Coriander Leaves Fresh	Salads, garnish for curries, chutneys, oriental sauces
Dill Leaves Fresh or dried	Pickles and vinegars, salads and dressings, soft cheeses, fish
Fennel Leaves, sprigs, stems Fresh	Fish, chicken, pork; stems placed under baking bread or grilling and roasting meats
Garlic Cloves Fresh	Dressings, casseroles, sautés; butters, dips, pâtés; soups; bread mixes
Hops Shoots, flowers Fresh	Young shoots and male flowers in salads; flowers in beer
Horseradish Root Fresh	In sauces and vinegars, especially with beef but also with poultry and fish
Lemon balm Leaves Fresh or dried	Wine cups, herb beers, teas; custards, sweet sauces; fish; mushrooms; soft cheese

Herb	Uses
Lemon verbena Leaves Fresh or dried	As lemon flavouring in cakes and fruit dishes; dried leaves as tea
Licorice Root Dried	As sweetener (mainly in medicines) and in confectionery
Lovage Leaves Fresh	Broths, soups, casseroles; chicken, ham, fish; avoid in pregnancy and kidney disease
Marigold Whole flowers, petals Fresh	Flowers in soups, stews; petals with grains, soft cheese, butter, salads
Marjoram Leaves Fresh or dried	Bouquet garni; widely used in savoury meat and vegetable dishes; desserts; beers
Mint Leaves Fresh or dried	Sauces and relishes; summer vegetables and fruit; teas and drinks
Oregano Leaves Fresh or dried	Widely used in savoury meat and vegetable dishes; stuffings; with pasta dishes
Parsley Leaves Fresh	Garnish for all savoury foods; butters and sauces; salads; bouquet garni
Rosemary Leaves, sprigs Fresh or dried	Lamb, pork, poultry; honey; fruit jellies; fruit juices and wine cups
Sage Leaves, sprigs Fresh or dried	Rich meats, stuffings, sauces, sausages; cheeses; teas, apple juice, hot milk
Salad burnet Small leaves Fresh	Salads, soft cheeses, stuffings; wine cups, cocktails
Savory Leaves Fresh or dried	Beans; cabbage, cauliflower; with flour and crumbs for coating; rich meats; eggs
Sweet cicely Leaves Fresh	For sweetening sour fruits; in salads, butters
Tarragon Leaves, sprigs Fresh or dried	Salads; eggs; chicken, lamb; vinegars; sauces, butters; fish
Thyme Leaves, sprigs Fresh or dried	All savoury dishes; bouquet garni; preserves; lemon and orange types with fruit
Woodruff Leaves, flowers Fresh or dried	As tea; for flavouring in wines and wine cups

CHAPTER FIVE

Herbs for Healing

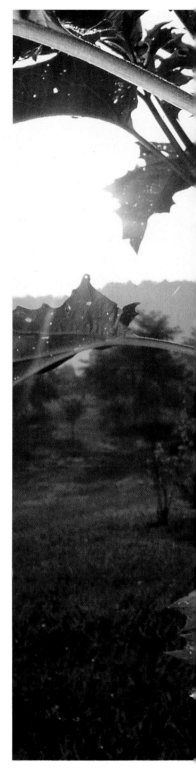

In this chapter we suggest possible herbal treatments for a range of common ailments, categorized according to each of the major systems of the body, such as the cardiovascular, respiratory, and nervous systems. You should use it in conjunction with the Glossary of Herbs (see pp. 26–128) which lists, plant by plant, the major medicinal and culinary herbs of the western herbal tradition, giving a detailed description of each one's constituents, its traditional uses, and its main therapeutic applications. Yet all this wealth of information about individual remedies and how they may be used to treat diseases fails to take account of a vital element – that of the essentially holistic nature of herbal medicine, for it is this that sets it apart from its orthodox counterpart.

The word holism was coined in 1926 by J. C. Smuts, to describe the tendency in nature to produce wholes from ordered groups of units. Herbal medicine is holistic in two ways – firstly, plant medicines are themselves essentially holistic and secondly, herbalists treat people holistically, taking the whole being of the patient into consideration, rather than just prescribing according to a specific disease. Although individual herbs may be evaluated by the chemicals they contain and their known pharmacological action, herbalists know from experience that the whole plant is greater than the sum of its constituent parts. This view is in marked contrast to that of the medical scientist whose aim is invariably to isolate and extract, from the intricate chemistry of the whole plant, a pharmacologically active ingredient or drug which can then be standardized and artificially synthesized in a laboratory, without any recourse to the perceived vagaries and inexactitudes of nature. Naturally, the modern professional herbalist values research into the chemistry of plants, for the information this imparts can often explain and verify the way a plant has been traditionally used and even sometimes point to new uses or pitfalls which have not hitherto been discovered. Herbalists positively revel in the chemical complexity of even the simplest plant, realizing that it is in this very multiplicity of chemical components that the strength of the herb lives and from this that it draws its healing virtue. It is this too that makes herbal medicine safe.

Some herbs are unsafe in certain circumstances. Consult the Glossary for cautions before use.

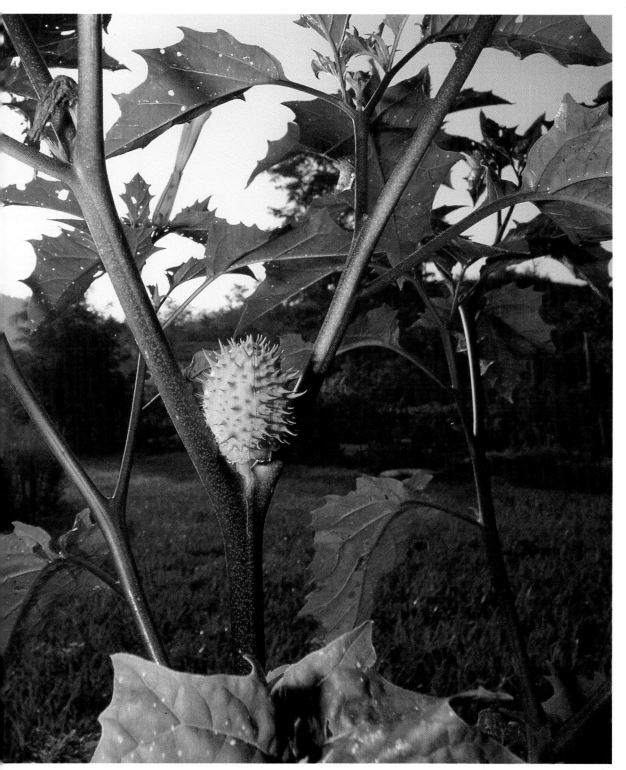

Thornapple, a powerful medicinal herb, growing in Tennessee

The natural balance of plant medicine

Scientists have tended to underestimate the fact that humans and plants have evolved side by side, and that consequently our systems have had many thousands of years to come to terms with the biochemistry of plants, by contrast with powerful modern drugs. Some seemingly less important components in plants display a so-called synergistic effect, for example, through which they can render an individual plant's active constituents more readily available in the human body. This is true of many vitamin C-rich plants, such as parsley, watercress, nettles, and rosehips, that also contain significant amounts of iron, which is much more efficiently absorbed by the body in the presence of vitamin C. Moreover, many plants which provide vitamin C also contain the yellow-coloured bioflavonoids like rutin and hesperidin which increase the bioavailability of vitamin C. These are natural balances of which the herbalist makes full use.

Some plant constituents buffer the action of other potent plant chemicals, so preventing possible harmful side-effects, a process we see in action in many medicinal plants. The Chinese herb ma huang (*Ephedra sinica*) is the source of the alkaloid ephedrine, which was for a time isolated from the herb and marketed by drug companies as a remedy for asthma. Once it came into widespread use, however, it soon became evident that the isolated drug had the disastrous side-effect of raising the blood pressure to dangerous levels, with the result that today it is hardly ever used to treat asthma. Yet in the whole plant there are some six other related alkaloids, one of which actually reduces the heart rate and lowers blood pressure. This medicinal plant has been widely used in China for thousands of years, with no undesirable side-effects.

A similar fate befell the plant *Rauwolfia serpentina*, famous for thousands of years in the ancient Indian ayurvedic medical tradition, and first mentioned in the *Charka Samhita*, an ayurvedic medical treatise dating from around 1,000 BC. From this plant was extracted the alkaloid reserpine which was hailed as a new wonder-drug for the treatment of high blood pressure. Before long, however, alarming reports began coming in from many doctors that patients to whom it had been prescribed on a regular basis had suddenly become subject to acute manic-depressive states. Today, reserpine is a more or less forgotten drug, abandoned due to these alarming side-effects. Yet a tea of the whole plant has for centuries been a famous Indian folk remedy for madness and hysteria. It was traditionally given to generations of Indian babies as a gentle sedative and Mahatma Gandhi himself regularly drank it for its calming effect. Aside from reserpine, the whole plant contains at least another 160 alkaloids, some of which have a balancing or buffering effect on reserpine.

These examples also illustrate how the very antiquity of herbal medicine has, for the most part, provided a built-in safety factor in the herbs we use, which have been tried and tested by countless generations of men and women through the ages. Every culture has its herbal tradition. Earliest written herbal records go back to the Ebers papyrus, written about 1,500 BC, although we know that official schools of herbalists existed in ancient Egypt as early as 3,000 BC. In China, one of the most famous herbals still in use today was reputedly written by the mythical Emperor Shen Nong whose reign ended about 2,700 BC. *The Shen Nong Pen Cao* (*Shen Nong's Materia Medica*) was in fact probably written by several authors in the first century BC. Later came the great Greek herbals, such as those of Dioscorides and Galen, whose books influenced the teaching of medicine for hundreds of years in Europe. Dioscorides' herbal, *De Materia Medica*, formed the basis of a famous Dutch herbal written by Deodens, and that of the Englishman John Gerard, herbalist to James I. *De Materia Medica* was still being used as a textbook in Turkish medical schools in the nineteenth century. How different things are today, when a medical textbook is out of date two or three years after publication.

The adaptogenic effect

The natural checks and balances inherent in medicinal plants are allied with the life-maintaining homeostatic mechanisms of the body. Chinese ginseng (*Panax ginseng*), for example, contains several saponins (hormone-like substances), some of which have a sedative effect and some of which are stimulating, so that ginseng has an overall adaptogenic effect, enabling someone taking it to withstand stress. Hawthorn berries have demonstrated a similar adaptogenic effect, lowering high blood pressure on the one hand while raising low blood pressure on the other.

Part of the skill of the herbalist lies in continuing this natural process, by combining plants together to render a complete herbal prescription more acceptable to the patient. Ginger and licorice, for example, are often included in herbal prescriptions to harmonize or blend other ingredients which might otherwise be rather hard on the digestive system. Laxatives like senna or cascara, which may cause griping if taken by themselves, are usually combined with aromatic herbs like mint, cardomom, or ginger to counter this tendency. Within a single prescription, two or more herbs may display apparently contradictory functions. A patient suffering from anxiety may be prescribed sedative herbs like hops and valerian, which are balanced by the addition of a more stimulating nervine like damiana to provide exactly the right measure of support for the over-stressed nervous system. Formulating individual prescriptions in this way is analagous

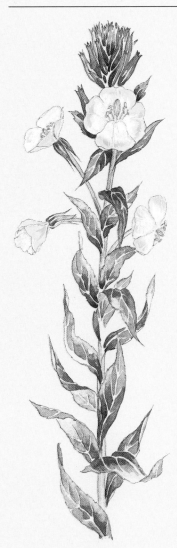

Evening primrose
The essential oil of this remarkable plant – the subject of innumerable scientific research studies (see p. 89) – has proved beneficial for a wide range of disorders, from PMS to rheumatoid arthritis and hyperactivity in children.

Green medicine

The vast majority of modern drugs in the West are wholly synthetic, laboratory-made chemicals. Even so, no less than 80 per cent of the medicines listed in the British Pharmacopoeia were plant-based at some time (like aspirin) and 30 per cent still are (like digitalis).

In the Third World, however, three-quarters of all medical needs are met by "off-the-tree", unrefined, unsynthesized herbal preparations. The chief advantages are cheapness, availability, and freedom from side-effects. Synthesis of basic compounds is often desirable (especially outside the indigenous areas) in order to improve efficacy and to prevent over-collection of the plants concerned, but sheer numbers of different medicinal plants – 6000 is an estimate, plus many others in local use which may not even be botanically identified – make systematic scientific study a daunting task. Apart from screening work in the USSR (whose extent is not well known in the West), only a few hundred herbal plants have been fully examined for drug potential.

Of the estimated ¾ million to 1½ million plant species on the earth, only about 300,000 have even been properly named and described, and even fewer have been thoroughly investigated for possible usefulness as food, medicine, or raw materials. Now, as the world's green places are being destroyed, not only are the plants vanishing – for ever – taking their secrets with them, but so also are the indigenous peoples who had knowledge of them.

One way of short-cutting costly and time-consuming field-work was advanced in the late 1970s by some American botanists who realized the immense wealth of herbarium collections. In some two thousand botanical gardens and museums round the world are specimens of almost all the quarter million species so far described. These herbarium collections have been assembled over the past two centuries and the specimen sheets often carry annotations on where the plant was collected, and what the finder was able to discover about its local names, lore and uses. These notes can greatly speed up the process of selecting live material for testing.

A scan of the 2½ million specimens in the Harvard University collections alone produced promising notes on 5000 species, most of which had not previously been recognized as having useful ingredients. Sometimes it is even possible to go further and perform spot-tests for particular chemicals on minute fragments of the dried specimen.

But however valuable the short-cut, there is no escaping the necessity for tracking down and evaluating the living plants. Among the most recent testimonies of this fact is current work on the Australian Moreton Bay chestnut (*Castanospermum australe*). This tree contains chemicals which scientists are analysing with the hope of finding a cure for AIDS. The information locked up in herbarium specimens, far from making growing plants redundant, provides more compelling evidence about why the attrition of the world's flora must be halted.

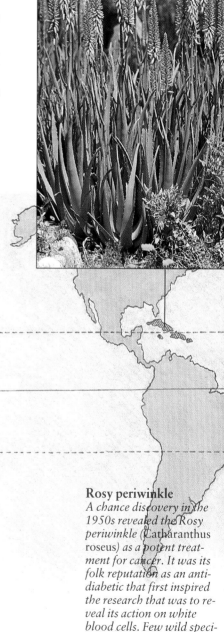

Rosy periwinkle
A chance discovery in the 1950s revealed the Rosy periwinkle (Catharanthus roseus) as a potent treatment for cancer. It was its folk reputation as an antidiabetic that first inspired the research that was to reveal its action on white blood cells. Few wild specimens of the plant remain in its native Madagascar.

Aloe vera

Today, aloe juice is a popular soothing lotion for sore, burnt, and irritated skin, and is now grown commercially in the Caribbean and Africa. The succulent aloe plant originated in the island of Socotra, off the horn of Africa, and was valued as a purgative by the ancient Greeks, who tried to conquer the island to procure specimens. Other tropical species unique to Socotra are now in danger of extinction before their medical potential can be assessed.

Feverfew

Feverfew (Chrysanthemum parthenium) is an example of an ancient remedy that modern research has turned into a spectacular medical success. Thorough clinical trials in the late 1970s found that feverfew relieved migraines in an overwhelming majority of cases, and users are now reporting beneficial side-effects such as relief from depression, nausea, and arthritic pain. Feverfew grows well in both Europe and the USA.

Quinine

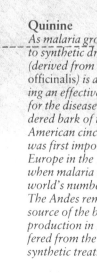

As malaria grows resistant to synthetic drugs, quinine (derived from Cinchona officinalis) is again becoming an effective treatment for the disease. The powdered bark of the South American cinchona trees was first imported into Europe in the 17th century when malaria was the world's number one killer. The Andes remain the main source of the bark, since production in Europe suffered from the boom in synthetic treatments.

to cooking, where ingredients are balanced one against another to make a harmonious and acceptable recipe.

The holistic nature of the herbalist's art

The second way that herbal medicine is holistic is in the herbalist's approach to the treatment of the patient. All traditional systems of herbal medicine share a common feature – namely their perception of disease an an imbalance or disharmony of the whole. Disease is not seen as an entity to be confronted, attacked, or eradicated. Instead, herbalists seek to resolve underlying imbalances, thereby resolving the disease itself. This is not the place for a detailed account of the various systems of herbal medicine. But briefly, Chinese medicine sees disease as a disharmony between the two universal forces of yin and yang, and Chinese herbs are described in terms of their yin or yang nature or the subsidiary categories of hot and cold. In this scheme of things, ginger, for example, is hot while rhubarb root is cold. Chinese herbalists still follow the advice given in *The Yellow Emperor's Textbook* (*Nei Jing*), compiled about the first century BC, that "hot diseases must be cooled, while cold diseases must be warmed". Ayurvedic medicine similarly categorizes herbs according to their temperature. Both systems teach that the taste of a herb (eg bitter, salty, sweet, sour, acrid, or pungent and astringent) is not incidental but is indicative of its properties, a variation on the theme of the Doctrine of Signatures (see p. 17), which played such an important role in western herbal medicine. Ayurvedic medicine teaches that herbs can strike a balance between the three primary humours, *vata* (air or wind), *pitta* (fire or bile), and *kapha* (water or phlegm), whose due proportion constitutes health. These same principles characterize the western herbal tradition which likewise defined its herbs according to temperature and humoral criteria. Modern herbalists similarly seek to restore balance and harmony within the body. Some follow the ideas developed in the USA in the last century by physiomedical herbal practitioners, who saw the need to correct in disease over-relaxed or over-contracted tissues or organs, using herbs which are astringent, relaxing, or stimulating as need be.

To herbalists of all traditions, however, the concept of the innate wisdom of body, mind, and spirit is paramount. Natural healing is founded on the basic principle that the human organism possesses the inherent ability to protect, regulate, adjust, and heal itself. This innate wisdom is often termed the vital force (*vis medicatrix naturae*). The ability to maintain a steady internal state, despite the onslaught of powerful external influences which threaten to upset our equilibrium, is known as homeostasis. During a herbal consultation the herbalist seeks to identify in which respect the vital force has been breached or

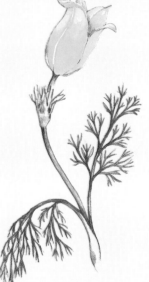

Pasque flower
A valuable plant in both the herbalist's and the homeopath's repertory (as pulsatilla), pasque flower is a particularly useful remedy for women's ailments. It is used to treat nervous exhaustion and gynaecological problems, and due to its antibacterial properties, to heal skin infections.

undermined. Such an assessment, which makes use of diagnostic techniques, equipment, and clinical tests common to orthodox doctors, plus careful questioning about the patient's past medical history, diet, and lifestyle, may lead the herbalist to the conclusion in one particular case that it is the nervous system which requires support while in another that it is the circulatory or immune system that needs help. Only by taking a full case history, which includes a careful observation and assessment of all aspects of the patient, can the picture become clear. The herbalist interprets the symptoms as a manifestation of the efforts of the vital force to return the body to health and so seeks to aid rather than suppress these attempts by the vital force to heal the body. The gentle, harmonizing effect of herbal medicines, which provide necessary trace elements, vitamins, and medicinal substances, are an ideal means to this end.

Recipes and dosages

Some of the prescriptions in this chapter are for self-help. Where more than one herb is used for a mixture, you will find the prescription given in parts, to enable you to make up the correct proportions. Generally you need at least an ounce (30 g) of herbs altogether so a small handful is a useful measure for one part. The basic method for making infusions and decoctions is given on page 135. The proportions of herb to water you should use are: 1 ounce (30 g) of dried herb to 1 pint (500 ml) of water for *infusion A*; 1 teaspoon of dried herb to a cup of water for *infusion B*; and ½ ounce (15 g) to 1 pint (500 ml) of water for *infusion C*. For a *decoction*, use 1 ounce (30 g) of dried root or bark to just over a pint of water. When making an *infusional decoction*, first decoct the roots or bark, then pour the whole decoction over the aerial parts to infuse for 15 minutes. Drink one cupful of an infusion or decoction hot, three times a day, unless otherwise stated.

When using local applications of *essential oils*, use a ratio of two drops of essential oil to a 5 ml teaspoon of vegetable oil. To make a *compress*, *poultice*, or *tincture*, see p. 135. For ailments requiring a tincture, take one teaspoon three times a day after meals. Do not take essential oils internally.

Note Please consult the Glossary for cautions on particular herbs, especially if you are under medication, menopausal, pregnant, or think you may be pregnant. Many of the conditions discussed in this section require medical diagnosis and attention. *Always* check with your doctor before attempting herbal treatments – especially if you are taking medication of any kind.

The respiratory system

We share the air we breathe with all other living creatures and every breath we take is a confirmation of the essential unity and interconnectedness of life. Air is a universal gift for which we neither have to forage nor to till. By a miracle of plant alchemy, solar energy, taken in by green leaves, acts to convert water and carbon dioxide into carbohydrate, releasing oxygen into the air.

Our respiratory system, through millions of years of evolution, is perfectly designed to extract this oxygen from the air. While we can go without food for many days and without water for just a few, without oxygen we perish within minutes, for the body does not store oxygen. Our cells need a constant supply, to burn carbohydrate and so provide the energy for life. This cellular use of oxygen, which gives off carbon dioxide as a waste product, is termed *internal respiration*. Since most of the billions of cells that comprise our being are internal, lying far away from the air, we need the respiratory and circulatory systems to ensure a constant supply of oxygen to them. The process of breathing in oxygen and breathing out waste carbon dioxide via our respiratory system – consisting of the nose, throat, larynx (voice box), trachea (windpipe) and lungs – is termed *external respiration*.

The lungs work like bellows. As we breathe in, the intercostal and diaphragmatic muscles lift the rib-cage and depress the diaphragm, and air rushes in through the nose and trachea to fill the lungs. As we breathe out, the chest wall and diaphragm relax, the lungs deflate, and carbon dioxide and water are released into the atmosphere. The lungs themselves consist of millions of microscopic sacs, called alveoli, enveloped by a network of blood capillaries. The total surface area of all the alveoli together is immense, about thirty times that of the skin, allowing the maximum amount of oxygen to diffuse through their thin lining and enter the blood vessels while carbon dioxide permeates through the opposite way.

The normal resting rate of breathing is about fifteen inhalations a minute, and at this rate, an adult pair of lungs holds about three litres of air. But deep breathing can double this volume, and exercise sees an enormous increase in the volume of air breathed in, about fifteen times that at rest. These simple facts and figures underline the importance of regular exercise and breathing techniques in promoting good health.

Traditional Chinese medicine ascribes to the lungs the function of controlling the Qi or the life-energy of the body. The Chinese believe that this life-energy, called "clean Qi", is extracted directly from the air we breathe. Perhaps for this reason, breathing techniques and ritual chanting are central features of many oriental spiritual practices like Zen meditation and yoga, and of traditional therapies like the ancient Chinese healing art of Qi Gong. Modern medicine also recognizes the importance of correct breathing for good health. Deep breathing exercises are an integral part of relaxation techniques to

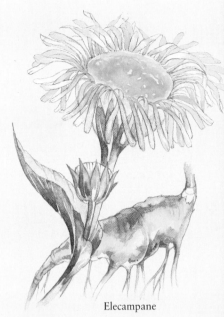

Elecampane

Expectorants

Expectorants help to expel excess mucus from the lungs, and in some cases act as a tonic for the entire respiratory system. Stimulating expectorants, such as elecampane, blood root, and white horehound, irritate the lining of the bronchials, so that phlegm is coughed up. Relaxing expectorants, such as coltsfoot and comfrey soothe bronchial spasm and loosen thick mucus secretions.

Demulcents

Demulcents contain a gummy substance known as mucilage that soothes irritated and sore bronchials and so reduces the spasms that cause coughing. Many demulcents have other, complementary actions. Licorice, for example, reduces inflammation and spasms and expels phlegm, as well as soothing the bronchials.

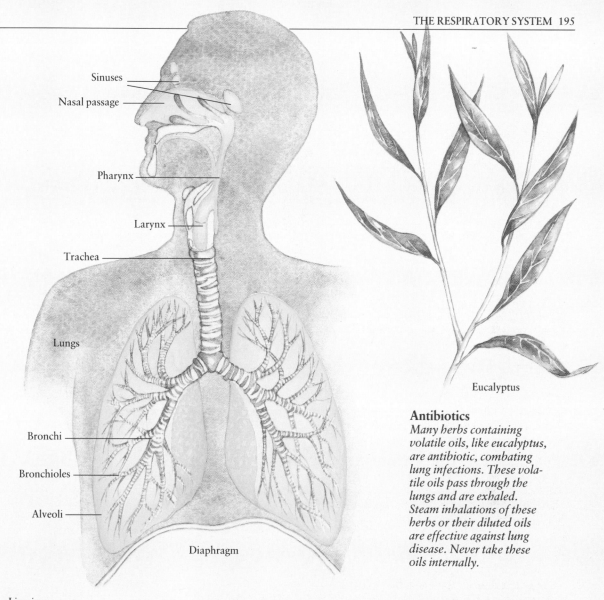

Sinuses

Nasal passage

Pharynx

Larynx

Trachea

Lungs

Bronchi

Bronchioles

Alveoli

Diaphragm

Eucalyptus

Antibiotics

Many herbs containing volatile oils, like eucalyptus, are antibiotic, combating lung infections. These volatile oils pass through the lungs and are exhaled. Steam inhalations of these herbs or their diluted oils are effective against lung disease. Never take these oils internally.

Licorice

counter stress and are now regularly taught to mothers-to-be because they encourage proper uterine contractions during birth and help to control pain. The value of singing too is now widely acknowledged. Dr M Judson writing in the *New England Journal of Medicine* has recommended that asthmatics take up singing because this makes use of about ninety per cent of the vital capacity of the lungs and so helps to prevent asthmatic attacks.

Lastly, we should not forget that the lungs are an important organ of elimination of waste products. Shallow breathing, smoking, or inhaling polluted air puts a strain not only on the lungs but also on other organs of elimination, such as the kidneys, bowels, and skin, as well as on the heart and circulation. Pollution and smoking rob us of the fresh air which is our lifeline and our birthright.

Disorders

The common cold

We all know from personal experience the symptoms of the common cold for which modern medicine has no answer. Colds are caused by a virus which replicates inside the cells of the host. Because of this, antibiotic drugs, which destroy bacteria outside cells, cannot touch a cold virus. Herbalists, however, concentrate on treating the person rather than the disease and so can provide effective treatment for colds. Here herbs are given to support and improve the function of the immune system which stands guard, repelling hostile viruses and bacteria. People who suffer frequent colds have a lowered vitality and immune response caused, perhaps, by a stressful lifestyle or irregular diet. Deficient vitality can be restored by herbal remedies, providing of course lifestyle and diet are improved.

At the first signs of a chill and/or sore throat take an *infusion* from the following common kitchen spices. 1 oz (30 g) fresh ginger, sliced, 1 stick of cinnamon, broken, 1 teaspoon coriander seeds, 3 cloves, 1 slice of lemon, 1 pt (500 ml) water. Put the ingredients in the water, bring to the boil and simmer for 15 mins and then strain. Drink a cupful of this hot, every two hours. Sweeten with organic honey to taste.

Another cold cure is to drink an *infusion* (B, see p.193) of equal parts of elderflowers, peppermint and hyssop. Footbaths are another effective method of treatment. Dissolve a tablespoon of mustard powder in 4 pts (2 l) of hot water. Bathe your feet for 10 mins, twice daily. You should also cover your head while you are doing this, to increase your body heat.

To clear the nose and throat, try this steam inhalation. Put a total of 8 drops of oil of lavender, eucalyptus or thyme (either separately or mixed) in a bowl and pour on 1 pt (500 ml) boiling water. Cover your head with a towel and inhale. **Note:** Do not use this treatment during pregnancy. For children, use half the amount of essential oil and do not give to infants.

You can also use commercial herbal preparations, such as Composition Essence. Add one teaspoon to a cup of hot water. For frequent colds, try taking Jade Screen Powder, available from Chinese pharmacies.

To prevent and treat colds, include garlic, onions, watercress, and cayenne in your diet and take 1–3 g of Acerola cherry Vitamin C per day.

Sinusitis

Sinusitis is inflammation of the four air-containing cavities in the skull. It usually occurs in an acute or chronic form after a cold. Like the nasal passages, the sinuses are lined with mucous membranes, which react to infection by producing mucus. This incapacitates infecting bacteria. Chronic sinusitis, however, may occur if one or more of the drainage passages from the sinuses to the nose becomes blocked. Chronic sinusitis can cause a dull pain across the face, temple, around the eyes or even headaches, all of which can become worse when bending down. If the maxillary sinuses above the cheeks are infected, this can produce toothache. Once the lining of the sinuses becomes swollen, the microscopic hairs or ciliae – which act as an escalator, sweeping the mucus and bacteria out of the sinuses and nasal passages – no longer operate. Once this happens, the lining of the sinuses can become permanently thickened, contributing to the retention of phlegm.

The herbal approach to these problems is both indirect and direct. The indirect approach sees upper respiratory disease within the context of the whole person. Sometimes, the overproduction of mucus can be a desperate attempt by the body to discharge waste material which is not being properly eliminated by the bowels, kidneys, and skin. In such cases, the herbalist may prescribe bitter digestive tonics to encourage regular bowel movements; or diuretic herbs which encourage kidney elimination of retained fluids and waste materials; or diaphoretic herbs which stimulate skin elimination.

A diet which reduces mucus production is also essential (see p. 199). In particular a fruit fast for two or three days can help clear a system clogged and over-burdened by toxic wastes. Hot lemon drinks reduce mucus production and so do garlic, onions and horseradish (grate the fresh root into cider vinegar or lemon juice and eat a little each day). You can also add mustard and aromatic herbs like oregano to your food. Extra zinc and Vitamin C will help build up the body's resistance to infection.

Sometimes, emotional factors like suppressed grief can lead to blocked upper respiratory passages. In these cases, a good cry can free this blocked energy and alleviate the problem. Some cases of chronic mucus production are due to allergy.

The direct approach makes use of herbs which specifically treat the upper respiratory system. There are, broadly speaking, four kinds. Herbs like mint, eucalyptus, thyme, pine, hyssop, lavender and rosemary, are all rich in volatile oils, which have an ascending nature. These herbs are ideal for treating problems in the upper part of the body. The oils are antibiotic, knocking out infecting organisms, and loosening sticky mucus – so opening up the nasal and sinus passages.

Astringent herbs are a second category of plants, useful for treating sinusitis. Herbs like agrimony, golden rod, bayberry bark, eyebright, and elderflowers contain tannins which tone the mucous membranes and dry up excess secretions. Herbs like echinacea, wild indigo and garlic form a third category. These herbs are antibiotic and counter upper respiratory infection. The fourth class of herb comprises soothing demulcents like marshmallow and mullein, which relieve irritation of the mucous membranes. One herb, golden seal, stands alone. This is of special benefit to mucous membranes throughout the body, but must only be used in small doses. If you suffer from sinusitis and catarrh, drink an *infusion/ decoction* (see p.193) of 1 part each of purple coneflower, golden rod, hyssop, elderflowers, eyebright, and peppermint, and ¼ part golden seal. If the nasal discharge is runny and clear, add two slices of ginger to this brew. A steam inhalant is one of the most effective ways to treat upper-respiratory mucus and sinusitis. You can either use a proprietary preparation, such as Olbas oil, or make your own. In a bottle, mix 30 ml of compound tincture of Benzoin (Friar's balsam) with 2.5 ml eucalyptus oil, 6 drops peppermint oil, 5 drops lavender oil and 5 drops pine oil. Shake well. Put a teaspoonful in a bowl and pour on 1 pt (500 ml) boiled water. Cover your head and the bowl with a towel or cloth and inhale. Mustard footbaths (see The common cold) can also be effective, and you can also wash out your nasal passages with 1 eggcupful of fresh beetroot juice, diluted in 1 eggcupful of water. It may look alarmingly like a prolonged nosebleed, but it can reduce mucus.

Sore throat

Herbal treatment is an effective way to treat a sore throat. An *infusion/ decoction* (B, see p.193) of one or more astringent herbs can be used as a gargle to ease the discomfort. Blackberry leaves, raspberry leaves, elderflowers, bistort root, five-finger grass or oak bark are all helpful herbs.

Particularly useful is a gargle of sage, cider vinegar and honey. Make an *infusion* (B, see p.193) and when cool, strain it and add a teaspoon of cider vinegar and honey. Gargle four or five times a day. Another useful gargle is made by mixing a teaspoon of *tincture* of myrrh, balm of Gilead or golden seal in warm water. Licorice and marshmallow, both soothing to the throat, make good additions to any gargle. If you have no herbs to hand, you can gargle with lemon juice and hot water or cider vinegar and hot water. You can also use plain salt and water, but don't swallow it, since it is emetic. If a sore throat persists, or is accompanied by a fever, see your doctor.

Tonsillitis

Strictly speaking, the word tonsil is used for any collection of lymphatic tissue anywhere in the body. We usually use it, however, to refer to the lymphatic tissue at the back of the tongue. This, like all other lymphatic tissue, produces lymphocytes, which protect the body from infection. Surgical removal should be a last resort.

Recurring tonsillitis calls for a general assessment of the body's ability to withstand infection. If the tonsils are swollen and inflamed, gargle as suggested for sore throats. In addition, take an *infusion/decoction* (A, see p. 193) of 1 part each of purple coneflower, ½ part thyme, and ¼ part golden seal. If a child runs a fever with inflamed tonsils, you should seek medical attention.

Laryngitis

Laryngitis is inflammation of the larynx or voice box or the vocal cords themselves. Such an infection will cause hoarseness or loss of voice altogether. If this is the case, rest your voice completely and use the steam inhalation formula suggested for sinusitis. Also, gargle with sage and cider vinegar. Any case of laryngitis that continues for more than a few days requires expert medical attention to exclude the possibility of a growth.

Cough

Coughing is a reflex response (Chinese medicine calls it "rebellious lung Qi") to anything blocking the airways. Usually this is mucus secreted by membranes lining the respiratory tract. Such mucus secretions help to protect the respiratory tract from any kind of irritant, trapping and flushing out hostile bacteria and viruses.

The herbal treatment of coughs aims to kill off bacteria, loosen and expel mucus secretions and restore lung function. Constant coughs and colds are a call to take herbs to strengthen the immune system (see The common cold). It is a bad idea to take suppressive cough mixtures. The most useful herbs for treating coughs are demulcents to soothe the irritation, such as marshmallow; expectorants, to expel the phlegm, such as coltsfoot; and antibiotic herbs to kill off bacteria, such as hyssop and thyme.

Any cough that lasts more than a few days, does not respond to treatment, or produces blood, should be investigated by a doctor, since it may be a sign of serious organic disease.

You can make a simple cough remedy by slicing a large onion into rings and putting them into a deep bowl. Cover the onion slices with organic runny honey and let it stand overnight. In the morning, strain off the mixture of honey and onion juice, which makes a simple cough elixir. Honey itself, which is often included in cough mixtures has antibiotic properties and is also expectorant. Take a dessert spoon of this mixture four or five times a day.

You can also make a useful cough mixture from an *infusion/decoction* (A, see p.193) of 1 part each of coltsfoot flowers, marshmallow leaves, hyssop and ½ part each of licorice root and aniseed. Simmer the infusion for 10 mins and strain. Sweeten the mixture with honey and drink a cupful hot, three or four times a day until the cough subsides.

Bronchitis

Bronchitis is an acute or chronic inflammation of the mucous lining of the bronchial tubes, the main airways carrying air from the windpipe (trachea) to the lungs. Chronic bronchitis is a serious disease which can lead to an early death. Emphysema, which often accompanies bronchitis, is damage to the elastic walls of the sac-like alveoli in the lungs. This is caused by constant coughing to try to dislodge the bacteria and mucus blocking the swollen bronchi. Microscopic hairs called cilia which line the airways act as a respiratory escalator pushing out particles of dust, soot, and bacteria. In chronic bronchitis the cilia become paralysed due to the constant secretion of viscid mucus. Smoking and to a lesser degree alcohol exacerbate this sorry state of affairs. It is a virtually impossible task to use herbs to treat someone who persists in smoking.

As when treating a simple cough, herbalists treat bronchitis by combining expectorant herbs, like squills, white horehound, coltsfoot, senega, elecampane, and blood root with those that have a soothing, demulcent action, like mullein, comfrey, marshmallow, flax seeds, licorice, violet leaves, and Irish moss. Antibiotic herbs, such as eucalyptus, are added to this mixture. Combine one or two herbs from each category in equal parts. Pour on 1 pt (500 ml) water, boil, then simmer for 15 mins before the herbs are strained off.

When treating acute bronchitis, add herbs to cause sweating, like yarrow, elderflower, and hyssop, to expectorant herbs, like white horehound and coltsfoot. Where the sputum is white and copious, and bronchitis gets worse in cold or damp weather, add sliced ginger root or a pinch or two of cayenne. If the phlegm is green (indicating infection), use garlic honey as a natural antibiotic. Cover four cloves of sliced garlic with 3 fl oz (100 ml) organic, runny honey. Leave overnight, strain off the juice, and take the garlic honey in teaspoonful doses several times a day.

Other antibiotic herbs which are good for the chest include thyme, pine and eucalyptus. To make a steam inhalation, pour 1 pt (500 ml) boiling water over 2 drops of the essential oils of each of the three herbs. Add a teaspoonful of tincture of benzoin and inhale the steam.

Asthma

Asthma is a condition in which the small bronchial airways temporarily constrict, so that it is difficult for the asthmatic person to exhale. This leads to breathlessness and wheezing.

Many asthmatics are allergic to house dust, animal fur, or various foods. They may also suffer from eczema and there is often a history of asthma in the family. If asthma sufferers get upset or exhausted, this may trigger an attack.

There are several herbs which can help to relax the bronchi and expel the mucus. The use of lobelia, ephedra and jimson weed is restricted. Other herbs, such as grindelia, pill-bearing spurge, sundew, coltsfoot, and skunk cabbage are generally available. It may be wise to add herbs to support the nervous system, such as wild lettuce, hops, chamomile, limeflowers, and skullcap. Licorice is a useful herb to add to asthmatic prescriptions because it is a soothing expectorant. It also supports the adrenal glands, which provide a natural cortisone – effective against stress and allergic reactions. Borage is also a soothing respiratory herb with a reputation for strengthening the adrenal function. You can make an *infusion* (A, see p.193) of equal parts of any of these herbs to ease the condition.

Our lungs are connected to our emotions in an obvious way – think about laughing or crying. If a person with asthma has difficulty in expressing his or her feelings, it is worth exploring why this should be. Bach Flower Remedies can help here (see p.235). Deep breathing can strengthen our connection to our feelings and will help improve asthma, if practised regularly. Other regular exercise, such as walking, swimming, yoga, or T'ai Chi, and relaxation classes, can also help to deepen and relax your breathing.

If you are asthmatic, look at your diet to see if you are sensitive to any foods. It may pay dividends to exclude, for a time, eggs, wheat, even gluten (found in wheat, oats, barley and rye), and dairy products. The early onset of asthma is sometimes triggered off by a child not being breastfed. Another source of concern is alcohol (wine and beer) and preserved fruit, which often contain sulphur dioxide. Many asthmatics react to as little as five parts of sulphur dioxide per million. It is wise to seek professional help for allergy detection since exposure to an allergen after it has been removed from the diet can produce a bad attack. Emergency treatments such as inhalers should be on hand to the sufferer in case of a bad attack.

Asthma is a serious disease. If this is your problem you should seek medical help.

The ear

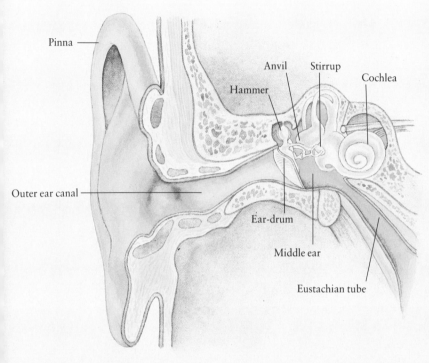

Pinna

Outer ear canal

Anvil

Hammer

Stirrup

Cochlea

Ear-drum

Middle ear

Eustachian tube

A highly intricate structure, the ear has three parts – the outer ear, the middle ear, and the inner ear. The outer ear consists of the funnel-shaped flap or pinna and the ear canal, which ends at the ear-drum or tympanic membrane. In the inner part of the ear canal are glands that secrete wax, which helps to entrap and drain out dust and bacteria. Behind the ear-drum lies the middle ear, comprising three bones, known as the hammer, anvil, and stirrup. These bones conduct vibrations from the ear-drum to the entrance of the inner ear. Inside the inner ear is the cochlea, a tiny coiled tube in which lies the organ of Corti – the organ responsible for analysing sound. Vibrations reaching it through the outer and middle ear are translated into electrical impulses and transmitted to the brain. The inner ear also helps to provide the brain with information about our balance and orientation, through its semicircular canals.

The ear, nose, and throat are linked by the Eustachian tube, which is why ear infections often originate in colds and throat infections. While herbal treatment can be very effective for disorders of the outer and middle ear, it is less effective for diseases of the inner ear. But there is much that we can do to ensure that our hearing ability lasts into old age – by avoiding prolonged exposure to, say, discordant sounds and by actively listening to beautiful music or to the sounds of nature.

Disorders

Earache is a worrying symptom and since it usually heralds middle-ear infection, it requires professional medical attention. If the condition is at all serious, antibiotics may be the only answer. But the regular use of antibiotics does nothing to treat the underlying cause of the problem.

If your child suffers from earache, it is important to strengthen his or her immunity to infection, by giving a wholefood diet with plenty of vitamin-rich fruit and vegetables and extra vitamin C and zinc during the winter months, provided, of course, that he or she is not allergic to these foods. Avoid foods which contribute to the production of mucus, such as refined carbohydrates and dairy products.

Herbal eardrops containing volatile oils and other herbs with antibiotic action can be applied whenever a child who is prone to ear infection gets a cold. However, before eardrops are used, it is important to ensure that the eardrums are undamaged. Be sure to check with your doctor before attempting treatment. When earache threatens, try a formula made up of 20 drops each of tincture of golden seal and eucalyptus oil, 10 drops of tincture of pasque flower, 5 drops each of tincture of myrrh and 30 ml of almond oil. Shake the mixture well and use two drops in the ear three times a day.

Alternatively, apply drops of garlic or mullein oil. Pack as many mullein flowers as you can into a bottle of olive oil. Place it on a sunny window ledge for a month. Then express the oil and store it in a dark bottle.

In addition, take an *infusion* (B, see p. 193) of 1 part each of mint, hyssop and chamomile, 2 parts of purple coneflower, and ½ part each of golden seal and dried pasque flower. To reduce the risk of ear infection, rub lavender oil diluted in olive or almond oil into the bony protruberance behind the ear and in front of the ear and the back of the neck.

The digestive system

Through the middle of our bodies runs the digestive tract, a hollow tube about twelve yards (11 m) long which, if it was extended, would reach higher than the high diving board of an Olympic swimming pool. The digestive tract is lined with mucous membrane, different parts of which secrete the digestive juices required to break down the food we eat into assimilable form. Vital digestive secretions are also supplied by the liver, the gallbladder (bile), and the pancreas.

When we have a meal, the food we have eaten, partially broken down by chewing and by the action of saliva, goes down the oesophagus to the stomach. After being further broken down by gastric juices, the food passes down into the small intestine. Here it is mixed with a range of digestive enzymes and with bile from the gallbladder. Part of it is absorbed into the bloodstream and transported by the portal vein to the liver while the indigestible part moves on into the large intestine, where water and electrolytes, such as sodium, are extracted. The remaining waste passes to the rectum for excretion.

The digestive tract is surrounded by a muscle coating, comprising both longitudinal and circular muscles. When circular muscle contracts, it produces a series of wavelike motions, called peristalsis, which propel food and fluid through the tract. The contraction of longitudinal muscle makes the tube enlarge, allowing food to remain longer in a particular part of the digestive system. In a state of health, the two poles of relaxation and movement exemplified by these muscular movements are balanced so that food and fluid remain in the tract just long enough for optimum digestion, and a bowel movement occurs at least once every twenty-four hours. Elimination is a vital function of the digestive tract, for in addition to voiding the residue of food and fluids, the intestines must also rid the body of other metabolic waste products. If this excretion is impaired, a build-up of toxic wastes will result.

The health of the colon, and its regular peristaltic movements and evacuation are dependent on a diet containing plenty of fibre or roughage which stimulates its rhythmical contractions. The functioning of the digestive system is also dependent on nervous control. When you eat a meal, the autonomic nervous system modifies the circulatory system so that more blood is sent to the digestive system. During exercise or stress, a reverse process carries blood away from the digestive tract to feed the muscles and brain and the digestive function is reduced. The nervous system also governs the secretion of hydrochloric acid in the stomach. During periods of stress, however, messages from the brain run directly via the vagus nerve to cause the secretion of extra acid in the stomach, and this can be a contributory cause of peptic ulcers. When treating digestive problems a herbalist therefore often uses remedies which relax the nervous system, as well as acting directly on the digestion.

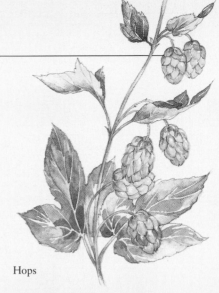

Hops

Digestive relaxants
Herbs like hops and chamomile operate at two levels. They relax an overactive and overcontracted stomach and bowel while sedating the central nervous system, so countering anxiety and stress.

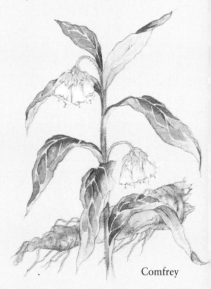

Comfrey

Digestive demulcents
Demulcent herbs like comfrey, marshmallow, slippery elm, and licorice soothe the inflammation and pain. Research on comfrey has shown it to reduce a local hormone-like activity which causes inflammation of the stomach lining.

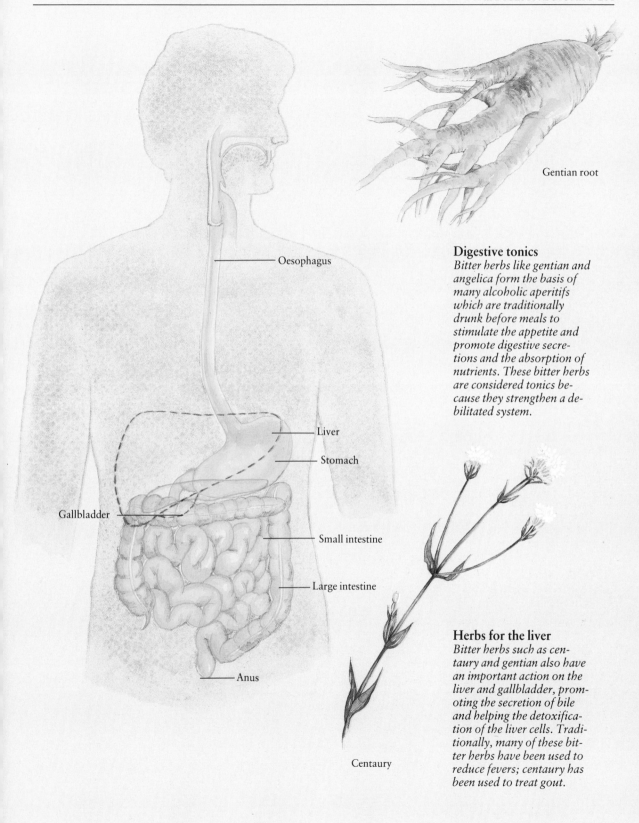

Gentian root

Digestive tonics

Bitter herbs like gentian and angelica form the basis of many alcoholic aperitifs which are traditionally drunk before meals to stimulate the appetite and promote digestive secretions and the absorption of nutrients. These bitter herbs are considered tonics because they strengthen a debilitated system.

Oesophagus

Liver

Stomach

Gallbladder

Small intestine

Large intestine

Anus

Centaury

Herbs for the liver

Bitter herbs such as centaury and gentian also have an important action on the liver and gallbladder, promoting the secretion of bile and helping the detoxification of the liver cells. Traditionally, many of these bitter herbs have been used to reduce fevers; centaury has been used to treat gout.

Disorders

Inflamed gums (gingivitis)

Inflammation of the gums is caused by poor oral hygiene and/or unwise eating. Foods which contain significant amounts of roughage clean the teeth and strengthen the gums too. An apple a day certainly will help to keep the dentist away! If the gums bleed or are inflamed, wash the mouth out with 1 teaspoon of *tincture* (see p. 135) of myrrh diluted in a cup of water or an *infusion* (B, see p. 193) of sage or marigold. Two drops of oil of thyme may be added to these mouthwashes. In addition, massage the gums each day with 1 teaspoon of eucalyptus oil diluted in an eggcupful of vegetable oil. Be careful not to swallow. It is also a good idea to take extra Vitamin C.

Indigestion

Indigestion is usually caused by bad eating habits. Eating irregularly, too much, too rapidly, eating when anxious or eating the wrong food can trigger feelings of bloating, heaviness, dull stomach pain or heartburn after a meal. The medical profession often prescribes antacids for indigestion to neutralize stomach acid. This unfortunately provokes the stomach to secrete more acid, so that digestion can take place. Herbs provide a more effective answer. *Infusions* (B, see p. 193) of fennel, mint, dill, chamomile, aniseed or lemon balm are all aromatic and relieve flatulence. These are usually taken after a meal. Bitter *decoctions* (see p. 193), like gentian or dandelion root, taken before a meal stimulate the appetite and digestive secretions and activity. Nervous tension may be eased by *infusions* (B, see p. 193) of chamomile and lemon balm, or hops.

Gastritis and peptic ulcers

Gastritis (inflammation of the stomach lining) and ulceration of the stomach or duodenum are essentially similar complaints, but ulcers require medical attention. The same elements that cause indigestion may be root causes of these allied conditions. Changing the diet, eating regularly and ensuring that stress is reduced is a vital part of the treatment. In addition, for gastritis take an *infusion/decoction* (A, see p. 193) of 1 part of meadowsweet, ½ part each of gentian and golden seal, and 2 parts each of comfrey and marshmallow.

A gastric or duodenal ulcer may respond to an *infusion/decoction* (A, see p. 193) of 1 part each of licorice, golden seal, marigold, and chamomile, and 2 parts each of comfrey and marshmallow.

Slippery elm powder coats the lining of the stomach and protects it against over-acid secretions. Mix the slippery elm powder with milk or water and eat a few teaspoons of it when you are in pain.

In general, eat little and often. Avoid food and drink that irritate the stomach, such as alcohol, fried food, pickles, spices, tea, and coffee. Even decaffeinated coffee increases stomach acidity.

Diarrhoea and constipation

Any change in normal bowel habit that suddenly occurs and lasts more than two or three days must be medically investigated.

Diarrhoea is usually caused by an infection or irritation of part of the digestive tract, e.g. gastroenteritis, and is often accompanied by nausea and vomiting. In such cases, vomiting and diarrhoea are natural physiological mechanisms to help the body rid itself of poisons. Once you have determined that there is no serious cause, you should allow the condition to run its course, taking care to replace lost fluids and electrolytes by drinking a solution of warm water and honey. Infants may quickly collapse after bouts of diarrhoea and vomiting, if lost fluids and electrolytes are not replaced. Get prompt medical help when babies are ill.

If diarrhoea persists, combine a teaspoon of a mixture of astringent

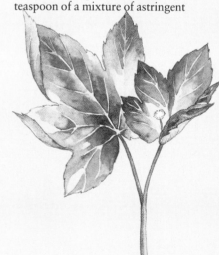

Golden seal
Through its powerful tonic effect on the mucous membranes, golden seal helps in the treatment of many digestive problems.

remedies, e.g. agrimony and five-finger grass, with a pinch of ginger and cinnamon powder. Garlic and echinacea can be taken as natural antibiotics. If diarrhoea is your problem, you should avoid cold drinks and cold food, since digestive activity is aided by warmth. Nausea responds well to spices like ginger, cardamom, cinnamon, and coriander. You could also try slippery elm tablets.

Constipation is usually the result of poor diet and lack of exercise. The long-term use of herbal laxatives like senna is to be avoided since the bowel can become habituated to their use. In general, there are two types of constipation: the flaccid type when muscular activity is weak, or the tense type when nervous and muscular tension inhibits bowel activity. The former condition can be relieved by regular exercise and abdominal massage and herbs which increase muscle tone and activity. A high-fibre diet is essential. To help this flaccid condition, try an *infusion/decoction* (A, see p. 193) of 1 part each of licorice, damiana, raspberry leaves, golden seal, rhubarb root, and ginger, and 2 parts of dandelion root.

An over-contracted gut – the tense condition – may respond to an *infusion/decoction* (A, see p. 193) which contains bowel relaxants. Use 1 part each of chamomile, ginger, valerian, peppermint, and 2 parts each of licorice, wild yam, and dandelion root. Relaxation exercises may also help to alleviate the underlying tension.

In both cases it is advisable to use psyllium seeds. The black variety are more effective than the white. Mix two teaspoons of seeds into a cup of warm water and stir well. Leave the cup for five minutes before stirring again. Swallow the contents which can be flavoured with a little lemon or grapefruit juice and honey which also helps to lubricate the bowel. Take a cupful from one to three times a day after meals. The seeds are an effective and gentle bulk laxative.

Irritable bowel syndrome (IBS) and colitis

Colitis is inflammation of the large intestine, characterized by alternating bouts of diarrhoea and constipation. The stools may contain mucus or blood if the disease is severe (seek medical help in these cases). A less serious condition is irritable bowel syndrome (IBS). Here diarrhoea or constipation and flatulence commonly occur without many signs of organic disease.

Food intolerance may be at the root of the problem. In one medical study published in the *Lancet*, two thirds of patients with IBS displayed food intolerance, and once these foods were removed from the diet, the condition improved. Suspect substances are coffee, strong tea, alcohol, cigarettes, dairy foods, eggs, and possibly even gluten, contained in the cereals wheat, oats, barley, and rye. These foods can be eliminated from the diet for a time, but this is probably best done with professional help. Herbs can be most helpful in treating colitis and IBS. If you suffer from severe colitis and your stools contain mucus or blood, you should seek medical help immediately.

Subsequently, take an *infusion/ decoction* (A, see p. 193) of 1 part each of wild yam, golden seal, and chamomile, 2 parts each of agrimony and American cranesbill, 3 parts of marshmallow and ½ part of acorus root until the problem subsides.

Worms

Worms are a common problem in children, especially when there are pets in the house. There are three types of worms that can infest the human body – threadworms, roundworms, and tapeworms. The latter is a dangerous parasite which requires professional medical treatment. The first two kinds, however, can be treated using a home herbal cure – but

seek medical help if they persist. Threadworms, which are about half an inch (1 cm) long, are the commonest of all parasites in children. They live in the large intestine and rectum, and cause rectal itching. They may also produce bad dreams, grinding of the teeth while asleep, constipation or diarrhoea, bad breath, dark rings under the eyes, nose picking, and an increased appetite.

Roundworms can measure about 10 inches (25 cms). Two or three may live in the intestine at any time. They cause similar symptoms plus abdominal pain.

If worms are suspected eat plenty of the kinds of foods that worms detest. These include raw onions and garlic; administer one or two chopped up garlic cloves in a spoonful of honey or simmered in a little milk, taken half an hour before breakfast. Pumpkin or melon seeds can be ground up or added whole to the breakfast cereal. Eating raw carrots in salads, chewing cloves, and eating pomegranates are a good idea. Add a little cayenne pepper to your cooking and eat slippery elm food (obtainable from health stores). Drink plenty of fennel, aniseed or mint tea. In general, avoid sugars and refined carbohydrates. Eat plenty of fresh fruit and vegetables.

Typical antihelminthic (worm expelling) herbs are those in the genus artemisia, namely wormwood, southernwood and tansy, and other bitter herbs, such as balmony (good for threadworms), centaury, gentian, hops, and the aromatic pennyroyal. These herbs are toxic and so should be used only under medical supervision. Do not take them during pregnancy.

If a child has worms, seek medical attention. You will have to worm the whole family, including pets.

Children will naturally object to the bitter-tasting worm-purging herbs. A simple expedient is to powder southernwood or tansy leaves in a coffee grinder and give a teaspoon of this to the child, either in capsule form or in something sweet, such as honey or molasses.

This recipe for a bitter brew to expel worms comes from France. It is for adults excluding pregnant women or those who are breastfeeding. Take 10 g (⅓ oz) each of wormwood leaves, southernwood leaves, tansy leaves, mint and gentian root, and add them to 2 pt (1 l) water. Bring to the boil and simmer for 5 mins. Leave to infuse for 10 mins. Drink a cupful on an empty stomach each morning before breakfast and before going to bed for a week. Repeat the following month if necessary. Examine the stools for worms which should be expelled during this period.

According to French folklore, the most effective worm treatments are when the moon is waxing, just before it is full. The worms are then said to be easier to dislodge.

Diverticulosis

A diverticulum occurs when mucous membrane lining the bowel protrudes through the muscle wall of the bowel. These pouches occur at points where the arteries pierce the bowel wall, or where the intestine wall is weak between the muscle fibres. Although diverticuli may occur anywhere in the digestive tract, they usually occur towards the end of the large intestine. Simple diverticular disease is characterized by cramping pains, usually in the left side of the abdomen, and irregular bowel movements. If food becomes lodged in the pouches, and inflammation occurs, the condition is known as diverticulitis. The symptoms may be much more severe and you may run a temperature, in which case, seek medical help.

Diverticuli are present in about twenty-five per cent of men and women over fifty. The problem is usually associated with lack of exercise and a diet low in fibre.

Please check the Glossary for cautions on particular herbs. If in doubt, consult a qualified practitioner.

Roughage, such as that found in whole cereals and vegetables, is vital to keep the digestive system healthy. Without it, the muscles of the colon have to work extra hard to move the less bulky faeces through the intestines. Over a period of years, this causes the muscles to lose their efficiency.

Psyllium seeds are an effective treatment for diverticuli (see Constipation). Also try an *infusion/*

Mullein
When used in conjunction with other herbs, mullein may be helpful in the treatment of diverticulosis.

decoction (A, see p. 193) of 1 part each of licorice, chamomile, peppermint, and ginger, 2 parts each of mullein and wild yam, and ½ part of acorus root. Do not attempt self-treatment during pregnancy.

The liver and gallbladder
The liver is the largest organ in the body. As the main storehouse and chemical factory of the body, it plays a vital role in maintaining health and overcoming disease. It is richly supplied with blood (about 3 pts or 1.5 l filters through it every minute). The hepatic artery brings fresh arterial blood to all the liver cells to provide oxygen for them to do their complex work. In addition, the portal vein brings all the products of digestion to the liver so that it can filter out and store substances like glucose and fructose as glycogen (a function it shares with the muscles). In this way the liver helps to regulate blood sugar levels. The liver also receives, via the portal vein, digested proteins as amino acids, and fats as fatty acids, which it metabolizes ready for use by the body. Equally important is the liver's ability to manufacture the blood-clotting proteins fibrinogen

down or detoxifies certain poisons, such as drugs or alcohol, deactivates hormones like oestrogens and steroids, and breaks down worn-out blood cells. At the same time the liver manufactures the fat-soluble Vitamin A and stores Vitamins B12, D, and K as well as iron. Last but not least the liver manufactures bile, producing about 2 pts (1 l) a day in adults. This is concentrated about ten times and stored in the gallbladder until we eat a fatty meal. The gallbladder then contracts and bile, which helps the digestion of fats, is ejected into the duodenum.

Remedies for the liver

Because of the central role of the liver in cleansing the body, it is sensible when treating chronic disease to regulate its functions by including one or two liver-acting herbs in your herbal mixtures. The herbal *materia medica* is rich in plant remedies for the liver such as dandelion root, barberry, boldo, fringe tree, gentian, and centaury. *Infusions* (B, see p. 193) of one or two of these herbs can be taken in spring as a liver tonic to help clear out the residue of heavy winter meals. For those who have been taking chemical drugs over a period of time, a liver-cleansing programme is essential.

A good liver-regulating remedy is a *decoction/infusion* (C, see p. 193) of 1 part each of barberry bark, Oregon grape root, gentian, rosemary,

artichoke leaves, licorice, and ginger, 2 parts of wild yam, and 3 parts of dandelion root.

Inflammation of the gallbladder and gallstones

Gallstones are formed because of too great a concentration of bile, especially cholesterol. If they lodge in the bile duct, they can cause severe colicky pain and the blockage may cause jaundice. Any inflammation or infection of the gallbladder is usually a consequence of gallstones.

For inflammation of the gallbladder take an *infusion/decoction* (A, see p. 193) of 1 part each of dandelion, Oregon grape, fringe tree bark, and wahoo, and 2 parts of marshmallow root until the condition improves.

Gallstones can be effectively treated using bitter herbal remedies like dandelion, Oregon grape, greater celandine, culver's root, and wahoo, combining these with relaxing and soothing herbs such as chamomile, crampbark, marshmallow, and slippery elm.

Note Treatment of these disorders should be done under the direction of a trained herbal practitioner.

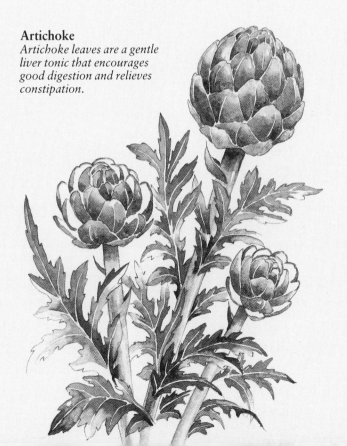

Artichoke
Artichoke leaves are a gentle liver tonic that encourages good digestion and relieves constipation.

The circulatory system

The heart is a highly efficient muscular pump, the powerhouse behind the circulatory system, by means of which blood is transported around the body. Every minute, the heart beats about seventy times, pumping the body's twelve pints of blood around in an endless circle. But it can greatly increase its output on demand, such as during exercise. While our western tradition links the heart chiefly with love, in Chinese medicine it is regarded as the house of the spirit (or *shen*) and of consciousness.

Arteries, which carry blood away from the heart, are the great highway along which all the nutrients necessary for growth, repair, and maintenance of the body's cells are carried. The arteries divide and sub-divide, eventually flowing into millions of microscopic capillaries which permeate all our tissues, with the exception of cartilage and the transparent tissue of the eye. The capillaries are the vital link between the arteries and veins, for it is through their permeable walls that nutrients are exchanged for waste products.

Blood leaves the left side of the heart, flowing through arteries which carry it to the various tissues and organs of the body. Deoxygenated blood, carrying waste carbon dioxide, drains from these structures, returning through the veins to reach the right side of the heart. The right side of the heart pumps this deoxygenated blood via the pulmonary artery to the lungs, where carbon dioxide is exchanged for oxygen. The newly oxygenated blood then flows through the pulmonary veins back to the left side of the heart to begin its circuit again. On its way, blood collects nutrients from the liver and intestines and waste is filtered from it by the kidneys.

Transport of oxygen and carbon dioxide between the lungs and tissues is dependent not only on the condition of the heart, arteries, and veins but on the health of the blood itself. Blood consists of red and white blood cells which float in a fluid called plasma. Plasma, which accounts for about half the blood volume, is a solution of salt, proteins, glucose, and other substances in water. Red cells, which account for almost all the other half of the blood volume, carry oxygen from the lungs to the tissues. White blood cells are part of the body's defence system, and multiply up to fourfold during an infection.

In western countries with a high standard of living, heart disease, strokes, and high blood pressure are responsible for more than fifty per cent of all deaths – and of this at least half are due to coronary artery disease. Britain has the worst record of heart disease of any country in the world. The majority of these cases are entirely avoidable, for they are the consequence of too little exercise, an inadequate diet too rich in fat and sugar, smoking, and high levels of stress. There are many ways in which herbal medicine can help in the healing of heart and circulatory disorders, but by far the wisest course of action is to take steps to prevent them developing at all.

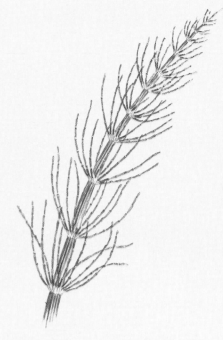

Horsetail
Horsetail contains silica, which strengthens the walls of the veins. Its astringent action also helps to tighten up varicose veins. This is a remedy which is best used fresh. Silica encourages the absorption and use of calcium by the body and also helps to guard against fatty deposits in the arteries.

Preventing cardiovascular disease

Exercise
You should take regular exercise two or three times a week. Such exercise should be aerobic, which means it makes a sustained (neither too gentle nor too intense) demand on the heart and lungs, and makes use of the large muscles of the body, like those in the legs. Regular aerobic exercise causes blood vessels to enlarge and become more elastic, and strengthens the heart muscle. Blood pressure and the resting heart rate also drop. If you are unused to exercise, begin gently.

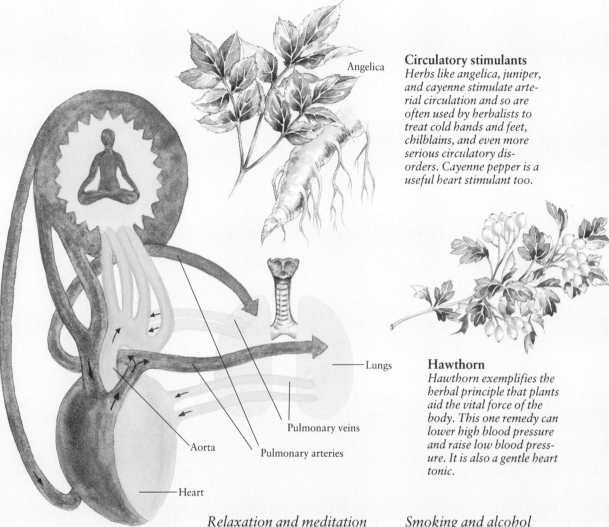

Angelica

Lungs

Pulmonary veins

Pulmonary arteries

Aorta

Heart

Circulatory stimulants

Herbs like angelica, juniper, and cayenne stimulate arterial circulation and so are often used by herbalists to treat cold hands and feet, chilblains, and even more serious circulatory disorders. Cayenne pepper is a useful heart stimulant too.

Hawthorn

Hawthorn exemplifies the herbal principle that plants aid the vital force of the body. This one remedy can lower high blood pressure and raise low blood pressure. It is also a gentle heart tonic.

Diet

Eat a high-fibre, low-animal-fat diet. Saturated animal fats can form fatty deposits in the arteries and prevent blood flow. If this occurs in the coronary arteries it may lead to angina and a heart attack. Avoid excess sugar and refined carbohydrates like sweet biscuits and cakes. Reduce salt, animal fats, and cholesterol-rich foods (which include red meat, dairy products and eggs) to a minimum.

Relaxation and meditation

Learn to relax and take up meditation. Modern coronary-care units have begun to adopt relaxation and meditation to teach patients with heart disease how to avoid undue stress. Research has shown that there are two basic personalities known as Type A and B. Type A people have a strong drive and tend to imagine they are indispensable. They find it hard to let up on work and may react angrily to anything that appears to thwart them. Type Bs are much more "laid back" and can relax from their work. Recent findings show that Type As have thirty-one per cent more chance of developing heart disease than Type Bs.

Smoking and alcohol

To protect your heart you need to stop smoking and avoid high alcohol intake. Nicotine acts to constrict the arteries, reducing blood flow, while the carbon monoxide in tobacco smoke reduces the amount of oxygen in the blood. Alcohol, in excess, contributes to the accumulation of body fat. In the USA, where there is increasing public awareness of the sense of such measures, deaths from heart disease have dropped by over twenty-five per cent.

Disorders

Angina

Angina, meaning pain in Greek, is the common abbreviation for angina pectoris, an often severe constriction of the chest. It is sometimes associated with pains in one or both shoulders or arms, which may also radiate to the back or jaw. The pain and constriction is usually increased by effort and relieved by rest. It may also be provoked by feelings of anger, anxiety, excitement, even by a meal or cold weather.

The symptoms are caused by reduced blood flow to the heart, usually the result of coronary-artery disease – the most common cause of death in the western world. For such a vital muscle, the heart seems relatively poorly supplied with blood vessels, since there are only two coronary arteries. Those who eat a lot of fat, take relatively little exercise and are subject to prolonged stress are particularly prone to the build-up of fatty plaque on the walls of the arteries (called atheroma, from the Greek word for porridge or gruel). This in turn causes fibrous tissue to be formed in the arterial wall and the aperture within the artery to narrow. Coronary artery disease is more common in men than in premenopausal women, and tends to run in families. There is an increased risk if there is a high level of cholesterol in the blood, high blood pressure, or in those who smoke or who live in soft water areas.

Anyone suffering from some or all of these symptoms *must* see a medical practitioner. Herbal remedies can have a significant long-term effect in helping to reduce cholesterol and opening up the coronary arteries to increase blood flow to the heart. These remedies, which include hawthorn, lily of the valley, limeflower, mistletoe, motherwort, crampbark and rosemary, should be prescribed by a qualified herbal practitioner. A Chinese herb which has a substantial reputation for helping to relieve angina is pseudoginseng root. Nervine relaxants like valerian and lemon balm can be used to calm the nervous system. Lemon balm was often used in medieval cordials, which were taken as medicines for the heart. The word "cordial" comes from the Latin, meaning "pertaining to the heart". The seventeenth-century English diarist, John Evelyn, wrote that "balm steeped in wine comforts the head and driveth away melancholy and sadness".

To prevent angina, follow the advice on diet and exercise given on p. 211. In particular, eat plenty of garlic, onions and leeks, which reduce cholesterol levels and blood pressure.

Arteriosclerosis

Arteriosclerosis is thickening of the arterial walls which tends to occur as a natural consequence of ageing. Atherosclerosis, a term often used interchangeably with arteriosclerosis, however, describes a preliminary process in which fat infiltrates the arterial walls, leading inevitably to arteriosclerosis. The hardening process can go a stage further, with calcification of the arterial walls, and the consequences of this can be dire. If the arteries to the kidneys are affected it can cause a rise in blood pressure. If those to the brain are involved, senility may occur, while atherosclerosis of the cardiac arteries can cause angina pectoris or even heart failure. Such a process also causes "shop window disease" or intermittent claudication, when poor circulation in the legs can cause severe leg cramps after even just a short walk.

Several factors can lead directly to arteriosclerosis, including chronic high blood pressure, diabetes and thyroid disorders. Smoking, the overconsumption of alcohol, animal fats, refined carbohydrates and even caffeinated drinks like tea and coffee can also play their part. A sedentary lifestyle and excess weight also significantly contribute to the problem.

If you suffer from arteriosclerosis, replace all animal fats with polyunsaturated fats. Recent studies also show that fish oils rich in EPA and DHA, which are precursors of hormones called prostaglandins, can effectively thin the blood. Soya lecithin in conjunction with B6 can help this process. Vitamin C with bioflavonoids and extra Vitamin E can also help to combat the disease. Foods which help resolve the condition are apple, lemon, globe artichoke, blueberry, cabbage, carrot, cherry, leek, onion, seaweeds, rye, watercress, soyabeans, sunflower seeds, and walnuts. Raw garlic taken regularly may be antisocial but can reduce the fatty sediment in the arteries very effectively.

Herbs which help to dilate the blood vessels, such as hawthorn, limeflowers, yarrow and mistletoe, can prove of considerable value. You could also try an *infusion* (B, see p. 193) of one of the following herbs: birch leaves, sage, horsetail, lady's mantle, and meadowsweet. Another useful remedy for this condition is a teaspoon of tincture of San Qi ginseng (Panax notoginseng), which effectively lowers blood cholesterol levels.

Varicose veins and haemorrhoids (piles)

Unlike the arteries, veins do not have a specialized pump like the heart to ensure efficient blood flow through them. Although arterial blood pumping into the tissues provides some pressure, veins rely mainly on the pressure of contracting muscles – particularly in the legs – to squeeze the blood through the valves in the veins back to the heart. Because deep

Please check the Glossary for cautions on particular herbs.
If in doubt, consult a qualified practitioner.

veins are often wrapped around the arteries, strong arterial circulation will sometimes milk the veins around them. Also, since the superficial veins are not supported by muscle and connective tissue as the deep veins are, some of these surface veins, with their relatively weak walls, may become swollen or twisted.

The healthy return of blood to the heart through the veins is aided by deep breathing as well as by muscular contractions. As you breathe in, blood is effectively sucked into your chest. So if you suffer from varicose veins, you should practise deep, abdominal breathing.

Varicose veins may be hereditary, but the problem is usually precipitated by lack of exercise, standing for long periods, pregnancy, tight clothing, constipation or excess weight. Varicose veins generally occur in the legs, but may also appear in the testicles where they are called a varicocele or in the rectum or outside the anus where they are called haemorrhoids or piles. Varicose veins are usually visible as swollen bumps or knots under the skin. The area around the damaged veins will often be warmer than surrounding tissue. Consult your doctor if the veins are painful.

Aside from deep breathing, regular exercise is also important, to encourage venous blood to make its way back to the heart. It is also wise not to stand for long periods of time and to avoid crossing your legs. Desk jobs can be equally bad, especially for piles. We spend about a third of our lives in bed, so if you have varicose veins, you could try raising the end of the bed so that your legs are higher than your head. Gravity can then work to keep venous blood flowing throughout the night. In the morning, spray the affected veins with cold water. This helps to tighten the tissues and improve venous return. Elastic support stockings are another way to relieve discomfort and swelling.

Many herbs help to improve varicose veins. Check the glossary for cautions. Those like horsetail and knotgrass, which are rich in silica, strengthen connective tissue, which supports the veins. These herbs are best taken fresh in an *infusion* (A, see p. 193), first blended into the water to make a colloidal solution. Nettles are also a good source of silica, and can be eaten as a vegetable when young, or in soups. Herbs containing bioflavonoids (particularly rutin), like hawthorn, yarrow, shepherd's purse (which is also astringent) and buckwheat all help to maintain the integrity of the walls of the veins, and can be taken as an *infusion* (B, p. 193). Rue, which as its name suggests, is rich in rutin, can be used externally as a cold *compress* (see p. 135) applied to the affected veins (discontinue if a rash appears). St John's wort can be used in the same way.

An important remedy for varicose veins is horsechestnut, which contains astringent tannins, flavonoids and saponins, which decrease the permeability of the vein walls. This can be applied externally as a compress. Another astringent remedy containing a high percentage of tannins is witch hazel, used externally as a cold compress. Inflamed veins can benefit from a witch hazel *decoction* (see p. 193). When it is cool, pour the liquid into an ice tray and leave it in the freezer compartment. When ice cubes have formed, wrap them in a cloth, crush them and hold the cloth to the affected area. Melilot can be taken internally as an *infusion* (B, see p. 193). The coumarins it contains are anti-inflammatory and improve lymphatic drainage, helping to take pressure off the veins. Another excellent remedy, which can be taken internally as a *decoction* of ½ oz (15 mg) to 1 pt (500 ml) water (see p. 193) to aid venous return is stoneroot – good for both varicose veins and haemorrhoids. Golden seal also aids venous return and relieves the portal circulation, reducing any back pressure on the veins in the legs. But never take it if you suffer from high blood pressure or are pregnant. Externally, marigold *compresses* (see p. 135) or calendula ointment can be soothing and healing, and an arnica *compress* (see p. 135) helps to relieve the pain. For the relief of painful haemorrhoids, you can apply pilewort ointment locally, or gently wash the area with a *decoction* (see p. 193) of witch hazel.

Varicose ulcers

If varicose veins deteriorate, tissue drainage may become stagnated, causing the skin to itch (varicose eczema). Worse, if it is knocked, it may break and become ulcerated. Varicose ulcers are slow to heal and require medical attention. Useful here are *poultices* (see p. 135) made from comfrey mixed with honey or marigold flowers. To encourage venous circulation, see varicose veins. To stimulate the lymphatic system and prevent infection, herbs like marigold, cleavers, and purple coneflower are prescribed for internal use.

High blood pressure

Most cases of high blood pressure are of unknown origin – so-called "essential hypertension". But any case of raised blood pressure needs investigation since it may be a sign of kidney or heart disease. Follow your doctor's recommendations.

Two major factors causing high blood pressure are stress and arteriosclerosis. Both are avoidable. Relaxation techniques and meditation can do much to alleviate stress and counselling sessions can help to come to terms with deep-seated anxieties. Diet can play a major part in reducing blood pressure. According to recent medical research conducted in

West Germany, vegetarians have thinner and less sticky blood than meat-eaters. Other medical studies have also shown that a vegetarian diet and taking regular exercise can significantly lower blood pressure.

If you suffer from high blood pressure, you would be wise to adopt a meat-free diet, consisting largely of fresh vegetables, whole cereals and fruit. In particular, try eating half a clove of fresh garlic a day – rolled into a piece of fresh bread and swallowed whole, or chopped into a salad dressing, for example. Celery also helps to reduce blood pressure. Avoid caffeine, which contributes to stress and tension. Instead of tea or coffee, drink water, grape juice (which has bloodpressure-lowering properties) and an *infusion* (A, see p. 193) of equal parts of hawthorn berries, yarrow and limeflower. If you suffer from nervous tension or headaches, add 2 teaspoonfuls of chopped valerian root to this herbal mixture. Rutin tablets taken regularly can also bring the pressure down. Buckwheat is rich in rutin so that this may be eaten, or a tea can be made from it and taken regularly.

If you suffer from high blood pressure, it is important to get rid of excess fluid from your body. To do this, during spring and summer, eat plenty of fresh dandelion leaves in salads. These are a good diuretic and have the added advantage of being rich in potassium. An *infusion* (A, see p. 193) of cornsilk is also an effective diuretic, with a reputation for lowering blood pressure. It naturally makes sense to avoid added salt, which causes fluid retention. Although it may sound severe, take no alcohol for the first three months of this experiment. Take regular exercise, which will also help you to lose weight. It may also help you avoid taking drugs.

Low blood pressure

Low blood pressure only becomes a problem when it is associated with poor circulation, dizziness, faints or general debility. It requires treating within the context of the whole person, but circulatory stimulants like ginger, horseradish, cayenne pepper, and angelica may be combined with other remedies, such as *infusions* (B, see p. 193) of hawthorn and Chinese angelica (dang gui). One remedy in particular, the flowering tops of broom, is used by herbalists to raise chronically low blood pressure.

Poor circulation and chilblains

Bad circulation can be treated by taking circulatory stimulants, such as prickly ash, angelica, and ginger, combining them with remedies that strengthen and dilate the blood vessels like yarrow, hawthorn and horsechestnut. Buckwheat tea and rutin tablets can also be beneficial. If you suffer from bad circulation, you could also try hand and foot baths using a *decoction* (see p. 193) of 2 oz (60g) of fresh ginger, sliced and 3 cinnamon sticks in 4 pts (2 l) water. Add 8 oz (250g) of epsom salts (magnesium sulphate crystals) and soak your hands in the morning and your feet in the evening for 8 mins. You can reuse the bath water for about four or five days, reheating it each time. Seek medical advice on circulation problems, which may be a sign of serious illness.

For chilblains, apply lemon juice, cayenne ointment or tincture of myrrh or arnica and wear plenty of warm clothes.

Anaemia

Anaemia is caused by the reduction of the oxygen-carrying potential of the blood, due to a lack of haemoglo-bin. This may cause symptoms such as pallor, breathlessness on exertion, fatigue, insomnia, dizziness, fainting, mental confusion and a lowered resistance to infection. There are many causes of anaemia and it is certainly not safe merely to assume that it is due to an iron deficiency. Other factors are lack of folic acid, or of B12 and/or protein. B12 may well be present in the diet but due to some derangement of the digestion it is not absorbed. Lack of B12 causes pernicious anaemia. Leukemia can inhibit the production of the red blood cells in bone marrow, causing anaemia. Abnormal production of haemoglobin (sickle-cell anaemia) or of the red blood cells (spherocytosis) can also cause anaemia. A common cause of anaemia is loss of blood, as in excessive or prolonged menstruation, or from internal bleeding due to such

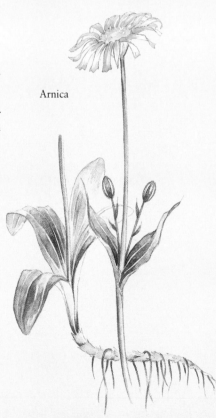

Arnica

conditions as haemorrhoids or ulceration of the gastrointestinal tract. Anaemia can also be caused by hypothyroidism and congenital blood disorders, such as thalassaemia. Women, especially when pregnant, are more prone to anaemia than men. Also at risk are the poor and the elderly.

Check with your doctor to establish the exact cause of anaemia before attempting treatment.

Vegetables, fruit and herbs such as parsley, nettles, watercress, blackcurrants, strawberries and rose hips are good sources of iron. It is remarkable how many plants that contain iron are also rich in Vitamin C which aids the absorption of iron. This demonstrates the natural balance to be found in foods and herbs. Take *decoctions* (see p. 193) of herbs, such as gentian, yellow dock, dandelion, nettles and centaury if you are deficient in iron. They will improve gastro-intestinal absorption of iron and generally strengthen the constitution. Folic acid requirements are increased in women taking the contraceptive pill, alcohol drinkers and by several common drugs, as well as during pregnancy. Richest sources are brewer's yeast, wheatgerm, fresh nuts, liver and green vegetables.

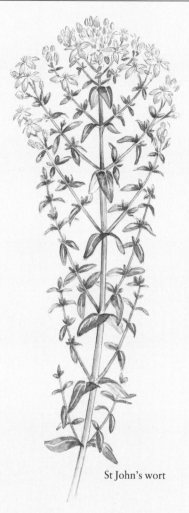

St John's wort

drink will help to restore the normal electrolyte balance if taken before bed: pour one teaspoon of cider vinegar and one of organic honey into a cup of hot water. Celery gives natural salt as well as potassium. Angelica or prickly ash tea will improve general circulation as will cayenne pepper added to food. If varicose veins are the problem, see pp. 208–209. Vitamin deficiency can also be a factor. It is worth taking extra Vitamin E and B if you suffer from chronic cramp. Doctors make use of quinine sulphate for the symptomatic relief of cramp. Some people have found that drinking tonic water, which contains a tiny amount of quinine, can be equally effective.

Cramp

There are many causes of cramp which may be due to an abnormal salt balance (either too little or too much), or a calcium deficiency. Constant stress, which causes chronically tense muscles can also be a factor, as can poor arterial or venous circulation or simple fatigue. It is important to establish the cause in order to treat this complaint effectively.

When you get cramp, do your best to extend and flex the joints of the affected limb. Gently massage the painful area, using warming and relaxing essential oils which stimulate

the circulation, such as chamomile, lavender or rosemary oil diluted in a little olive oil (see p. 193). A hot *compress* of cramp bark is another possibility and some of the oils mentioned can be added to increase its effect. Alternatively, a hot ginger *compress* (see p. 135) will also stimulate the circulation. Chronically bad circulation can be reinvigorated by ginger or mustard footbaths (see p. 196). Stress can be helped by using nervine herbs such as wild oats and skullcap. Calcium levels can be maintained by taking sesame seeds and sesame-seed paste (tahini) in the diet, or drinking horsetail, comfrey or nettle tea, or by taking kelp tablets. The following

The musculoskeletal system

We tend to take our body shape very much for granted. Yet throughout our lives the muscle and bone which largely determine our appearance are constantly being renewed. And the health of our musculoskeletal system is affected not only by how we use it – by our posture, walk, and way of moving – but also by our diet and metabolism, by how well we assimilate and eliminate our food.

The skeleton, comprising bone and cartilage, gives support and protection to the rest of the body. In conjunction with the muscles, it also allows us to move around. The marrow in our bones is a factory in which red blood cells are formed, and the bones themselves are storehouses of the essential elements, calcium, phosphorus, and sodium.

The strength of our bones is largely dependent on the work we ask of them. The greater the weight they bear and the more they bend, the more active are the osteoblasts or bone-forming cells. Bones subjected to continuous loads and strain generally grow thick and strong, while bones not used at all, such as those in plaster casts, waste. There is now medical evidence that aerobic exercise can slow down or even reverse the tendency of bone to become decalcified and brittle as we grow older.

Muscles, aside from their obvious power to enable us to move, also help to maintain our posture and are responsible for a large part of our body heat. Like bones, muscles enlarge and grow stronger when called upon to do regular work. Conversely, the muscle fibre of sedentary people becomes permeated by fat. In the majority of people, muscles form almost half the body weight. So if you learn to relax your muscles, you are effectively learning to relax the whole body. For movement to occur, some muscles have to relax while others contract. In other words, muscle relaxation is as vital as contraction, and much ill health and musculoskeletal degeneration later on in life occur because of our inability to relax.

Chronic muscle tension is often based on emotions that have been inwardly repressed instead of being outwardly expressed. Emotional tensions are often translated into muscular contraction. Anyone suffering from disorders such as arthritis, muscular rheumatism or lumbago needs to look at how much their disease is due to inner tension and at what they can do to learn to relax.

Many musculoskeletal disorders respond quickly to the manipulative therapies, chiropractic and osteopathy, or to massage, shiatsu, rolfing, or acupuncture. And chronic bad posture can be rectified by such methods as the Alexander Technique. However, some musculoskeletal problems are often directly attributable to poor tissue supply or drainage, or to over-relaxation or contraction of the muscles. Here, different kinds of herbal remedies come into their own.

Alterative herbs
Where there is a build-up of toxins in the tissue, a herbalist uses alterative herbs, like burdock, blue flag, echinacea, yellow dock, sarsaparilla, poke root, figwort and nettles. These cleanse the tissues and eliminate toxins. To ensure that these waste materials are voided from the body, alterative herbs are usually combined with herbal diuretics.

Relaxants or tonics
Some disorders respond well to remedies such as crampbark, valerian, mistletoe, skullcap, or lady's slipper, which relax or tone nerves and muscles.

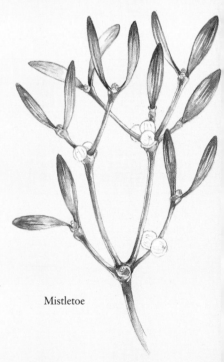

Mistletoe

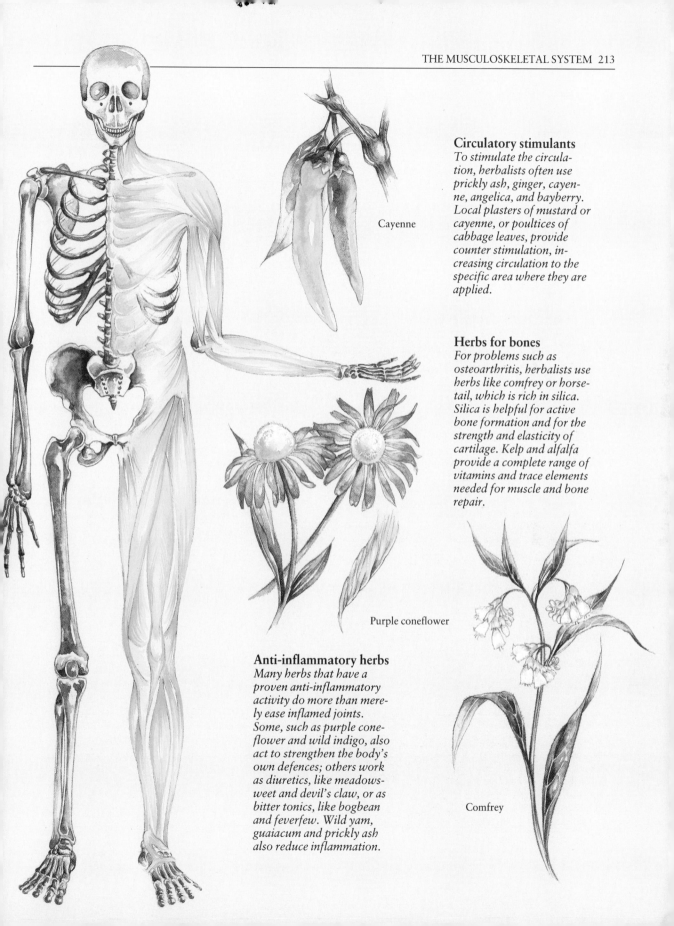

Cayenne

Circulatory stimulants

To stimulate the circulation, herbalists often use prickly ash, ginger, cayenne, angelica, and bayberry. Local plasters of mustard or cayenne, or poultices of cabbage leaves, provide counter stimulation, increasing circulation to the specific area where they are applied.

Herbs for bones

For problems such as osteoarthritis, herbalists use herbs like comfrey or horsetail, which is rich in silica. Silica is helpful for active bone formation and for the strength and elasticity of cartilage. Kelp and alfalfa provide a complete range of vitamins and trace elements needed for muscle and bone repair.

Purple coneflower

Anti-inflammatory herbs

Many herbs that have a proven anti-inflammatory activity do more than merely ease inflamed joints. Some, such as purple coneflower and wild indigo, also act to strengthen the body's own defences; others work as diuretics, like meadowsweet and devil's claw, or as bitter tonics, like bogbean and feverfew. Wild yam, guaiacum and prickly ash also reduce inflammation.

Comfrey

Disorders

Arthritis

Arthritis is inflammation of a joint while rheumatism is an indefinite term used to describe the same problem. There are many different kinds of arthritis and it is important to identify which kind one is dealing with before beginning treatment. The two main kinds are osteoarthritis (sometimes called osteoarthrosis), and rheumatoid arthritis. Although they both cause pain, stiffness and degeneration of the joints, these are two quite separate diseases.

Osteoarthritis is usually caused either by damage to a joint, from a sports injury, for example, or by general wear and tear. In some cases, it is precipitated by obesity, due to extra stress on the joints. The development of bony nodules (known as Heberden's nodes) on the last joints of the fingers is often an early indication of this disease.

While men are more likely to contract osteoarthritis before forty-five, women are more prone to it after this age. After the menopause the oestrogen levels in women drop, making them more susceptible to the action of the parathyroid hormone which causes loss of calcium from the bones. As a result, some women lose more calcium while asleep than they absorb from their diet during the day. However, with a proper diet and a happy and fulfilling life, including regular exercise, this decalcification, called osteoporosis, need not occur.

Rheumatoid arthritis is one of the auto-immune group of diseases, in which the body's defence system goes haywire and attacks its own tissues. In this case, a rogue antibody, which can be found in the blood, is responsible for the inflammation, swelling, pain and stiffness of the joints. Unlike osteoarthritis, rheumatoid arthritis may affect many joints, often with a symmetrical swelling involving the same joint on both sides of the body. The swelling and pain may flit from joint to joint and the sufferer may also run a temperature. In some people small nodules appear just beneath the skin in characteristic areas – just under the elbow, for example. Rheumatoid arthritis is a chronic disease, marked by exacerbations and remissions. Women are three times more likely to contract the condition than men, and it can occur at any age. In children, it is known as Stills disease. Statistics show that those who have a close relative with rheumatoid arthritis run four times the risk of developing the disease themselves.

Another kind of arthritis is gout. The excruciating pain of this disease is caused by the accumulation of thousands of uric acid crystals in the joints, particularly that of the big toe. Gout usually runs in families because of an inherited inability to deal with a product of cell breakdown called purines. Recent research at Oxford University which studied the magnetic field of the human body made the interesting discovery that many gout sufferers also fail to break down fruit sugar (fructose). This leads directly to raised uric acid levels. Fruit and wine, particularly sweet wines, such as port, contain large quantities of fructose, and table sugar also breaks down into fructose and glucose. If you suffer from gout, try to avoid them at all costs. Over-eating, stress and trauma also trigger this disease. Stress greatly increases the breakdown of body cells, which raises uric acid levels. Certain orthodox drugs, particularly diuretics, can also provoke attacks.

The herbal approach to these forms of arthritis is similar but not identical. The fundamental principle is to treat the patient and not the disease. The practitioner has to weigh up the particular imbalances – mento-emotional, hormonal, nutritional, circulatory, nervous or other – present in each patient. It is then possible to give a herbal prescription which is "made to measure" rather than "off the peg".

Dietary measures are important in the treatment of all kinds of arthritis. If the bone and cartilage are to be repaired, it is vital that all the vitamins, trace elements and other necessary nutrients are present in the diet. So a balanced, wholefood diet is essential. As with gout, some foods may aggravate arthritis. These include red meat and pork, citrus fruit and sour or acid

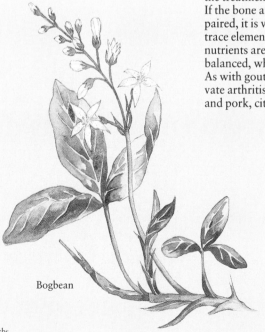

Bogbean

fruit, such as plums, rhubarb, gooseberries, strawberries, and red- and black-currants. Pickles and malt vinegar are also best avoided, and spinach (which like rhubarb contains oxalic acid), can cause painful joints. It is also wise to replace stimulants, like coffee or strong tea with caffeine-free herb teas or spring water. Anyone who has rheumatoid arthritis should investigate their diet for food sensitivities or allergies which may disrupt the immune system. All arthritis sufferers, particularly post-menopausal women, need to maintain a high calcium intake. Provided there is no allergy to dairy products, a cup of warm milk before bed, together with plenty of green leafy vegetables and some sesame-seed paste (tahini), should ensure an adequate calcium intake.

Because rheumatoid arthritis is more common in women than men, particularly after the menopause, herbs which balance the hormonal system, like wild yam, black cohosh, sarsaparilla and licorice, are often prescribed. Seek your doctor's advice before attempting such treatments.

Anti-inflammatory herbs (see p.213), such as bogbean, are important in all forms of arthritis. To reduce inflammation, make a *decoction* (see p. 193) of devil's claw and take this three times a day for six weeks. If gout is your problem, try an *infusion/decoction* (A, see p. 193) of 1 part each of burdock root, purple cone-flower, birch leaves, centaury, devil's claw and ½ part of celery seed. Alterative herbs and diuretics will also help to remove wastes and toxins deposited in the tissues over many years. When treating rheumatoid arthritis, the herbalist may include specific remedies like licorice and wild yam to support the adrenal glands which are a source of natural anti-inflammatory hormones.

Arthritis may be triggered by chronic states of anxiety and tension. Here, herbs which relax and nurture the nervous system can be helpful,

such as crampbark, lady's slipper, wild oats, skullcap and vervain. These will also help to relieve pain.

Local remedies such as capsicum plasters or cabbage and comfrey poultices (see p.135) are useful to stimulate the circulation and encourage healing. Stimulating essential oils, like mint, thyme, rosemary and eucalyptus, in a vegetable oil base, can be gently rubbed into inflamed joints (see p. 193). If the circulation is poor, circulatory stimulants like prickly ash and ginger are called for.

Backache and sciatica

It is important to establish the cause of backache before treating it. It may be due to poor posture, muscular tension, kidney or urinary infection, gynaecological problems, diseases of the bone such as arthritis, or even growths. Consult your doctor for a proper diagnosis. The possibility of a growth should not be overlooked.

If you suffer back pain, avoid lifting heavy weights, standing for long periods, wearing high-heeled shoes or boots, and carrying shoulder-bags.

Many cases of backache are best treated by gentle osteopathic or chiropractic manipulation or the attentions of a trained physiotherapist or acupuncturist. Poor posture can be remedied by learning the Alexander or Feldenkrais techniques or by practising yoga. Herbal remedies can be a valuable adjunct, or sometimes a first line of treatment. To stimulate and relax muscles in spasm, and so allow misaligned bones to fall back into place, ask someone to gently massage your back, with a massage oil or liniments (see p. 134). These should contain relaxing volatile oils such as lavender, chamomile, or geranium, or include herbal extracts of crampbark or cayenne pepper. Herbal plasters containing these and other herbs are another traditional way to give relief from back pain. Spinal nerve pain may be treated by applying St

John's wort oil to the affected part. Applications of oil of wintergreen (see p. 193) are analgesic and anti-inflammatory and can also be used for sciatica and back pain. If the kidneys are weak, resulting in low back pain, take an *infusion* (A, see p. 193) of equal parts of bearberry, cornsilk, horsetail and half a part of lady's slipper. You should consult a doctor if you have weak kidneys.

The urinary system

Consisting of the kidneys, ureters, bladder, and urethra, the urinary system's main function is to produce and excrete urine and thus control the body's water and chemical content. The kidneys are among the body's most important organs – without their constant hard work, we would be poisoned by our own waste products. In traditional Chinese medicine, the kidneys are said to house the primary energy of life, the so-called kidney *jing*, which ultimately determines our longevity and health. In addition, according to the Chinese, the kidneys are responsible for the maintenance of a healthy internal environment or homeostasis of the body, which the Chinese characterize as a harmonious balance between yin and yang.

Each kidney is composed of about a million tiny units, called nephrons. Blood enters the kidneys via the renal arteries and is then filtered out and conveyed to the ureters to be voided as urine, whilst valuable substances, such as glucose and amino acids, are reabsorbed and go back into the bloodstream via the renal veins. The importance of the kidneys rests as much with what they reabsorb as with what is voided as urine. About ninety-eight per cent of the water and most of the nutrients are reabsorbed. Waste products such as urea, which is formed from the breakdown of protein, are passed into the urine and so voided from the body. Urine collects in the pelvis of the kidneys and passes along the ureters to the bladder, where it is stored until urination occurs. During urination, urine is expelled through the urethra. A healthy adult loses about 5 pints (2½ l) of water a day. Of this, 3 pints (1½ l) is passed as urine, while the remaining 2 pints (1 l) consist of moisture lost via the bowel, in perspiration, and through breathing. These figures highlight the important part played by the urinary system in eliminating waste produces and toxins.

As well as regulating the body's water and salt content, specialized cells in the kidneys are responsible for controlling the acid/alkali balance of the body. The kidneys are also able to monitor and raise the body's blood pressure by means of the hormone renin. Via a complex pathway, this hormone causes the arteries to constrict and blood pressure to rise. High blood pressure may in fact be a sign of underlying kidney disease. In addition, the kidneys produce erythropoietin which stimulates bone marrow to make red blood cells.

Herbs for the urinary system are not only beneficial for urinary disorders, but also help the body's cleansing mechanism as a whole. You should never undertake a herbal cleansing programme, however, unless your kidneys are functioning properly. The use of deep-acting alterative herbs, which stimulate the sloughing off of waste material by the body's tissues, is likely to provoke a damaging crisis if kidney elimination is inadequate. It is usually advisable to start by using gentle diuretic remedies, which strengthen the kidneys and encourage metabolic debris to be excreted effectively in the urine.

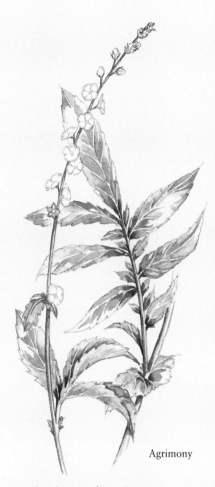

Agrimony

Astringent diuretics
Many herbs help to increase the flow of urine, but a number of diuretics have other, complementary functions. Astringent diuretics, like agrimony and horsetail, help to stop bleeding from the urinary tract (a symptom which always calls for medical investigation).

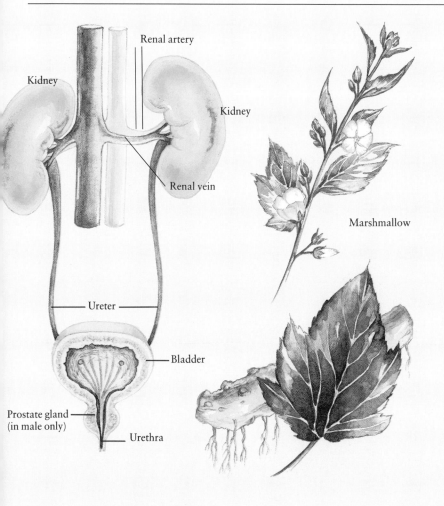

Kidney

Renal artery

Kidney

Renal vein

Ureter

Bladder

Prostate gland
(in male only)

Urethra

Marshmallow

How herbs are diuretic

Some herbal remedies, such as lily of the valley and broom, work by virtue of their action on the heart, since an increased cardiac output enhances the efficiency of kidney filtration. Others contain substances which cannot be reabsorbed from the kidney tubules, for example mannitol from couch grass and the volatile oils in juniper and buchu. Due to osmosis, these also increase the flow of urine. Although herbs containing volatile oils act as effective urinary antiseptics, an infected kidney or urinary tract may be further irritated by herbs containing strong volatile oils, such as juniper. Caffeine in coffee, tea, and cola and the allied substances theobromine and theophylline in tea dilate the blood vessels in the kidney and so have a diuretic effect.

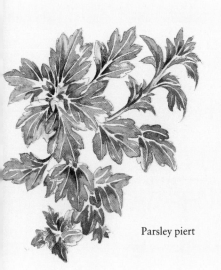

Parsley piert

Antilithic and demulcent diuretics

In addition to increasing urine flow, herbs, such as parsley piert or gravel root have an antilithic effect, eliminating urinary stones or gravel. Other diuretics, like marshmallow, cornsilk and couchgrass, are demulcent and soothing, and so are good for treating an inflamed urinary tract.

Disorders

Cystitis

Cystitis is inflammation of the bladder. Sufferers are all too familiar with the symptoms which may include scalding urine, a dull pain in the lower abdomen, and a frequent urge to pass water. The urine itself may be cloudy because it contains pus or blood and it may also have an unpleasant smell. If untreated, cystitis can be serious or even fatal, so consult your doctor before attempting self-medication.

Cystitis can occur at any age and is about twenty times more common in women than men. This is because the urethra is much shorter in women than in men, so allowing infective organisms easier access to the bladder. Such "ascending" infections are usually announced by discomfort at the urethral opening and as the condition progresses, the irritation travels upwards. These infections are usually caused by the rod-shaped bacterium called *Escherichia coli* (*E. coli* for short). This is a normal bacterium found in the bowel. Some people, it seems, have more *E. coli* in their bowels than others and after a bowel movement these can be wiped on to the urethral opening. Less commonly, infection from the bloodstream and the kidneys descends into the bladder. These "descending" infections are usually heralded by backache, headache, tiredness, and pains in the abdomen.

If you suffer recurrent attacks of cystitis there are several common-sense precautions you can take. Be sure to wash the perineum (the area between the urethra and anus) after every bowel movement and in the morning and evening. Never use powder, cream, antiseptic, or vaginal deodorants since they can irritate the sensitive tissue of your urinary tract. Wear cotton underclothes, change them every day, and wash them with a soap powder instead of biological washing powders. Also, avoid wearing tights which prevent the air from circulating.

Women can guard against attacks of cystitis by avoiding internal tampons, as the cotton wool may contain additives which can injure the sensitive lining of the vagina.

To fight the infection that causes cystitis, you need to make your urine more acid or alkaline. When an attack starts, you can make it more alkaline by taking a teaspoon of sodium bicarbonate (baking soda) in a little water twice a day, but ignore this advice if you have any kind of heart trouble. A vegetarian diet and avoiding acid foods like vinegar, pickles, rhubarb and gooseberries will also help to keep your urine more alkaline.

Cystitis can be triggered by sexual intercourse, if the sensitive lining of the vagina is damaged. KY jelly or comfrey ointment can reduce the risk of bruising. Always pass an effective amount of urine within 15 mins of making love and then wash in water mixed with a teaspoon of witch hazel *tincture* or calendula *tincture* (see p. 135). The urine will flush out any germs which have passed into the bladder during intercourse. Men should wash before intercourse, particularly if uncircumcized. During attacks of cystitis, try to rest as much as possible and use hot water bottles wrapped in towels to help relieve the discomfort.

To reduce the inflammation, drink plenty of water and an *infusion/decoction* (A, see p.193) of 1 part each of marshmallow root, cornsilk, couch grass, horsetail, and bearberry and ½ part of buchu. Take this 4 or 5 times a day.

To soothe the urinary tract, try this recipe for barley water. Boil 4 oz (100 gm) whole barley in a little water, then strain off the water. Now pour 1 pt (500 ml) of water over the cleaned barley and add ½ oz (15 g) of peel of a well-washed lemon. Simmer until the barley is soft, remove from the heat and allow to cool until lukewarm. Strain, add a little honey and drink several cups a day.

Kidney stones and gravel

The causes of kidney stones and gravel (ie smaller deposits) are sometimes obscure but the following factors appear to contribute.

An infection of the urinary tract can cause cellular debris to act as a focus or "seed" on which crystals can form. Bacterial action makes the urine more alkaline, resulting in the deposit of phosphates, which form calcium phosphate stones.

Profuse sweating or a low fluid intake can make the urine more concentrated, causing urinary salts to solidify and stones to form. If you have stones, try to drink 4 to 6 pts (2–3 l) of fluid a day. Drink 1 pt (½ l) of fluid before going to bed, to ensure that washing out continues throughout the night. You should drink enough to ensure that your twenty-four hour urine output is never less than 3 pts (1½ l).

Excessive uric acid, as in gout, increased excretion of calcium by the kidney, combined with an increased insolubility of calcium in the urine, can also cause stones to form. Long-term confinement to bed or even a chronic lack of exercise may encourage mobilization of calcium from the bones into the blood and so increase calcium levels in the urine. Similarly, steroids can increase blood and urine calcium levels. An inherited disposition and excess weight can also predispose you to kidney stones.

There are three different kinds of kidney stone: uric acid stones, calcium oxalate stones, and calcium phosphate stones. If you find gravel in your urine, take it to your doctor to have it analyzed. Once you know what kind of stone it is, you can take appropriate action. If the stones are formed from uric acid, the urine will be acid. You can check the acidity with pH papers bought from any chemist. To dissolve these stones, eat an alkaline diet, including potatoes, vegetables and fruit (not citrus). Reduce your protein intake, since eating protein tends to increase uric-acid levels. In particular, avoid liver, kidneys, sweetbreads, fishroe, sardines, and sprats. Also, drink alkalinizing mineral water.

If the stones are formed from calcium oxalate, avoid foods containing oxylates, such as spinach, rhubarb, beet, parsley, sorrel, and chocolate. Those who have a tendency to form oxylate stones often secrete too much calcium in their urine, which reacts with oxalic acids to form the stones. For this reason it is also advisable to restrict dairy products which are rich in calcium. Drink mineral waters that are rich in magnesium to increase the solubility of calcium. Both Vitamin B6 and folic acid are thought to restrict the amount of calcium formed in the body.

Calcium phosphate stones are usually formed when there is a urinary infection. In such cases, the urine is alkaline, so if your doctor confirms you have this kind of stone, eat foods to acidify the urine such as meat, fish, and eggs. Once again, however, avoid dairy products.

To dissolve and wash out stones of all kinds, try an *infusion/decoction* (A, see p. 193) of 1 part each of hydrangea, parsley piert, pellitory of the wall, couch grass, cornsilk and cleavers, and 2 parts each of gravel root and marshmallow root.

Prostate disease

The prostate gland is an accessory organ of the male reproductive system. The gland is normally about the size of a chestnut, but if it becomes inflamed or enlarged, it may exert pressure on the urethra, through which it passes. Or it may block the outlet to the bladder, so obstructing the flow of urine. If this happens, it can cause interrupted or difficult urination (so-called dribbling incontinence) or urgent or frequent urination, especially at night. There may

be pain on urination too. Urine trapped in the bladder may become infected and cause cystitis, and backward pressure can lead to kidney infection. The high level of urea retained in the blood can sometimes be a cause of mental confusion.

There are three types of prostate disease: prostatitis, benign enlargement of the prostate, and cancer of the prostate. Prostatitis is infection of the prostate gland either from urinary infection or venereal disease or from some blood-borne infection. Here the main symptom is painful urination and groin or back pain. There may also be a fever. Qualified medical help should be sought but you can alleviate the condition by taking an *infusion/decoction* (A, see p. 193) of 1 part each of bearberry, golden rod, gravel root and couch grass, and 2 parts each of echinacea and horsetail.

Benign enlargement of the prostate gland is extremely common – in North America and northern Europe half the men over sixty suffer from it. It seems to be partly triggered by sedentary work and delay in passing water. In some cases, however, the enlargement is related to changes in the relative amounts of oestrogen and androgen caused by the ageing process. Any prostate problem calls for a rectal examination by a qualified practitioner and, in some cases, blood and urine tests. Enlargement of the prostate gland can be helped by long-term herbal treatment. Some herbs work directly on the prostate, while others aid the male hormone balance.

If you have enlargement of the prostate gland, take a handful of pumpkin seeds each day. They contain a male hormone-type component and zinc which both benefit the prostate. Extra Vitamin E and zinc can also help. Take plenty of exercise and herbal sitz baths containing a strong *infusion* (see p. 193) of equal parts of each of the following herbs: horsetail, juniper, couch grass, and bear-

berry in equal parts. Use 2 oz (60 g) of the mixture to each 1 pt (½ l) of water. Some herbs work directly on the prostate; others aid the male hormone balance. For hormonal problems, try an *infusion/decocotion* (see p. 193) of 1 part each of sarsaparilla, false unicorn root, damiana, hydrangea, and solidago, and 2 parts each of sabal and couch grass.

A small number of enlarged or inflamed prostates may be cancerous. This fact underlies the need for a proper medical investigation.

Bedwetting (enuresis)

Children who wet the bed may do so for emotional reasons. They may feel insecure due to the arrival of a new baby, a change of school or because of the parents' marital problems. In these cases, the child needs love and reassurance. Sometimes bedwetting occurs because of lack of nervous control of the bladder. In this case, give an *infusion* (B, see p. 193) of 1 part each of horsetail, St John's wort, cornsilk, wild oat, and lemon balm. Give half a cup three times a day, and try to give the last dose well over an hour before bedtime. Also give 500–1,000 mg of oil of evening primrose daily and add pumpkin seeds and wheatgerm to the diet. Set up a gentle reward system to help remove any psychological block. Get your child to put a red star on a calendar for each dry night. A dry week gets a gold star. Also try not to give any drinks after six o'clock at night, and massage St John's wort oil into the base of the spine before bedtime.

Kidney disease

Because the kidneys are such a vital organ, it is inadvisable to practise self-help medicine if you suspect kidney disease. In such cases seek help from a qualified practitioner.

The female reproductive system

Since ancient times, women have used plant medicines to regulate and reduce the pain of menstruation and to make childbirth easier and less painful. Modern scientific analysis confirms the validity of this, since many of the herbal remedies used for these purposes contain steroidal saponins, which closely resemble human hormones. Indeed, for many years, extracts of the wild yam were used to provide the raw material from which the contraceptive pill was manufactured (see p. 56). For centuries prior to this, North American Indian women had used the wild yam for its effects on the reproductive system – to ease menstrual cramping and prevent miscarriage.

Since the female reproductive system is more complex than its male counterpart, it more often requires the gentle support of herbal remedies. The system operates according to an approximate twenty-eight day cycle. During the first half of this cycle, the uterus prepares for pregnancy, making itself ready to receive a fertilized egg or ovum released from one or other of the ovaries around the fourteenth day of the cycle. The process of pregnancy itself only proceeds, however, if the ovum is fertilized on its way to the womb. In the days leading up to ovulation, the cells of the lining of the womb (the endometrium) proliferate so the lining thickens. This process continues after ovulation until the lining is about 6 mm thick. The lining is richly supplied with blood vessels which constrict if fertilization of the ovum does not occur. This cuts off the blood supply to the lining, causing it to be shed and menstruation to occur, a process which takes about five days. At the end of menstruation the cycle starts again.

The menstrual cycle is controlled by hormones – chemical messengers secreted by the pituitary gland and the ovaries. After menstruation, the level of the hormone progesterone is low. The pituitary gland secretes follicle-stimulating hormone (FSH) which stimulates the development of the ovum and the secretion of the hormone oestrogen by the graafian follicle, the outer casing of which contains the ovum. Oestrogen causes thickening of the lining of the womb. About the ninth day of the cycle, the pituitary gland secretes another hormone, luteinizing hormone (LH), into the blood. Under the influence of LH, the mature follicle ruptures, expelling the ripe ovum, a process called ovulation. It also causes the formation of the yellow corpus luteum in the ruptured follicle. The corpus luteum secretes progesterone which, together with oestrogen, prepares the lining of the womb to receive a fertilized egg. If fertilization does not occur, around day twenty-five progesterone and oestrogen secretion ceases and blood levels of these hormones fall dramatically. No longer supported by the female hormones, the lining of the womb degenerates and is shed during menstruation. Once again, the low level of progesterone acts as a feedback mechanism to stimulate the pituitary to secrete FSH.

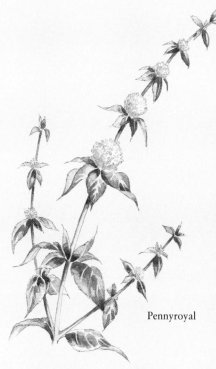

Pennyroyal

Pennyroyal
Pennyroyal has been used since ancient times to promote menstruation often with fatal consequences. Many women have died trying to procure abortions by using pennyroyal oil.

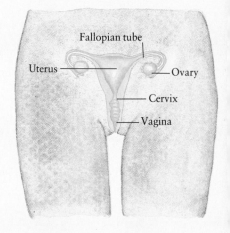

Fallopian tube

Uterus

Ovary

Cervix

Vagina

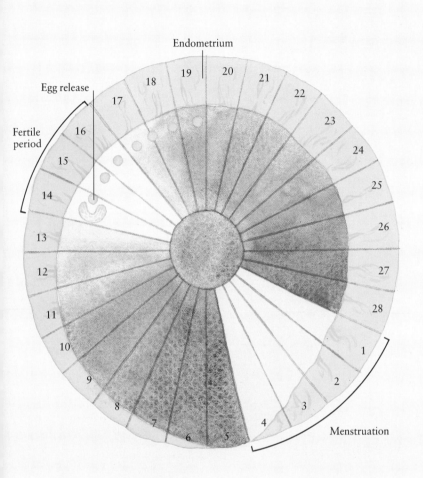

Endometrium

Egg release

Fertile period

Menstruation

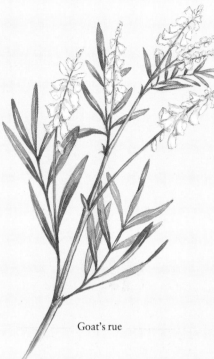

Goat's rue

Galactagogues

Many herbs display hormonal properties and some, like goat's rue, have traditionally been used to stimulate milk production. These herbs not only increase the amount of milk, but also improve its quality. Some galactagogues, like fennel and aniseed, have essential oils which pass to the baby in diluted form through the mother's milk. This in turn helps the infant's digestion.

Cranesbill

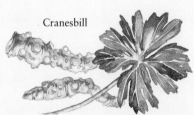

Astringents

Remedies like cranesbill and raspberry leaf have a wide range of uses because of their astringent tannins, which tone up the mucous membranes and muscles of the reproductive tract, and reduce leucorrhoea and excess bleeding. (It is important always to have these symptoms checked out by a doctor.)

Disorders

Premenstrual syndrome

Premenstrual syndrome (PMS) affects about 40 per cent of women of menstruating age, and includes physical, mental, and emotional symptoms. Note: Since PMS symptoms resemble those of pregnancy, always consult your doctor before attempting herbal treatment.

With PMS, the main aim of herbal treatment is to redress the hormone imbalance. One remedy alone, oil of evening primrose, has been outstandingly successful in easing PMS, particularly breast swelling. The oil provides gamma linoleic acid (GLA), from which the body may manufacture the hormone-like prostaglandin PGE1. The recommended dose is 3,000 mg a day taken for 10 days prior to the period. The benefits can be enhanced by simultaneously taking Vitamin B6, Vitamin E, calcium, and zinc.

Research at the University of Göttingen has shown that chaste tree appears to stimulate the pituitary gland to secrete hormones which in turn encourages the corpus luteum to produce progesterone and oestrogen. Herbalists recommend that ½ teaspoon of the *tincture* (see p. 135) be taken before breakfast for several months. False unicorn root, which contains hormone-like saponins is another helpful remedy. Take 2–3 cups of a *decoction* (see p. 193) of this herb every day.

There are also remedies for specific symptoms. For a headache, try an *infusion* (C, see p. 193) of 1 part each of chamomile, pasque flower and valerian, and 2 parts each of skullcap and vervain, and drink one cup 2–3 times a day. For fluid retention, drink an *infusion* (A, see p. 193) of cornsilk and reduce your salt intake.

Herbalists distinguish between two kinds of painful periods. It may be an over-active or excess (sthenic) condition, characterized by intense cramps which subside when the menstrual flow starts. Dark red or purple blood clots may be present.

Alternatively, it can be an under-active or deficient (asthenic) condition. Here the pain comes on during or after menstruation and the flow is scanty or pale in colour. If you suddenly start suffering from painful periods, you should visit a doctor.

For the excess type, herbalists may use a mixture of pasque flower, lady's slipper, chamomile, blue cohosh, crampbark, black haw, wild yam and motherwort.

For treating the deficient type, the herbalist may use a mixture of prickly ash, Chinese angelica, false unicorn root, squaw vine, motherwort, vervain, and borage.

If you suffer painful cramps, you may get relief from an *infusion* (A, see p. 193) of 1 part of crampbark, chamomile and wild yam and ½ part of prickly ash.

Excessive or prolonged periods (menorrhagia)

If you have constant heavy periods you should consult a doctor or gynaecologist. It may indicate a serious complaint or may simply be caused by an IUD. In cases where the cause is not clear, a herbalist may use herbs which tone up and astringe the uterus and so stop the bleeding. These include agrimony, beth root, white deadnettle, shepherd's purse, cranesbill, and raspberry leaves.

Absent periods (amenorrhoea)

If periods are absent you may be pregnant or, if you are over thirty-eight, the possibility of menopause should be considered. If neither applies, then gentle herbal remedies may stimulate the resumption of menstruation. Herbalists use false unicorn root, pennyroyal, motherwort, blue cohosh, Chinese angelica, mugwort, cinnamon, and ginger.

Threatened miscarriage

If you think you are in danger of a miscarriage, consult your doctor or obstetrician immediately. If the foetus is poorly developed, no herbal treatment can prevent a miscarriage. If a weakness in the mother threatens the foetus, herbs can help to sustain the pregnancy. Herbs used by herbal practitioners to prevent miscarriage include wild yam, false unicorn root, black haw, and squaw vine.

Childbirth

During the last three months of pregnancy, you can drink two herb teas which tone up the uterus and ease childbirth. These are *infusions* (B, see p. 193) of either raspberry leaf or squaw vine. Alternatively make an *infusion* of equal parts of the two herbs.

During the birth, if your contractions are weak, try sipping an *infusion* (B, see p. 193) of either blue or black cohosh, which will help to strengthen uterine contractions. Talk to your doctor or midwife about this treatment before the birth.

Breast-feeding

Many breast-feeding problems occur because the baby is not properly latched on to the breast.

To soothe sore or cracked nipples, apply comfrey, marigold, or chickweed ointment. You could also use a cold *poultice* (see p. 135) of chopped cucumber or freshly gathered chickweed.

To stimulate or enhance milk supply, try an *infusion* (B, see p. 193) of any of the following herbs: vervain, borage, goat's rue, blessed thistle, dill, fennel, aniseed, chaste tree, or raspberry leaves.

To stop milk production, try a stronger *infusion* using 2 teaspoons of sage to a cup of boiling water.

Please check the Glossary for cautions on particular herbs.
If in doubt, consult a qualified practitioner.

Menopause

The menopause marks the end of a woman's child-bearing age. Usually occurring in the early fifties, this is when menstruation ceases.

Many women experience the change of life with little or no discomfort. Undoubtedly, taking regular exercise, eating a balanced, wholefood diet and leading a happy and full life with the support of an understanding partner can help to minimize any discomforts. However, some women do experience health problems related to the drop in oestrogen and progesterone that occurs at this time. These symptoms may include hot flushes, depression, palpitations and a drying up of the natural secretions of the vagina, making sexual intercourse painful. The usual orthodox medical answer to these problems is hormone replacement therapy (HRT). But it is worth trying a herbal hormone-balancing mixture rather than resorting to HRT.

To balance the hormones, make a *decoction* (see p.193) of 1 part of each of the following herbs: false unicorn root, black cohosh, blue cohosh, chaste tree, blessed thistle, wild yam, squaw vine, and ½ part of licorice.

Hot flushes can be controlled by drinking a mixed *infusion* (B, see p. 193) of sage and motherwort (a teaspoon of each). Vitamin E (around 400 IU a day) can also help.

A mixture of Vitamin E oil and comfrey ointment can be applied directly to the vagina. Making love regularly contributes to a healthy vaginal membrane.

For depression at menopause, try *infusions* (B, see p. 193) of any one of the following herbs: wild oats, St John's wort, vervain, borage, lemon balm, motherwort, rosemary, or skullcap. Palpitations can respond to an *infusion* (B, see p. 193) of equal parts of valerian, lemon balm, hawthorn, and motherwort. In both cases, consult your doctor before attempting herbal treatment.

Thrush

Thrush is infection by *Candida albicans*, a yeast which lives in all of us. The problem occurs when this yeast gets out of control and infests the mouth and throat, the whole of the digestive tract and the genito-urinary system. Candida can even invade the bloodstream and other body tissues. If allowed to run riot, candida can cause a variety of physical and even mental symptoms, since it sometimes manufactures the toxic substance, acetaldehyde.

Since *Candida albicans* thrives in moist, warm, damp areas, women may be particularly prone to vaginal thrush especially during pregnancy.

Vaginal thrush makes itself felt by intense itching and soreness and a thick white discharge. Infestation of the digestive tract can cause abdominal bloating, pain, and diarrhoea. Thrush in the mouth or throat can lead to swollen glands and a sore throat as well as a sore mouth and tongue.

Another group particularly prone to thrush are diabetics, in whom higher than normal levels of blood sugar and the presence of sugar in the urine can create ideal conditions for candida to multiply. In general, candida infestation is on the increase. This is probably due in part to the wide use of antibiotics and steroids. These knock out other natural yeasts in our system which keep candida under control, and tend to undermine the strength of our immune system, which can combat candida. Even those who do not take antibiotics may receive them at second hand, for example by eating meat that is contaminated with antibiotic residues.

The other factor in the explosion of candida-induced problems is poor diet. To prevent and relieve thrush, try to avoid sugar and sweet food and drinks, cutting out cakes, biscuits and all refined starches. It is also essential to exclude for a time food and drinks carrying yeast spores or those made by fermentation. These include

mushrooms, vinegar, soya sauce, cheese (cottage cheese may sometimes be tolerated), dried fruit, malted products, and alcohol. Replace yeasted with unleavened bread.

Some foods actually help to control candida. Cold-pressed olive oil, for example, contains oleic acid which prevents the growth of yeast infection. Garlic is also anti-fungal and unsweetened, live yoghurt can help to prevent and treat thrush. A lactobacillus supplement, available from health-food stores, also supplies friendly yeast which can control thrush.

Herbs such as marigold, golden seal, rosemary, hyssop, thyme, and fennel all have anti-fungal properties. These can be *infused* (using infusion B) or *decocted* (see p. 193).

For vaginal thrush, make the same infusion or decoction and add a few drops of the essential oil of either thyme, oregano, hyssop, tea tree, or cinnamon to the brew. Use it as a douche or to soak pads, which you can then apply to the vulva to soothe the itching or burning. In such cases, it is essential to avoid wearing tights or nylon pants which can cause an ideal environment for yeast to multiply. Alternatively try a chamomile sitz bath or a bath of salt and water. For a chamomile bath, make an *infusion* (A, see p. 193), allow it to cool and add it to the bath water, which should also be cool. Bathe for a few minutes. You can also apply live, sugar-free yoghurt to the sore areas.

For thrush in the mouth and throat, make a mouthwash with astringent herbs like witch hazel, bistort, or sage. Make an *infusion* (B, see p. 193), allow to cool and add two drops of thyme oil to each cup. Alternatively, use a teaspoon of tincture of myrrh or calendula diluted in a cup of water. You can also gargle or wash your mouth out with pure lemon juice diluted in an equal amount of water. A general disinfectant is a *decoction* (see p. 193) of purple coneflower tea.

The nervous system

Today it is commonly understood that disease is as likely to be caused by the mind (or psyche) as by the body (or soma). Psychological problems may be manifested on a physical level while, conversely, physical problems may have ramifications in the psychological sphere. Nowhere is the interconnectedness of the human structure and the reciprocal relationship between mind and body so evident as in the nervous system.

The nervous system is made up of nerve cells called neurones, which consist of a cell body and a long fibre called an axon. What we call nerves are in fact bundles of these fibres. Some axons are very long, running from the spinal cord to the feet, for example. Nerve cells can transmit messages from one to the other, enabling us to process information from the world outside and to regulate our inner world.

There are two main parts to the nervous system – the central nervous system, which comprises the brain and spinal cord, and the peripheral nervous system. Within the peripheral nervous system are the voluntary or somatic nervous system and the involuntary or autonomic nervous system. The voluntary or somatic system comprises 43 pairs of peripheral nerves which emerge from the central nervous system. There are two types of peripheral nerves – sensory or afferent nerves which conduct sensory information to the spinal cord and brain, and motor or efferent nerves which transmit instructions from the brain to the body. The brain and spinal cord thus receive, process, and act on information received from the peripheral system.

The autonomic nervous system governs such reflex activities as digestion, respiration, and blood circulation. It comprises two parts, the sympathetic and parasympathetic nervous systems. The sympathetic nervous system consists of nerves issuing from the spinal cord, in the chest region: the parasympathetic nervous system consists of two groups of nerves, one group emerging from the cranial region, the other from the bottom of the spinal cord, in the lower back region. The sympathetic system prepares us for action in the face of possible danger – for the "fight and flight" response. When we sense danger, the sympathetic nervous system facilitates those body functions that aid muscular activity while reducing those which hinder muscle efficiency. Thus digestive functions are reduced and saliva flow ceases, producing a dry mouth; the skin becomes pale as blood is withdrawn to feed the muscles; sweat glands step up their secretion to cool the body down; heart rate and breathing quicken; and pupils dilate, to improve eyesight. The parasympathetic system acts to redress the balance once the crisis has passed, slowing down breathing and heartbeat and relaxing the muscles. Today, these body responses are often unnecessarily triggered by the strains and tensions of modern life. Fortunately, however, there are many herbal remedies for the nervous system which act to counter this stress.

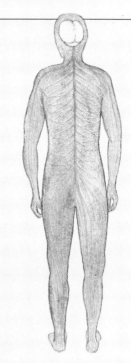

Categories of herbs
There are two main types of herbs for nervous disorders – relaxants and restoratives. Nervous stimulants have a more limited use. Excessive use of stimulants stresses the nervous system.

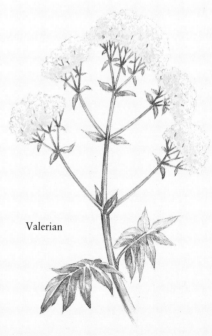

Valerian

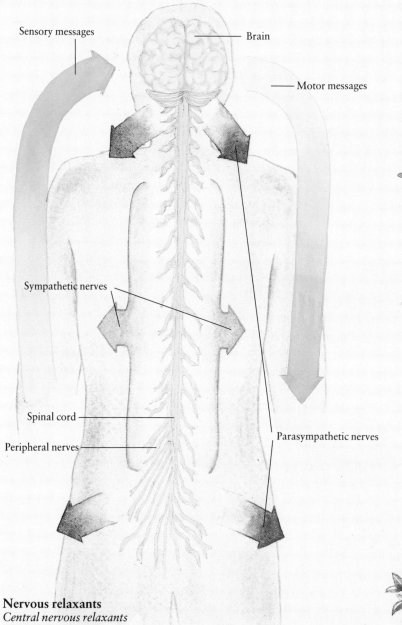

Sensory messages

Brain

Motor messages

Sympathetic nerves

Spinal cord

Peripheral nerves

Parasympathetic nerves

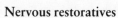

Vervain

Nervous restoratives
Examples of these are vervain, skullcap, wild oat, and ginseng. Nervous restoratives such as these are useful to take when your nervous system is debilitated or run down, for example after a long illness.

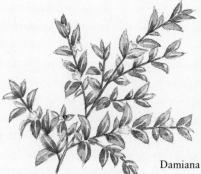

Damiana

Nervous relaxants
Central nervous relaxants abound, for example passion flower, valerian, crampbark, hops, and chamomile. The latter two also act locally to ease an over-contracted digestive system. Herbs containing volatile oils can directly affect the limbic system of the brain via the olfactory cortex – which explains the effectiveness of aromatherapy.

Nervous stimulants
Coffee, tea, and cola all contain caffeine, which is a central nervous stimulant. Damiana also tends to stimulate the nervous system. The use of stimulants like these on a long-term basis is to be avoided, however, since they will rapidly deplete the body's energy reserves and lead to exhaustion.

Disorders

Migraines and headaches

Migraines are intense, usually one-sided headaches, sometimes signalled by a distortion of vision and often accompanied by nausea and vomiting and a sensitivity to light. Such headaches occur, it seems, when arteries in the brain first constrict and then become flaccid. At the height of an attack swollen arteries on the face and head can sometimes be seen, and may be tender to the touch.

Migraines can be effectively treated using a combination of dietary measures, herbs, and relaxation techniques. Migraine sufferers are often high achievers and perfectionists who need to learn how to adopt a more "laid back" lifestyle.

Some women experience migraines around the time of their period. In these cases there is usually a hormonal imbalance (see p. 220).

If you suffer from migraines, try eating a fresh leaf of feverfew (see p. 43) between two slices of bread, once a day as a prophylactic. In addition, you can drink an *infusion* (A, see p. 193) of 1 part each of chamomile, hawthorn, hops, and peppermint, 2 parts each of wood betony and skullcap, and ½ part of pasque flower. Other herbs which you may add to your infusion are limeflower, valerian, rosemary, and vervain.

Local applications are also useful. Mix 10 drops of rosemary or lavender oil into an eggcup-ful of vegetable oil and rub gently onto the affected area. Mint leaves, moistened and applied to the temples, can also be useful. An *infusion* (A, see p. 193) of peppermint or chamomile can also help the nausea and the headache.

Certain foods are known to act as triggers for many migraine sufferers. If you suffer from migraines try avoiding the following foods and see if there is an improvement: coffee, tea, cocoa, chocolate, yeast-extract, oranges, bananas, hard cheeses, alcohol, cream, pickles, pilchards. In addition, adopt a largely vegetarian

diet. Do regular relaxation exercises, and avoid getting up later at weekends than usual, since this can sometimes precipitate a migraine.

Insomnia

Nothing, perhaps, is more likely to destroy the quality of life than an inability to sleep properly. There are many reasons why we may not sleep well. As we grow older, we usually need less sleep and provided we are happy and busy, the extra working hours we gain can be extremely useful. Taking a nap during the day can also account for a shortened sleep at night. Sometimes there are specific problems which account for insomnia, such as painful joints or a thyroid condition. Certainly, it is unwise to eat a heavy meal late at night or to drink caffeinated drinks before going to bed. Most commonly, however, insomnia is a reflection of a high level of tension during the day. Relaxation and meditation as well as regular exercise can help to calm an over-stressed nervous system.

Whatever the cause of the insomnia, it is best to avoid sleeping pills at all costs since they can undermine your general health when taken over a long period. They are addictive, too, and many people experience withdrawal symptoms when trying to wean themselves off them.

Herbal remedies offer a safe and non-addictive alternative to sleeping pills. Try drinking an *infusion* (B, see p. 193) of a teaspoon to a cup of boiling water of chamomile or limeflower. Alternatively, you could try an *infusion* of 2 teaspoons of the following mixture in 1 cup of boiling water, half an hour before going to bed: 2 parts each of passionflower and skullcap, 1 part each of valerian and hops, and ½ part of licorice.

You can also try taking a relaxing herbal bath. Make a muslin bag and fill it full of herbs or lavender and tie

Ginseng
Ginseng contains substances that both calm and stimulate the nerves.

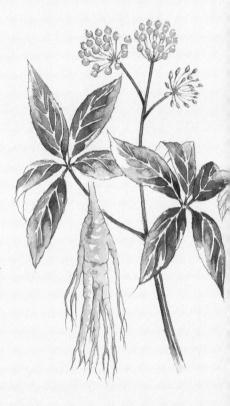

the bag on to the hot tap so that the hot water runs through it. Before you get into the bath add a strained infusion of the same herbs you have in your muslin bag to top up the potency of the herb bath. Just make sure that you don't go to sleep in the bath!

Another effective sleep aid is two teaspoons of cider vinegar and one of honey, mixed into a cup of hot water. It may be that the other trace elements in this mixture have a soothing effect on the nervous system and therefore induce sleep.

Anxiety

Chronic anxiety is a background to much ill health and is often a response to stress. Twentieth-century lifestyles tend to provoke sympathetic nervous arousal – the "fight or flight" mechanism – without allowing an outlet for this adrenalized state. For this reason, anxiety is described as "fear spread thin" and calls for herbs which restore and relax both the central and the sympathetic nervous systems. Chamomile, limeflower, hops, valerian, and lady's slipper are all relaxing herbs which when *infused* (B, see p. 193) can calm an overstressed nervous system. *Infusions* (B, see p. 193) of vervain, skullcap, and wild oats can also be used to strengthen and support the nervous system. Massages using *essential oils* (see p. 193) of lavender, rose, or neroli can also reduce the stress level. Try also the Bach Flower Remedies (see p.235). Meditation, relaxation exercises and counselling can be an enormous help in relieving the symptoms and the underlying causes of the anxiety.

Depression

If you suffer from depression, consult your doctor. Severe depression may have organic causes and may require medical treatment.

Herbal remedies can do much to counter the physical exhaustion and debility that often underlies this condition.

Make use of herbs which strengthen and support your nervous system, such as wild oats, ginseng (available as capsules or tablets from a health food store), damiana, vervain, skullcap and wood betony. Lemon balm, rosemary, St John's wort and borage are particularly appropriate to raise the spirits. These can be taken as *infusions* (B, see p. 193). Also good for depression are *essential oils* (see p. 193) of bergamot, orange,

lemon, jasmine, neroli, and rose, used as a healing massage oil.

Regular counselling can bring greater understanding of the deep causes of depression and help to inspire a positive self-image which is lacking in depression. Regular exercise is also an effective measure against depression, since it stimulates the production of potent mood-elevating hormones, known as endorphins, which can help to improve your outlook.

A wholefood diet is essential to provide a range of nutrients to feed your nervous system. You may also find it helpful to take brewer's yeast, which is rich in the B vitamins that help to blow away the blues. It is also worth trying the Bach Flower Remedies (see p.235).

Neuralgia (nerve pain)

Nerve pain is often a prayer for nutrition to the affected part, so all the physiological factors that contribute to health have to be considered. A purely symptomatic treatment which merely aims to block the pain will not solve the problem.

A herbal practitioner will assess whether the affected area is over-contracted or over-relaxed and flaccid. If the area is over-contracted, a herbalist might prescribe herbal relaxants, such as crampbark, valerian, hops, wild lettuce, and lady's slipper.

Local treatments with *compresses* (see p. 135) of these herbs or lobelia plasters, which are only to be prescribed by trained herbal practitioners, can be beneficial. If, however, the affected area lacks tone, a herbalist might use such remedies as St John's wort, wild oat, damiana, skullcap, and vervain. Remedies like ginger, angelica, and hawthorn can encourage the arterial blood supply to the area and ginger *compresses* (see p. 135) can also be useful if the area is cold and flaccid. Lymphatic and venous drainage can be encouraged

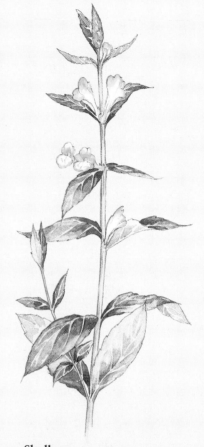

Skullcap

Skullcap, which acts as a tonic, a sedative and an anti-spasmodic, helps to strengthen and support the nervous system. It has been successfully used to treat a wide range of nervous disorders, including migraines, depression, anxiety, insomnia, and neuralgia.

by using cleavers and marigold. St John's wort oil, used externally, is specific for painful and damaged nerves, and is particularly useful for sciatica. Herbal baths containing some of the herbs mentioned and hot or cold *compresses* (see p. 135) can also be soothing for nerve pain. But in every case, consult your doctor to determine the underlying cause.

The eye

Light is essential to life, and our eyes connect us directly to it. As it enters the eye light is focused by the lens and then passes to the sensitive receptor cells of the retina, at the back of the eyeball. Here the electromagnetic wave patterns of light are converted into nerve impulses and sent via the optic nerve to the brain where they are interpreted as images. Light is as necessary for our mental health as for our physical wellbeing. Recent research has identified a particular type of depression, appropriately labelled SAD (seasonal affective disorder), which is induced by lack of light, as in the dark winter months of the northern hemisphere. It has also been discovered that teardrops produced by crying contain minute amounts of potent endorphine hormones which act like powerful opiates to calm us down and make us feel better. Such findings merely confirm what we have always known, that the eyes are the windows of the soul. The sparkle or glint in the eye is the first thing a herbalist looks for to show that a patient is on the mend.

We use our eyes throughout our waking hours, but hardly spare them a thought unless they go wrong. Yet correct use of the eyes is essential if we wish to avoid failing eyesight later on in life. The value of eye exercises has been known in yoga practice for thousands of years. In China today, schoolchildren routinely start their day with eye exercises and we would be wise to follow suit. Begin the day by splashing cold water on to your eyes. Afterwards, sit quietly and roll your eyes to the right, then to the left. Without moving your head look up and down, left and right, and horizontally and diagonally. Cup your hands over your closed eyes and imagine you are looking at deep black velvet for about half a minute. You will find this most restful for your eyes. Exercise your eye muscles by altering your focal length. Look at a pencil held at the end of your nose and then into the distance out of a window. This is a good exercise for city-dwellers and those whose work involves reading or staring at computer screens, who are deprived of the healing and strengthening effect of gazing at distant horizons. Finally, try to remember from time to time during the day to "colour" or "shape" your world, for seeing does not necessarily imply looking. Do this by becoming aware of the colour and shape of the objects around you. You will be surprised how much more vivid the world becomes.

Herbs can be successfully used to treat disease affecting the superficial areas of the eye, such as the eyelids and conjunctiva – the transparent membrane covering the eyeballs. But more serious problems affecting the inner eye or the optic nerve, such as glaucoma, iritis, detached retina, cataract, and the other various causes of blindness, are not so easily rectified by herbal medicine. This is not to say, however, that in these cases some good cannot be done by improving the health of the whole person.

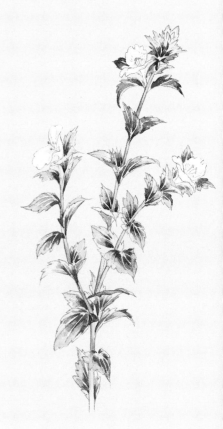

Eyebright
Culpeper may have been ex-aggerating in his claim for eyebright that "if the herb were as much used as neg-lected, it would spoil half the spectacle-makers' trade." But certainly it is an excellent remedy for eye problems, used externally as a compress or as a sterile eyewash.

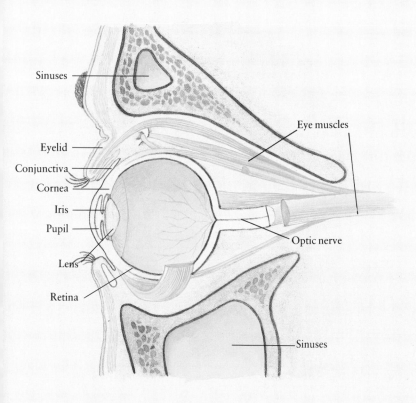

Sinuses

Eye muscles

Eyelid

Conjunctiva

Cornea

Iris

Pupil

Optic nerve

Lens

Retina

Sinuses

Disorders

Conjunctivitis and blepharitis

Conjunctivitis is inflammation of the conjunctiva, the mucous membrane which coats most of the eyeball and the eyelids. Acute conjunctivitis is generally caused by infection from bacteria or a virus, but may be triggered by an allergic reaction, as in hayfever. Chronic conjunctivitis may be as a result of infection or exposure to polluted air in inner cities. And it sometimes occurs in the elderly if the eye secretions dry up. One kind of viral conjunctivitis called "trachoma" or Egyptian opthalmia, prevalent in the Third World, may lead to blindness. Blepharitis is inflammation of the eyelids, caused by infection.

Both problems can usually be safely treated with eyebright and marigold flower eyebaths (see Tired, strained eyes). A weak *decoction* (see

p. 193) of golden seal, using ½ teaspoon of the root boiled in 1 ½ cups of distilled water, is also effective. **Note:** Always sterilize the eyebath before using it and use a new solution for each eye.

If your child has inflamed eyelids (blepharitis), encourage him or her to wash the hands frequently and not to rub the eyes, since this can cause infection. This problem usually responds well to a cold *poultice* (see p.135) made from the pulp of baked or stewed apples, or to ordinary tea, used as an eyebath. Consult your doctor before attempting self-treatment of eye inflammations.

Tired, strained eyes

If you suffer from tired eyes, rest them as much as possible. Try to avoid working or living under neon strip-lights and in smoky atmos-

pheres, and keep reading, watching TV and driving at night down to a minimum.

Bathe tired eyes with *infusions* (B, see p. 193) of eyebright, using distilled water and a sterilized eye bath. Cover the mixture and leave it to cool. Use a fresh brew each time you bathe your eyes, and change the herbal wash for the second eye to avoid passing the infection from one eye to another. You can also drink eyebright tea, though distilled water is not necessary. Alternatives to eyebright are *infusions* (B, see p.193) of elderflowers, marigold flower petals, plantain leaves, raspberry leaves, cornflowers, fennel seeds or just plain rosewater, available from most chemists.

You will find it restful and soothing to place a couple of fresh slices of cucumber, one over each closed eye, while lying quietly in a darkened room for about 15 mins. Get a friend to change the cucumber slices after 5 to 10 mins. Eat plenty of Vitamins C, B, and A (carrots which contain a precursor to Vitamin A are particularly good for the eyes). To relieve puffy eyelids and reduce swellings under the eyes, apply a *compress* (see p. 135) of grated raw potato to your closed eyes. Swelling under the eyes can be due to insufficient kidney elimination, so you may also benefit from drinking an *infusion* (B, see p. 193) of cornsilk or couch grass. However, for this condition you should also seek medical help.

Styes

Styes are inflammation of the small glands at the base of the eyelashes which secrete a lubricating fluid. The infection is usually a sign that the sufferer is generally run down. Apply a *compress* (p. 135) of warmed fresh parsley or marigold-flower petals directly to the stye, and eat blood-purifying herbs, such as garlic, purple coneflower, and burdock.

Please check the Glossary for cautions on particular herbs.
If in doubt, consult a qualified practitioner.

The skin

The elastic nature of the skin is perfectly designed to guard the sensitive underlying tissues and organs against physical or chemical damage, as well as protecting against the destructive effects of harmful bacteria or excessive sunlight. It also prevents the loss of precious body fluids. What is less obvious is that the skin is itself an active and vital organ whose proper functioning is essential to our survival.

Temperature regulation, for example, is mainly managed by the skin. If the body becomes too cold, blood vessels in the dermis (the deeper layer of skin underlying the epidermis) constrict, thereby retaining heat in the interior of the body. At the same time, smooth muscles also in the dermis may cause shivering, which raises the body temperature. If the body becomes too hot, the blood vessels in the dermis dilate, allowing blood to reach the surface of the body, where it can lose heat to the outside atmosphere. If there is a greater need for cooling, the sweat glands excrete sweat on to the surface of the skin which, as it evaporates, cools the body down.

Adult skin contains several million sweat glands. Each day we secrete about a pint (0.5 l) of sweat, but if we take vigorous exercise or find ourselves in warm surroundings, the sweat we excrete can amount to about eight quarts (9 l). Our sweat glands also fulfil many of the basic functions of the kidneys in that they, like the kidneys, excrete nitrogenous wastes, water, and mineral salts, as well as other toxic substances. For this reason, the skin has sometimes been called the third kidney. If the kidneys fail to function properly, a heavier demand is made on the sweat glands. Conversely, should the sweat glands be ineffective, an added burden falls on the kidneys. For herbalists, diaphoretic herbs (herbs which induce sweating), such as catnip, yarrow, or elderflower, have always been an important tool, to help the body rid itself of toxic encumbrances. Sweat itself, aside from eliminating wastes, forms a protective acid mantle on the skin, which kills off harmful bacteria.

The skin is also a sense organ, for it is richly supplied with microscopic nerve endings which act as antennae, informing the brain about heat or cold, touch, pressure, and pain. Since it is our point of contact with the outside world, when we fail to accord with our external surroundings – either in physical terms, as when we are exposed to polluted air, or emotionally – skin disease may result. It should not be overlooked that the epidermis develops from exactly the same section of the embryo that gives rise to our nervous systems.

In fact, our skin is a mirror of our general well-being, and treating skin diseases therefore requires an overall evaluation of the sufferer's health. Mere application of an ointment is unlikely to achieve a cure in the long term. Indeed, it is more likely to do damage by suppressing the symptoms, for it is in the nature of skin to bring to the surface problems which would otherwise do damage at a deeper level.

Disorders

Acne

Acne is chronic inflammation of the sebaceous glands, characterized by blackheads, papules, pustules, and cysts. Most common among adolescents, the disease often disappears spontaneously in the early twenties. The affected areas are usually those where the sebaceous glands are naturally large, namely the face, the chest, the back and sometimes the upper parts of the arms. The sebaceous glands produce an oil, called sebum, which usually maintains the suppleness of the skin. Acne is related to the activity of the sex hormones. When they are highly active, in adolescence for example, the sebum becomes thicker and more profuse. Sebum reaches the surface of the skin by draining along the hair follicles. Sometimes, however, these follicles and their ducts atrophy, but

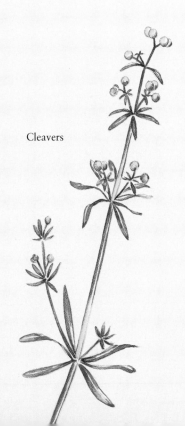

Cleavers

the sebaceous glands continue their production. In this case, excess sebum accumulates and plugs the follicle. The visible end of this plug becomes discoloured, producing a blackhead. Papules are raised, red spots which indicate inflammation of a blocked sebaceous duct. Pustules or whiteheads occur as the infection develops, while cysts are infections beneath the skin. *Corynebacterium acnes* is the bacterium which is normally responsible for the secondary infection which can eventually cause scarring. Certain medicines, namely iodides, corticosteroids, androgens, and some drugs used to treat epilepsy, may increase the likelihood of acne.

To control acne, the diet should consist mainly of fresh vegetables and fruit. Avoid refined carbohydrates, sugar, fried foods and animal fats, including cheese and butter, but do include cold-pressed vegetable oils. Chocolate, sweets, crisps, and other junk foods, are also likely to make the skin worse. It is wise, too, to avoid coffee and alcohol, as well as shellfish and kelp, which are rich in iodine. A high-fibre diet will ensure regular bowel movements, to maintain elimination of toxic wastes.

Scientists have demonstrated that Vitamin A is especially helpful for acne, so try to drink one or two wine glasses of carrot juice a day. If you have a juicer, mix carrot juice with cabbage, apple, and beetroot juice, all of which will benefit your skin. Zinc is necessary for stored Vitamin A in the liver to be released into the blood so if you suffer from acne, take 15 mg of zinc a day and eat pumpkin seeds which are rich in zinc. Oil of evening primrose is another valuable supplement while extra rosehip tablets will provide extra Vitamin C, to help fight skin infection. Wheatgerm, rich in Vitamin E, can help to balance out hormone production. Vitamin E, either by itself or mixed with comfrey can be applied to heal scarred skin once the inflammation has resolved.

In addition to these measures, take *infusions* and *decoctions* (C, see p. 193) of herbs that help to purify the blood, such as dandelions, nettles, yellow dock, burdock, cleavers, Oregon grape root, and blue flag. To control infection of the skin, take herbal antibiotics like purple coneflower and wild indigo. Some women notice that their acne gets worse just prior to a period, when their oestrogen levels drop and the progesterone hormone is in relative excess. Androgen excess is a male problem in puberty too. *Infusions* (C, see p.193) of a mixture of herbs, such as false unicorn root, sage, wild yam, and Chinese angelica, help to control such hormonal excesses. Never use these treatments if pregnancy is suspected.

Since acne is caused by blockage of the follicles by sebum, use a steam facial to help open the pores. Pour 1 pt (500 ml) boiling water over one tablespoon of either lavender, chamomile, elderflowers, limeflowers, yarrow, or lady's mantle. Allow the herbal steam to wash the grease from your face for about 8 mins. Gently wipe the blackheads with clean cotton wool afterwards.

To clean greasy skin, mix equal parts of fresh lemon juice to rosewater or elderflower water or distilled witch hazel. Alternatively, add lemon juice to oatmeal and water or clean the skin with warm milk or yoghurt. But these external applications are only effective if the acne is treated internally too.

Warts

Warts are caused by a virus that is mildly contagious and spread by contact. Genital warts, for example, may be spread by venereal contact. Warts on the soles of the feet are known as verrucas, although this is a medical term for warts anywhere on the

body. If you suffer from warts, strengthen your general vitality (see Eczema). Not long ago many country districts boasted a wart charmer who could magic away warts. You could try one of the following wart-charming remedies. Apply dandelion sap to the wart for 10 days. Or wash it with 1 teaspoon of tincture of Thuja, diluted in a cup of water, every day for 10 days. You could also try macerating the rind of two lemons in cider vinegar for 10 days, and painting the wart with the mixture. Onions and garlic may also help. Crush a clove of garlic and tape it to the wart. Be very careful to protect the skin around the wart from blistering by covering it with protective plaster. For an alternative remedy, cut an onion in half, scoop out the middle, and fill it with sea salt. Paint the wart daily with the juice that flows from the onion.

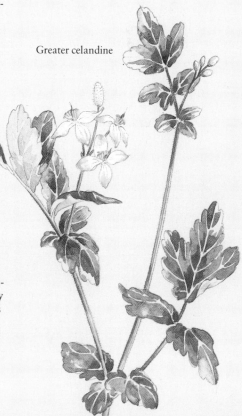

Greater celandine

Boils and carbuncles

A boil is a local inflammation of a hair root or a cut due to staphylococcal infection. A cluster of boils is known as a carbuncle. If you are constantly suffering from reinfection of this kind, reassess your diet and lifestyle and make changes to enhance the body's resistance. You should also seek medical help. It is sensible to look out for a particular septic focus in the body that may be undermining the general health, such as a dental abscess. Use *infusions* (A, see p. 193) of herbs such as purple coneflower to boost the immune system, combined with those that fight infection, such as wild indigo, myrrh, burdock, sweet violet, dandelion root, garlic and thyme. Hot poultices help to draw a boil and cause it to discharge. You can make an effective poultice by mixing slippery elm powder with water to make a paste. Add a few drops of lavender or eucalyptus oil to the water for antibacterial power.

Psoriasis

Psoriasis is a relatively common skin disease affecting up to 4 per cent of the white-skinned population. It is characterized by dry, silvery scaling, often affecting the limbs and scalp. Beneath the scale, the skin is pink or red and may be itchy. The root cause is unknown, but the immediate problem is gross over-production of the epithelial cells which constitute the superficial layer of skin. This outer layer of skin sloughs off too quickly, revealing an unprotected deeper layer. Psoriasis is associated with arthritis and changes in the health of the nails. It tends to run in families and often comes and goes.

The essential pattern of psoriasis is over-activity of the external layer of the body. Many sufferers lead stressful lives, characterized by a restlessness and over-activity that is mirrored by their skin. In some cases, psoriasis first occurs after a bad

shock, which results in adrenocortical hormone disturbance. If you suffer from psoriasis, take definite measures to reduce stress by practising regular exercise and relaxation techniques or meditation. Herbal remedies which relax and strengthen the nervous system, such as skullcap, vervain, wild oats, passionflower, chamomile, and hops, can be included in a herbal prescription to treat psoriasis to good effect. Licorice may help to support the adrenal glands and a Bach Flower Remedy (Star of Bethlehem) can also be taken if appropriate.

To counteract the dryness of the skin, take *infusions* (C, see p.193) of herbs that enrich the blood. These include sarsaparilla (also helpful for balancing the hormones), Oregon grape root, burdock, queen's delight, yellow dock, red clover, nettles, and blue flag. Chinese angelica, dang gui, is a useful blood tonic too.

Because the skin exfoliates so fast in psoriasis, severe cases may result in a strain on the circulatory system, which can eventually affect the heart. Herbs which support the heart and circulation, such as hawthorn and motherwort, are helpful. Remedies which increase peripheral blood flow, however, such as diaphoretics and circulatory stimulants, should not be used. Alcohol, which dilates the peripheral blood vessels, must also be strictly avoided.

External applications can help the dryness of the skin. Apply the *essential oil* (see p.193) of lavender mixed with olive oil. Another application is made from the *essental oils* (see p. 193) of lavender or bergamot oil mixed with equal parts of St John's wort oil and comfrey oil. Comfrey ointment and oil of cade (Juniper-Tar ointment) can also sometimes help, and coal-tar shampoo sometimes improves psoriasis of the scalp.

Also, use fine-milled oatmeal soaps, instead of those which dry out the skin. A yarrow bath, made from an *infusion* (see p. 135) of 2 oz (60 g) of yarrow in 2 pts (1 l) water poured

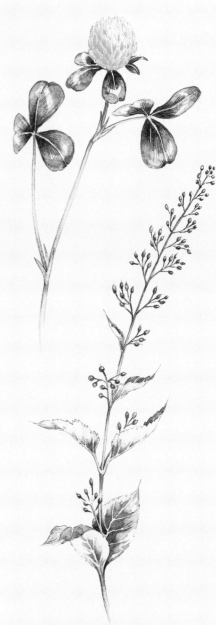

Red clover and figwort
Figwort and red clover both help to treat skin complaints by cleansing cells and blood of toxic accumulations. They soothe itching and irritation in such conditions as eczema and psoriasis, slowly achieving their effect over a matter of weeks.

into the bath water, or a sea-salt bath can sometimes be soothing. Psoriasis usually occurs on body areas shielded from light and is more active in winter. Sensible sunbathing can help to alleviate this condition.

When the skin flakes off constantly, substantial quantities of nutrients are lost. If you suffer from psoriasis, take extra vitamins and minerals to supplement those lost through the skin. Also drink a glass of fresh carrot juice twice daily for extra Vitamin A. Kelp tablets provide valuable trace elements and minerals which may be depleted. The *International Medical Digest* (April 30, 1965) gave details of successful treatment of psoriasis by Russian medical scientists using Vitamin C, B12, and folic acid. According to the *New York Journal of Medicine* (November 15, 1980), psoriatic skin contains abnormally high levels of cholesterol. 155 patients were treated with lecithin and of these 118 (76 per cent) were controlled or improved. Lecithin, nature's washing up liquid, helps to clean out fatty deposits, like cholesterol, from the tissues. Eat soya and sunflower oils, which contain good quantities of lecithin.

Eczema

Eczema is a non-contagious inflammatory disease of the skin. It is characterized by a rash which is sore, often dry but sometimes weeping, and invariably itchy. There are so many causes of eczema that finding the best treatment demands detective work and a considerable amount of patience.

One common kind of eczema is known as contact dermatitis. This is caused by contact with an irritant, which either damages the surface of the skin, or penetrates more deeply into it and sets up an allergic reaction. To prevent and treat this kind of eczema, avoid contact with strong or caustic chemicals. Detergents or biological washing powders can leave an irritating residue in clothes and some make-up, face creams, and nail varnish may also inflame the skin. Common chemical allergens are nickel and chromium, often found in jewellery, buckles, and straps. Some people have an allergic reaction to rubber so that protective gloves can make matters worse. The common house-dust mite is frequently to blame, and vacuuming fitted carpets and mattresses can control this problem. Wool and nylon may irritate the skin so use cotton instead and do not encourage children with eczema to sleep with soft toys. Animal dander from household pets can also bring sensitive skin out in a rash.

Eczema can also be caused by nutritional deficiencies and the skin will quickly return to normal once the deficiency is made good. Infantile or children's eczema may, for instance, be due to lack of gamma-linolenic acid (GLA), present in breast milk but absent in cow's milk. Always consult your doctor on skin ailments in babies or children. Including cold-pressed vegetable oils such as sunflower and safflower in the diet will also help. Vitamins A, B, C, and E are all necessary for healthy skin. Drink carrot juice every day for a good dose of betacarotene, a precursor of Vitamin A. A supplement of Vitamin B6 can sometimes heal dry flaky skin. Eating kelp will also help to provide necessary trace elements and minerals. If you suffer from eczema, avoid fried food, alcohol, junk foods, and foods and drinks which contain sugar, artificial colouring and flavouring. Eat instead a wholefood diet with plenty of fresh vegetables and fruit.

Some eczemas are due to sensitivities to common foods. If you suspect this to be the case, try excluding various categories of food from the diet for three or four weeks to see if the skin improves. Common culprits are dairy products, eggs, wheat, tomatoes, oranges, marmite, pork, chocolate, fish (especially shell-fish), peppers, and aubergines. Fruit rich in natural salicylates such as strawberries can also cause a skin flare-up.

Another kind of eczema is common in older people and comes with hardening of the arteries which prevents the blood from nourishing the skin. Alternatively, if the veins are in poor shape and fail to drain an area, a stagnant pool can develop, leading to varicose eczema (see p. 206–211).

The main herbal treatment for eczema is internal. Take *infusions* or *decoctions* (B, see p.193) of alterative herbs, such as yellow dock, burdock, red clover, figwort, fumitory, heartsease, purple coneflower, and nettles. Such herbs help to nourish and cool the blood and skin. Combine them with *infusions* (B, see p.193) of herbs that help the nervous system, which may be under stress, including oats, skullcap, and vervain. Add herbs that support the adrenal glands, such as licorice and borage. Avoid cowslip, which may cause an allergic reaction.

External treatments can be used simultaneously. To oil dry skin, use the *essential oils* (see p. 193) of lavender or chamomile, added to almond or olive oil. External applications of the oils of evening primrose, Vitamin E, or jojoba can also be effective. Some skins also respond well to oil of cade (Juniper-Tar ointment). To nourish the skin, add oatmeal to the bathwater and use oatmeal soap. Some eczema sufferers gain relief from epsom salts (magnesium sulphate) or sea salt added to the bath water. To reduce inflammation, try a *poultice* (see p.135) made from watercress, comfrey root or leaf, or chickweed, mixed with fine oatmeal. A coltsfoot-leaf poultice can also soothe the skin. Itchy skin will sometimes respond to a *compress* (see p.135) made from a cold *infusion* (B, see p.193) of plantain-leaf or dock-leaf. A few drops of essential oil of chamomile in aqueous cream makes a soothing ointment.

The herbal first-aid cupboard

For most medicinal uses, herbs that you have grown yourself, using proper organic methods (see pp. 242–79), are the best. If you cultivate and harvest herbs correctly, their active constituents will be preserved and they will be free from the pollutants that can be found in plants that are grown commercially using modern methods and chemical fertilizers. But there are some commercially available herbal preparations that have such valuable healing properties that it makes sense keeping a stock in the home. This is particularly true of preparations that are used in first aid, where you will need instant access to remedies.

It is a good idea to familiarize yourself with the most useful herbs for first aid, so that you can act promptly if one of the family has a minor accident. Herbal remedies can provide quick, effective relief for a whole range of mishaps, from wasp stings to minor burns and sprained ankles.

On the opposite page are details of a range of these herbal medicines. The two most important categories are those used in healing minor cuts, wounds, and burns (such as marigold, witch hazel, and arnica), and those with antiseptic properties (such as clove oil, eucalyptus oil, and lavender oil) that are invaluable for combating infections. In addition, there are also useful remedies for calming the nervous system and helping conditions such as emotional shock or insomnia (including the Bach Rescue Remedy).

As well as the herbs and remedies featured opposite, you may like to keep a supply of herbs handy for common ailments such as colds, flu, and stomach upsets, for it is always best to treat illness promptly. Among the most useful are composition essence for colds, chamomile for relaxation, and lemon balm for insomnia.

Alongside the herbs and herbal preparations that you need near at hand, you should have the basic equipment common to any medicine chest: scissors, bandage, sterile absorbent gauze, lint, and waterproof plasters. In addition there are several non-herbal items that are effective as first aid in conjunction with herbal remedies. Sodium bicarbonate (sold as bicarbonate of soda) can be made into a cooling paste for burns and bee stings. Arrowroot or talcum powder is useful for mixing with powdered cayenne pepper for chilblains (see p. 238). Cider vinegar makes an adequate substitute for aloe vera when treating poison ivy rash (see p. 238).

Note: Always consult your doctor if wounds and cuts are deep, if burned skin is broken, or for any conditions that do not quickly respond to treatment.

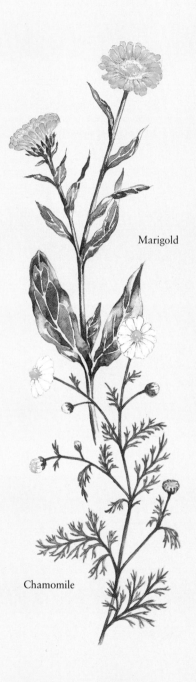

Marigold

Chamomile

First-aid herbs
Marigold and chamomile are excellent first-aid herbs. Marigold is good for cuts and sores, chamomile for insomnia.

Marigold

Available as tincture of calendula, this is one of the most effective healing remedies for small cuts and cold sores. Alternatively, you can buy calendula ointment, which is also a useful healing preparation. An infusion of marigold flowers is also used to heal cuts and to relieve sunburn.

Witch hazel

This is one of the most widely used first-aid remedies, valued for its astringent and blood-clotting actions. It is available as distilled witch hazel. You can use it in a compress for minor burns and sprains or apply it directly to the skin in cases of insect bites, nosebleeds, and cuts.

St John's Wort

As an oil this is a useful remedy for burns and minor wounds. As a compress it helps heal deeper cuts.

Aloe vera

The best way to make use of the healing powers of this plant is to grow one on a sunny window sill. You can then break off a leaf and rub the inner pulp directly on to the skin, to relieve sunburn or poison ivy. If you cannot obtain a plant, try some of the commercially available creams and ointments containing aloe vera gel. These vary in quality, however – some are adulterated, and harsh solvents may have been used in the extraction of the gel, so take advice from a medical herbalist if you are unsure.

Comfrey

In the form of an ointment or an infusion, comfrey helps to heal bruises and cuts. It encourages the growth of scar tissue after cuts.

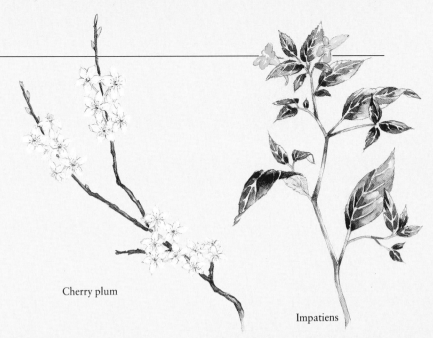

Cherry plum

Impatiens

Arnica

This plant is highly valued in both herbalism and homeopathy for sprains and bruises when the skin is not broken. It is also available in several other forms – as a tincture and in ointments.

Slippery elm

This plant is sold in several different forms. As slippery elm food it is good for the digestion (see p. 202), but the most valuable form for the first-aid cupboard is slippery elm powder. You can use this in a poultice to help bring boils to a head.

Clove

Clove oil is a traditional remedy for the pain associated with toothache. Because of its antiseptic property, it is also useful in the treatment of cuts.

Eucalyptus oil

This antiseptic oil is used in aromatherapy and herbalism to treat cuts and boils. It is also a good inhalant for colds and coughs.

Composition essence

Including elderflower and peppermint, this is a good remedy for colds and flu.

Lavender oil

An important oil in both herbalism and aromatherapy, lavender is well known for its antiseptic, antibacterial and wound-healing properties (see pp. 150–1).

Chamomile

It is worth keeping a supply of the dried herb to make relaxing teas for insomnia. You will also find it useful for other disorders (see p. 49).

Lemon balm

This is a good herb for children, particularly for stomach upsets and other ailments where a relaxing effect is required (see p. 68).

Rescue Remedy

This is a composite of five of the flower remedies discovered by Dr Edward Bach and used widely by herbalists, homeopaths, and other natural therapists. Most of the remedies are extracts from the flowers and buds of plants. Although no one knows exactly how the Bach Flower Remedies work, many practitioners and patients have experienced enormous benefits after using them for emotional problems. The Rescue Remedy is particularly recommended for emotional shock.

First aid

The chart on the following pages gives commonsense first-aid treatments and herbal remedies for a range of common problems. Read any cautions in the first column, carry out the basic recommendations in the second column, and choose a herbal remedy from the third. If the caution points out a potentially serious or chronic problem, seek professional advice as quickly as possible. You should also consult a qualified therapist if your first-aid and herbal treatments do not bring about an improvement.

Disorder	First aid	Herbal treatments
Sprains and bruises Sprains result from over-stretching or tearing of the ligaments around joints, most commonly the wrists or ankles. 　CAUTION Severe bruising may be accompanied by serious internal haemorrhage, and painful joints may be fractured. Always seek medical advice.	Support the sprain with a bandage around the affected joint. If you suspect a fracture call for medical assistance. If you bruise easily you may be short of vitamin C, which you can take together with rutin tablets.	Bruises and sprains both respond well to compresses of witch hazel, comfrey, or arnica. In the latter case make the fluid for the compress by diluting half a teaspoon of arnica tincture in half a pint of water and wash the bruised or sprained area. The common garden daisy (*Bellis perennis*) is in the same family as arnica and an infusion of daisies can also be used as a compress for bruises (the old name for daisy was bruisewort). Ice-packs are also useful, and diluted witch hazel can actually be poured into an ice-try and frozen before use. 　If you have nothing else, bind a cabbage leaf over any bruised or painful area.
Minor cuts CAUTION If cuts are gaping or there is any risk of infection such as tetanus, seek medical help.	To stop cuts bleeding, apply pressure for a few minutes. 　If the sides are gaping open, bring them together firmly with your finger and thumb. Bind the wound with surgical tape then cover it with a dressing and bandage. 　If the cut is relatively minor, it is best left uncovered.	Cuts can be bathed with an infusion of marigold flowers. Diluted tincture of marigold (calendula) will do as well. Alternatively, use distilled witch hazel, applying it to the cut on cotton wool. It helps to stop bleeding and promotes healing. 　Also antiseptic and healing is diluted oil of clove, lavender or eucalyptus, which can be applied with cotton wool. If the cut is deeper, use a compress of St John's wort or apply St John's wort oil. 　Scar tissue can be encouraged to heal by applying comfrey ointment and Vitamin E oil daily.

Disorder	First aid	Herbal treatments
Minor burns and scalds If the burn or scald has affected a small area and damaged only the outer layer of skin, then you can safely treat it at home. Seek medical advice in the case of electrical burns. CAUTION Do not puncture blisters. If a burn becomes more painful or infected seek medical attention.	Cool the affected area by immersing it in cold (but not ice-cold) water for at least ten minutes or until the pain has gone. Alternatively, you can use a cold compress. Once the pain has gone, cover loosely with a clean, dry dressing. Avoid fluffy material which can stick to the burn. If it is a chemical burn, remove any clothing splashed with chemicals and flush the affected area with running water.	Apply lavender oil to the burnt area – 6 drops to an eggcupful of olive oil – or use St John's wort oil. Break off a leaf of the aloe vera plant, which can be grown as a house plant on a sunny window ledge. Alternatively, make a compress by wetting a gauze in distilled witch hazel and gently bind it to the site of the burn. An infusion of comfrey, cooled and applied as a compress, is another effective remedy. Comfrey ointment can also be applied.
Nosebleeds CAUTION Nosebleeds which occur after a blow on the head can be a sign of a fractured skull. Seek medical help at once.	Grasp the soft part of the nose firmly, using your thumb and index finger and hold for about 10 minutes. When the bleeding stops, don't blow your nose or sniff, as this could dislodge the blood clot and start the nose bleeding again.	Apply distilled witch hazel to the nasal passage with cotton wool. In addition, apply a cold compress to the back of the neck.
Fainting and shock CAUTION Emotional shock is quite different from "medical shock", which can follow a serious injury and requires urgent medical attention. If someone faints and does not regain consciousness after a few minutes, place him or her in the so-called recovery position and summon medical assistance.	If someone feels faint, get him or her to sit down with the head between the knees. If the person has actually fainted, gently raise the legs so that they are higher than the head to encourage blood to flow back to the brain. When the person regains consciousness, give small sips of water. Loosen any tight clothing and ensure that the person gets as much fresh air as possible.	Use the composite Bach Flower Remedy known as Rescue Remedy, which is excellent for shock. If the patient is unconscious you can still use this remedy: apply a drop or two on to the pulse points. If the person is conscious, put four drops in a glass of water and get him or her to sip it slowly. Alternatively, get the person to sip a glass of water in which has been mixed no more than five drops of arnica tincture.
Splinters CAUTION Don't dig deep into the skin for splinters and never ignore splinters, for they can go septic. Always seek medical assistance if the splinter is large, especially if there is glass.	Use antiseptic to gently wash the area around the splinter. Then try to pull the splinter out with tweezers. If the splinter does not project out of the skin, sterilize a sewing needle by heating the point in the clear part of a flame. Allow it to cool, then use it to ease the splinter out.	Use a slippery-elm poultice made with slippery-elm powder, which allows even stubborn splinters to be drawn out quickly and easily.

Disorder	First aid	Herbal treatments
Sunburn CAUTION Extensive sunburn requires medical attention.		The best sunburn treatment is to apply the juice of the aloe vera plant to the affected area. Also effective is a compress of fresh cucumber juice or a marigold infusion. Failing this, try applying fresh, live yoghurt (plain and unsweetened), or a solution of sodium bicarbonate, to the affected area.

Bites and stings
Bees leave their barbed stings behind in the skin, unlike wasps.
    CAUTION Bee and wasp stings affect some people seriously. If this is the case seek medical assistance at once.
    To repel insects, apply to the skin citronella, lavender or tea tree oil all diluted in a little olive oil.
	Remove bee stings with tweezers sterilized by running the ends through a flame. Hold the sting near the skin, taking care not to grip the poison sac. If you don't have any tweezers, try "brushing" it away with a needle held parallel to the skin. Holding the affected area under cold water may reduce the pain.	A bee sting may be washed using sodium bicarbonate applied as a past to the site.
		    Wasp and mosquito bites you can treat by applying lemon juice, witch hazel, or cider vinegar, or crushed plaintain leaves. Alternatively, apply a sliced onion or some onion juice to the affected area.
		    Lavender or cinnamon oil rubbed on to the affected area will help to remove the discomfort of a bee or wasp sting or an insect bite.

Poison ivy CAUTION Don't scratch – scratching spreads the poison.	As soon as possible, wash the skin thoroughly with household soap and water. Scrub the skin well.	Squeeze the juice of the aloe vera leaf on to the affected area, or bathe it with cider vinegar.
Chilblains CAUTION Circulation problems can be a sign of serious illness. Check your symptoms with your doctor.	Wear plenty of warm clothes and take regular exercise to improve your circulation.	Mix powdered cayenne pepper with talcum or arrowroot powder. Dust your feet with this before putting on your stockings or socks. Use hot footbaths of ginger (1 oz or 20 g) and cinnamon (2 sticks) to 2 pt (1 l) of water. To this add 1 tablespoon of magnesium sulphate crystals. Water prepared in this way can be retained and you can use it again for four or five days.
Toothache CAUTION You should consult a dentist if you have toothache – the remedy described, right, is not a substitute for proper dental treatment.	Avoid alcohol as this will exacerbate the pain.	If the pain is caused by a cavity, apply a piece of cotton wool soaked in oil of cloves directly to the site. CAUTION Do not swallow.

Disorder	First aid	Herbal treatments
Diarrhoea	If there is an infection of the digestive tract, diarrhoea may be the body's way of eliminating toxins. So let the condition run its course, giving a solution of warm water and honey regularly to replace lost fluids. This is important for infants, who may collapse after diarrhoea and vomiting if lost fluids and electrolytes are not replaced. Seek medical help if this happens.	Combine a teaspoon of a mixture of astringent remedies, such as agrimony and tormentil, with a pinch of ginger and cinnamon powder. Garlic and purple coneflower can be taken as natural antibiotics. If the diarrhoea persists, see your doctor.
Earache CAUTION Earache may be a symptom of a serious middle-ear infection, particularly if it occurs in children. Seek medical assistance for earache.	Fill a hotwater bottle with warm water, cover it with a cloth, and apply it to the ear.	There are a number of herbal remedies for earache, mostly consisting of eardrops containing volatile oils and herbs with an antibiotic action. For further details, see p. 199.
Motion sickness This is a disorder of the vestibular part of the middle ear, caused by a discoordination between messages received by the brain from the eyes (which may indicate that the world is still) and the ears (which tell the brain it is moving).	If you are suffering from motion sickness on a boat, go out on deck and look at the horizon; this will confirm via your eyes that the world is moving underneath you. If you are in a car, avoid reading and look out of the window.	Chew a piece of fresh ginger root or crystallized stem ginger.
Hayfever Hayfever is caused by an allergy to pollens.	Try eliminating wheat from your diet during the hayfever season. It is also worth cutting out dairy products for a while to see if there is any improvement. Extra vitamin C and zinc in the diet may also help to counteract hayfever.	Take an infusion (1 teaspoon to a cup of water) of one of the following herbs: elderflowers, mint, eyebright, pill-bearing spurge, golden rod, or wood betony. You can also try nettles, which are now available freeze-dried in capsules. Use the following steam inhalant: mix 30 ml of compound tincture of Benzoin (friar's balsam) with 2.5 ml eucalyptus oil, 6 drops peppermint oil, 5 drops lavender oil and 5 drops pine oil. Shake well. Put a teaspoonful of the mixture into a bowl, pour on 1 pt (500 ml) of boiled water, cover your head and the bowl with a towel or cloth, and inhale.

Disorder	First aid	Herbal treatments
Cold sores (herpes simplex) Cold sores are caused by a common virus of the chickenpox family that in another form may cause either genital herpes or shingles (herpes zoster).	Improve your general resistance by taking plenty of vitamin C-rich fruit and vegetables. Avoid foods (such as peanuts and chocolate) that are rich in the amino acid argenine, which may have the effect of triggering an attack of cold sores. A supplement of the amino acid L-lysine is said to restrict attacks.	Drink herb teas made from burdock, yellow dock, and dandelion root. Boost the immune system by combining these with herbs such as echinacea, astralagus, and licorice. Locally, apply directly to the cold sore a diluted tincture of myrrh, marigold, or golden seal.
Boils and carbuncles A boil is a local inflammation of a hair root or cut, due to infection. A cluster of boils is known as a carbuncle.	Constant reinfection of this kind calls for a general reassessment of diet and lifestyle to enhance the body's resistance. Alternatively, look for a particular septic focus in the body, such as a dental abscess or chronically diseased tonsils, which may be undermining your general health.	Use herbs that boost the immune system, such as echinacea and astralagus, with those that fight infection, such as wild indigo, myrrh, burdock, sweet violet, dandelion root, garlic, and thyme. A hot poultice applied locally will help to draw a boil and cause it to discharge. Mix hot water with slippery elm powder to make a paste. Add a few drops of lavender or eucalyptus oil to the water to give the poultice antibacterial power.
Corns Corns are areas of hardened skin on or between the toes. They are nearly always caused by pressure or friction from badly fitting shoes. If you have bad corns, you should arrange to visit a chiropodist.	Get better-fitting footwear and if possible walk barefoot for a time every day.	Paint the hard skin daily with fresh lemon juice or apply calendula ointment regularly.
Bunions A bunion is inflammation and swelling of the joint of the big toes with the result that the toe is sometimes pushed towards the others. The usual cause is badly fitting shoes.	Get better-fitting footwear.	Apply a poultice of comfrey leaves or marigold flowers to the affected joint or use a daily footbath of an infusion of equal parts of comfrey leaf, marigold flowers, chamomile, and meadowsweet. You may also paint the bunion daily with fresh lemon juice.

PART THREE

Growing Herbs

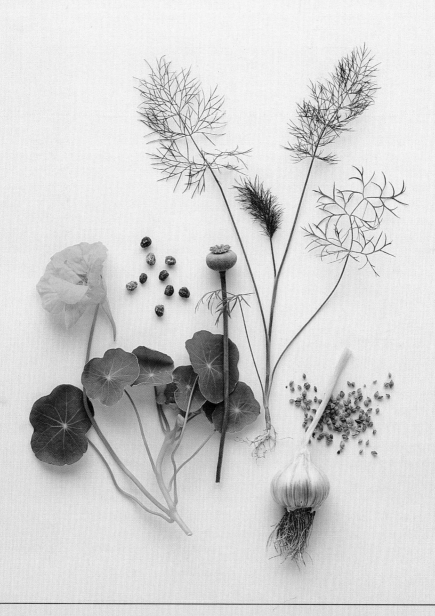

CHAPTER SIX

Herb Gardening

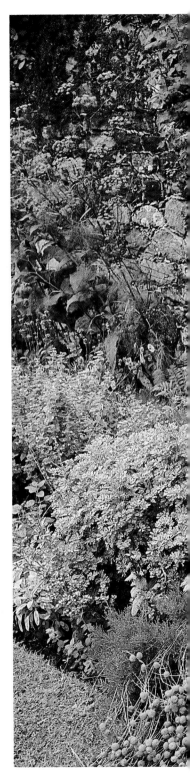

To obtain the best quality herbs exactly when you want them it is wisest to grow them yourself. Fortunately, herbs are among the easiest plants to cultivate. Some, like dandelion, are often thought of as garden weeds, while others, like mint, are difficult to restrain once they are established. And you do not need a lot of space to cultivate herbs – many will grow in a window box or in pots on a sunny window ledge, and some can even be grown indoors as houseplants. This chapter concentrates on herbs that grow best in northern latitudes, since the majority of the most useful herbs are hardy, though some, such as sweet bay, need protection from the frost. Most of these herbs will also do well in the south. In addition, there are a few exotic herbs, such as aloe vera, where the virtues of the fresh plant are so great that is worth growing them indoors; you can use a sunny window ledge if you do not have a greenhouse. If you have a cold frame, this can provide a good place to put seedlings that have germinated indoors, to accustom them gradually to conditions outside.

The best possible way to grow herbs is by organic methods, using natural products to foster a healthy soil. This has several advantages. First, because only natural composts and fertilizers are used, the soil remains "clean" – free from chemical pollutants which may be passed on to the plant. This is especially important in herb cultivation, because such pollutants will alter the biochemistry of the plant and may affect its action on the body. Second, organic cultivation creates a healthy soil, which in turn leads to healthy, vigorous plants. And third, organic methods are labour-saving, reducing activities such as digging and weeding to a minimum.

As well as being healthy for the user, herbs are also good for the garden. Many of the aromatic herbs attract bees and other pollinating insects to the garden; and some herbs, especially those native to clay soils, have large, strong root systems that help to break up the soil. These properties are self-evident to the observant gardener, but there are other actions that are more subtle and less easy to verify. Many herbs are reputed to keep particular garden pests at bay, while some are thought to benefit the growth of other plant species when they are cultivated nearby. These are virtues that it is worth bearing in mind

Not all herbs are safe to handle. Consult the Glossary for cautions before planting.

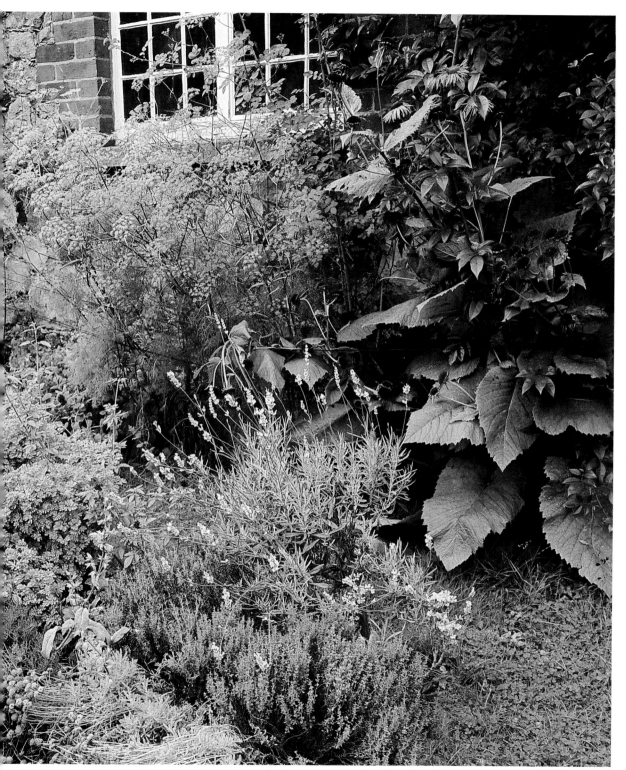

An assortment of medicinal and culinary herbs in an English garden

when planning a garden. It can be beneficial, for example, to inter-plant herbs and vegetables, rather than putting all your herbs together in a bed of their own. Rosemary, for example, is thought to repel certain flies; hyssop is reputed to enhance the crop yield of vines.

The garden ecosystem

All life-forms are interdependent. Plants – in the garden as in the wild – are no exception to this rule. In addition to their basic environmental needs – sun, air, water, and soil – they need the help of every class of living organism to complete their life cycle: insects make pollination possible for many species (see p. 12); birds and animals assist seed dispersal; soil organisms help to make the necessary nutrients available; and all of these creatures depend for food or shelter on the plants they support. In the garden, you have the chance to nurture these systems, to make your garden a healthy ecosystem in its own right.

Garden plants form an interface between the natural and the human worlds. It is at the level of the soil that you can have most influence over the garden ecosystem – and the best way to feed the soil is to garden organically, using simple, natural composts and fertilizers that assist the cycles of growth. The plants themselves return nutrients to the soil in a steady rain of leaves, twigs, and petals. By means of compost, you can help the dead plant give its own substance back to the earth, so that the whole cycle restarts. Composting the soil does more than introduce nutrients directly. It also helps to break up the soil, producing the more aerobic conditions favoured by most plant roots – and by a host of organisms that improve the soil in turn. The best known of these are earthworms. They help in breaking up the soil further and in processing nutrients – studies carried out on worm casts show that they contain several times more available nitrogen, phosphorous, and potassium than the surrounding soil. Composting will also increase the number of microscopic organisms, which help the gardener by making the nutrients in the soil available to the plants.

Another way to encourage these creatures is to plant leguminous crops, such as clover, which are particularly good hosts. Legumes develop bacterial nodules on their roots which make nitrogen available in the soil to other plants. The also act as hosts to mycorrhizal fungi, which live partly in the soil, partly in the roots themselves. These fungi take carbohydrates from the plants and give back other nutrients that the plant requires to manufacture protein in return. All the soil organisms require organic matter to thrive. In a soil treated continuously with chemical fertilizers, soil bacteria and fungi are not present in sufficient quantities to support the plants, resulting in a "dead" soil and plants which must be fed chemically. An organic soil is the only one that will sustain a balanced ecosystem in the garden.

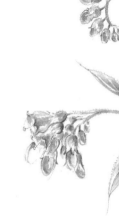

Comfrey
This is one of the most useful plants to grow in the garden. It gives a good yield in rich soil, but self-sown seedlings can be invasive.

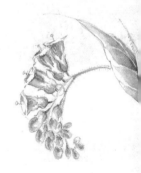

Healthy soil
The top humus layer consists of organic material – decomposing plant and animal remains – that gives the soil its fertility. Below this lies the dark topsoil in which the plant grows. This gives way in turn to the underlying subsoil of sand, stone, chalk, or clay.

Nutrient cycles and health

The recurring cycle in which de-caying leaves and stems feed organ-isms in the soil, which make available nutrients that in turn feed the grow-ing plant, has a significance that ex-tends far beyond the garden. Organi-cally grown plants are generally heal-thier than their chemically grown counterparts: organic conditions en-courage the absorption of nitrates.

This means that pesticides are seldom required – any pests and diseases that do occur can be dealt with naturally (see p. 267). The result is that organi-cally grown herbs and vegetables are not contaminated by pesticides, un-like those grown chemically, making them healthier for the gardener as well as for the environment of the garden as a whole.

Compost

This needs three main ingre-dients to recycle waste effi-ciently: a good air supply to encourage soil organisms to multiply and heat up the heap, killing off weed seeds and disease organisms; an activator to supply nitrogen; and moisture.

Companion planting

Combinations of different plant species, growing together, can form mutually beneficial associations (see pp. 268–9).

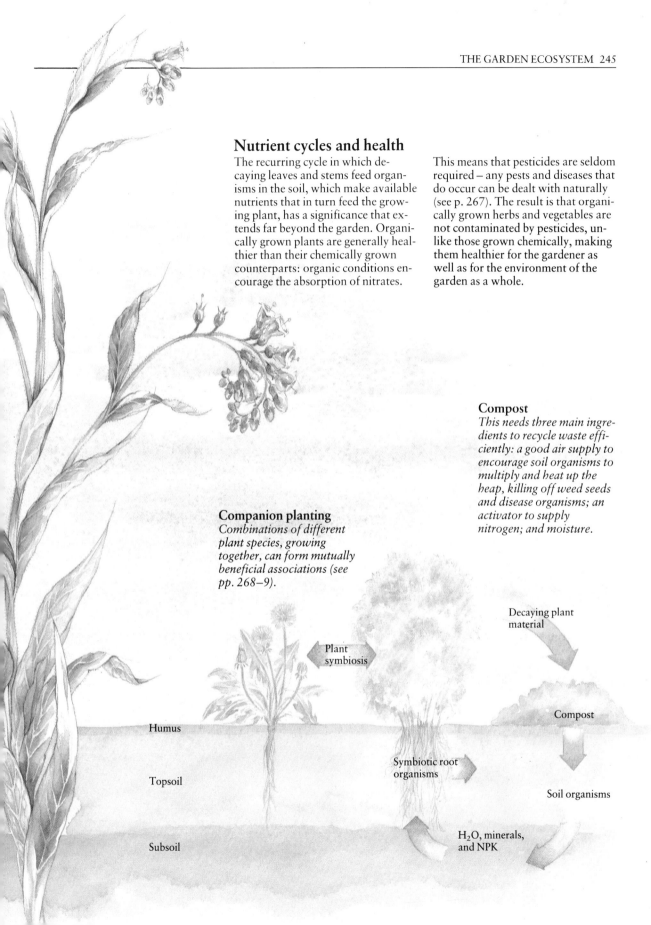

Plant symbiosis

Decaying plant material

Compost

Humus

Topsoil

Subsoil

Symbiotic root organisms

Soil organisms

H_2O, minerals, and NPK

The organic soil

The soil holds the secret to healthy plants. One of the first principles of organic gardening is to make the best use of the soil in your garden. This means matching plants to the soil types they prefer (see pp. 248–9), and caring for your soil by feeding it so that it gives you the best possible results (see pp. 264–5). Soil is a collection of individual particles, varying in size according to type, and the spaces between them – the pore spaces – containing life-giving air and water. To us the most obvious characteristic of the soil is its mass – the whole collection of particles composing the soil; but plant roots are more concerned with the nature of pore spaces – how big and how many – into which they can penetrate and from which nourishment is derived.

Soils are classified according to the size of their individual particles, from the tiny particles of clay (smaller than 0.002 mm in diameter) to the larger grains of sand (as large as 2 mm in diameter). But you do not have to measure soil particles to find out what soil types are present in your garden. In practice, what you first need to know is how easy the soil is to break up and how rich in nutrients it is likely to be. You can tell a good deal by simply looking at your soil, putting a fork into it, and crumbling some between your fingers. Is it heavy and difficult to work or friable and easy to dig? Is it dark and rich or light and sandy? Looking below the surface by digging a hole will show you more – exactly how well drained the soil is, the depth of the topsoil layer, and how easily roots can penetrate. If the topsoil is dark in colour, it should contain plenty of the organic matter necessary for successful gardening. A lighter coloured topsoil will be lower in nutrients. If your soil is crumbly in texture, it will have a stable, open structure that will prevent waterlogging, keep the air circulating, and allow it to warm up faster. A soil such as clay, in which the particles stick together in large masses, will get waterlogged easily and will need breaking up. Plants native to heavy soils (see p. 248) have strong root systems that help break up the soil.

If you want to analyse your soil in more detail, a useful method is to mix a sample in water. The elements will separate out so that you can see what type of soil you have (see opposite). The nature of the soil can vary within a garden, so you should take samples from different areas.

Soil acidity also influences the nature of your soil. An acid soil may be short of calcium, or contain too much aluminium or manganese, or the power of the roots to take up essential foods such as phosphate may be reduced. Alkalinity can be reduced by a dressing of organic manures or compost. You can test the acidity level of the soil with one of the kits available commercially, or with simple litmus paper strips (see opposite).

When you have established the characteristics of the soil in the different parts of your garden, you can start to match plants to soils as closely as possible, or modify the soils where necessary.

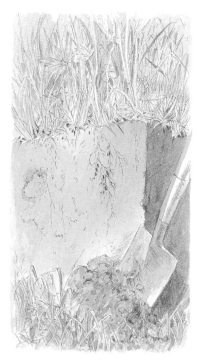

Taking a soil profile
After rain, dig a hole 12–18 ins (30–45 cm) deep in a place where some plants are growing. Look at the depth of the topsoil layer and at what sort of subsoil you have underneath. Check whether rainwater has drained away or whether the subsoil is waterlogged. You should also notice how deeply the roots have penetrated. If they have gone down deep into the subsoil, you are likely to have a soil in which your herbs will thrive; otherwise you may need to improve soil conditions with applications of compost and by growing deep-rooting plants.

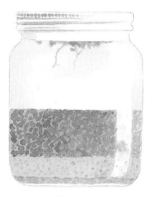

Clay soil

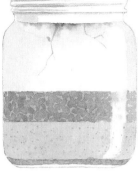

Medium soil

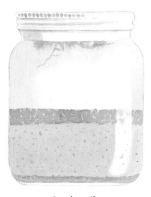

Sandy soil

Soil samples

Put a sample of soil into a screw-top jar, add water, and shake well. When the sample has settled, you will see how the stones, sand, and clay separate out and the organic material floats on the surface. A good soil is rich in organic matter with a balance of clay and sand.

Soil acidity

A particularly important feature of soil is its acidity level. This is measured as a pH value on a scale from 0 to 14. Acid soils have pH values below 7, a neutral soil has a pH of 7, and alkaline soils a pH greater than 7. A neutral soil is ideal, though most herbs will tolerate any level between pH 6.5 and pH 7.5. Various soil-testing kits and meters are available to help you check this, together with simple strips of pH test paper, which are very easy to use. But they can be misleading. The acidity level of your soil may vary from one part of your garden to another. In addition, certain plants, such as bluebells, influence soil acidity, and you will probably also affect the level yourself by the type of material you apply to your garden. Adding lime to the soil will raise the pH level, making it more alkaline; the addition of organic fertilizers reduces alkalinity. But other materials also have an effect on pH. For example, sphagnum moss peat has a pH level of 3.5–4, but sedge peat has a pH of 5.5.

pH scale		
0	ACID	
1		
2		
3		
	pH 3.5	Sphagnum moss peat
4		
	pH 4.5	Sandy soil
5		
	pH 5.5	Coarse loam soil / Sedge peat
6		
	pH 6.5	Heavy clay soil
7	pH 7	Neutral soil
8		
	pH 8.5	Fine loam
9		
10		
11		
12		
13		
14	ALKALINE	

Acid-tolerant plants

Arnica (*Arnica montana*)
French sorrel (*Rumex scutatus*)
Curled dock (*Rumex crispus*)
Dandelion (*Taraxacum officinale*)
Foxglove (*Digitalis purpurea*)
Heather (*Erica sp.*)
Honeysuckle (*Lonicera periclymenum*)
Juniper (*Juniperus communis*)
Pennyroyal (*Mentha pulegium*)
Sweet cicely (*Myrrhis odorata*)
Thyme (*Thymus vulgaris*)
Wood sorrel (*Oxalis acetosella*)

Alkali-tolerant plants

Centaury (*Centaurium erythraea*)
Chickweed (*Stellaria media*)
Chicory (*Cichorium intybus*)
Cowslip (*Primula veris*)
Elder (*Sambucus nigra*)
Juniper (*Juniperus communis*)
Lily of the valley (*Convallaria majalis*)
Lungwort (*Pulmonaria officinalis*)
Pasque flower (*Anemone pulsatilla*)
Rose (*Rosa sp.*)
Salad burnet (*Sanguisorba minor*)
Solomon's seal (*Polygonatum sp.*)
Thyme (*Thymus vulgaris*)
Wood sorrel (*Oxalis acetosella*)
Wormwood (*Artemisia absinthium*)
Yarrow (*Achillea millefolium*)

Soils and plants

Herbs are tolerant plants. Most species will survive in a range of soil types, but you will get the best results if you grow plants in the soil types of their natural habitat. The soils described on this page cover the most important herb habitats.

Chalky soil

Soil that forms over chalk is light and well drained. Because of the underlying rock it is also usually rich in calcium and alkaline in character, with a pH level as high as 8. Although you can increase the nutrient content of this soil by adding compost, it is difficult to lower the pH level significantly. If you have chalky soil and find that some plants do poorly, try making a raised bed (see pp. 252–3) with a less alkaline. Plants from chalk uplands often have long, penetrating roots that bring water and minerals from deep down in the rock though some have shorter, thicker roots.

Light, sandy soil

A soil with a high percentage of sand is likely to be well drained and, because nutrients get washed away as the moisture drains through, it will also have low fertility. Sandy soil often has a pH level slightly lower than normal. Though this is a poor soil for vegetables and most garden plants – you may have to use a plant food in addition to building up the soil nutrients with compost – the many herbs from places such as the Mediterranean and Middle East will thrive here.

Loam

A loam soil is rich in nutrients and has a good overall balance of clay, sand, and silt. Some loamy areas become wet and unworkable during winter and spring, but you can usual-ly improve the drainage by pushing a fork deeply into the soil at regular intervals. A well drained loam is ideal for herb growing, since it allows water to penetrate to the roots while also fostering the more open and aerobic conditions that they need in order to go deeper and break up the soil still further. The majority of herbs that do not require moisture-retentive or light soil will grow well here. The plants listed below do particularly well in loam.

Moist loam

This rich soil contains plenty of organic material, but is poorly drained and retains some water throughout the year. You can improve the drainage by forking through the soil, and by growing deep-rooted plants that break up the subsoil. This is a useful soil for the herb gardener – a wide range of herbs favour it and herbs whose natural home is heavy soil also do well.

Clay

Clay soil contains a predominance of tiny particles, which stick together in large masses. The soil bakes hard in summer and is heavy and sticky in the winter. Working compost into the first few inches will help make it better drained and easier to cultivate. The herbs that thrive on clay have deep penetrating roots that break up the heavy soil and are not affected by baking – burdock, for example. As well as the plants listed below, many others will tolerate clay.

Wet, marshy soil

This type of soil retains moisture at all times either because it is very poorly drained or because it is only just above the water table, so that the water has nowhere to drain. A number of herbs are native to wet, marshy areas. Most have lush, green foliage that grows prolifically, taking advantage of the high nutrient levels usually found in this type of soil.

Herbs and soil types

Chalk	Moist loam
Catnip, chicory, hyssop, juniper, lavender, lily of the valley, lungwort, marjoram, motherwort, pasque flower, rosemary, salad burnet, summer savory, wild marjoram	Angelica, bergamot, comfrey, elecampane, French sorrel, lady's mantle, lemon balm, meadowsweet, mints, parsley, skullcap, soapwort, sweet cicely, sweet violet, valerian
Sandy	**Clay**
Alfalfa, anise, arnica, borage, centaury, Roman chamomile, coriander, cumin, evening primrose, fennel, foxglove, lavender, pleurisy root, tarragon, thyme, wild carrot, wild marjoram, winter savory	Bergamot, burdock, coltsfoot, comfrey, lesser celandine, mints, wormwood. Provided that the topsoil is good and the drainage reasonable, loam and moist loam plants will also tolerate this soil
Loam	**Marshy**
Basil, bay, betony, blood root, burdock, caraway, catnip, chervil, chives, coltsfoot, coriander, dill, foxglove, fennel, lady's mantle, lovage, parsley, rosemary, rue, sage, tansy, thyme	Bogbean, golden seal, gypsywort, horsetail, iris, marsh mallow, meadowsweet, skullcap, sweet flag, valerian

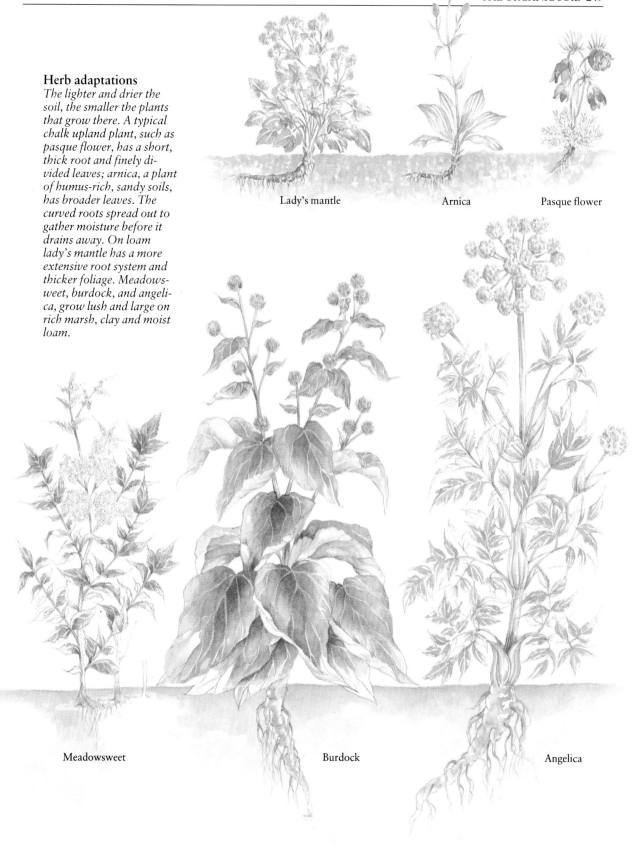

Herb adaptations

The lighter and drier the soil, the smaller the plants that grow there. A typical chalk upland plant, such as pasque flower, has a short, thick root and finely divided leaves; arnica, a plant of humus-rich, sandy soils, has broader leaves. The curved roots spread out to gather moisture before it drains away. On loam lady's mantle has a more extensive root system and thicker foliage. Meadowsweet, burdock, and angelica, grow lush and large on rich marsh, clay and moist loam.

Lady's mantle

Arnica

Pasque flower

Meadowsweet

Burdock

Angelica

The site

Before introducing herbs into your garden you should survey the whole site in some detail. Make a simple plan, and mark on it the north/south aspect and the main areas of shade. Divide these up into light (or intermittent), medium, and dark (or permanent) shade. Mark in features, such as banks and depressions, hedges, trees, and screens, and note any variations in the soil type (see pp. 246–7). Your survey will show you the best places to plant different herbs, and the best sites for features such as rock gardens and raised beds.

Herbs are essentially wild plants so it makes sense to grow them in conditions as close as possible to their natural environment. They derive from a wide range of habitats all over the world and therefore vary in the type of site they prefer. Many of our most familiar culinary herbs come from dry sunny areas such as the Mediterranean. As a general rule these plants, which include rosemary and marjoram, have small leaves; those from temperate climates have larger, fleshier foliage. Within these broad groups plants have particular preferences – cool shade, damp areas, or well drained soil. But herbs are adaptable, and many will do quite well outside their native habitats. A practical solution is to create a main herb bed in a sunny part of the garden and use other areas for herbs that prefer special conditions. Most woodland plants do well in open ground, but do not like being baked by the sun in the warm months. Grow them near shrubs or behind a screen of annuals such as sweet peas if you do not have a suitable area of shade. Herbs from a damp environment will grow in moisture-retentive soil that does not dry out in summer.

Other places you can use for herbs include areas of rubble and south-facing slopes (for herbs that enjoy good drainage and those of Mediterranean origin); and shaded banks (good for many of the woodland herbs). If you have a large, exposed garden, avoid areas open to icy north and east winds which can kill plants such as rosemary and lavender.

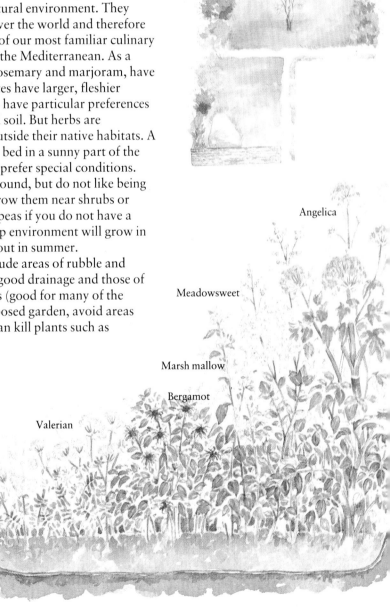

Angelica

Meadowsweet

Marsh mallow

Bergamot

Valerian

Damp bed
If you do not have a damp area, you can create moist conditions in your garden by laying a sheet of polythene under 12–18 ins (30–45 cm) of soil. Pierce the sheet to allow the moisture to drain slowly, and run a dripping hose into the area to give moisture. Plant bergamot, marsh mallow, meadowsweet, angelica, and valerian here.

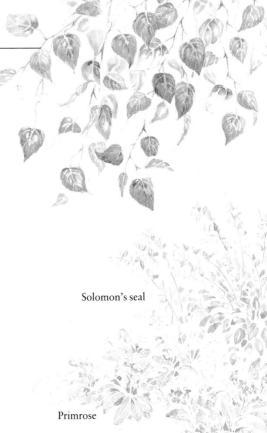

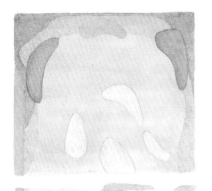

Open and sunny

Shaded

Damp

Wild garden

Well drained

Planning the beds

Mark the main features of your garden on a plan and then sketch in the sunny and shady zones, together with the damp and well drained areas. You will then be able to see the best sites for herb growing. In the example, left, the main herb bed could go in one of the sunny places, the area next to the pond would make an ideal damp bed, and one of the shady areas near trees could be used for planting woodland herbs. In addition, you could make use of south-facing beds near the house for sun-loving Mediterranean herbs, or create a wild garden amongst the shrubs on the left.

Solomon's seal

Primrose

Lungwort

Shaded bed

Give woodland herbs some shade near trees or shrubs. Some of the most useful herbs that enjoy shade are mint, lily of the valley, woodruff, sweet violet, lungwort, primrose, and solomon's seal.

Sweet violet

Dill

Fennel

Sage

Marjoram

Woodruff

Main herb bed

The best site for this bed is in a sunny area, accessible to the house. The soil should be well drained but should have enough humus to keep it moist in summer. Most culinary herbs (such as sage, coriander, rosemary, basil, marjoram, and thyme) will grow well here. (For full growing requirements see pp. 273–81).

Basil

Thyme

Lavender

Lily of the valley

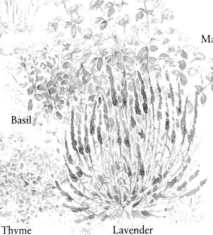

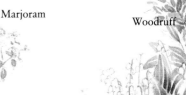

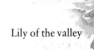

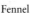

Rock gardens

Specially constructed herb beds can give you greater control over the herb-growing environment. You can introduce better soil and improve the drainage. A sunny, well drained rock garden, for example, is an ideal habitat for many herbs, especially those from the Mediterranean, such as rosemary, sage, and oregano. A raised bed without rocks offers niches for alpines and trailing species in the walls, larger plants in the bed itself, woodland plants in the shade provided by the taller species.

If your soil is heavy, build your rock garden on top of the existing soil; with lighter soil you can dig to a depth of 1 ft (30 cm) so that the rockery is roughly level with the surrounding soil. Start with a 6 ins (15 cm) layer of rubble, add a 3 ins (8 cm) layer of gravel, and cover this with a 3 ins (8 cm) layer of soil consisting of 3 parts topsoil, 2 parts peat,

and 1½ parts grit or sharp, gritty sand. Finish off with attractive stones or old red bricks.

Growing herbs in gravel

A gravel path is a good place to grow herbs, but prepare it carefully to ensure good drainage. Dig the soil out to a depth of 12 ins (30 cm) and fill the trench with a 6 ins (15 cm) layer of rubble; next add a layer of upturned turf, followed by a 2–3 ins (5–7 cm) layer of the soil mix used in the rock garden (see left). Top up the trench with a layer of gravel or stone chippings. Herbs from dry, southern climates will thrive here and will usually seed themselves readily – fennel, creeping and bushy thymes, winter and summer savory, sage, rosemary, marjorams, lavender, marigold, borage, tarragon, blessed thistle, German chamomile, hyssop, horehound, catnip, clary, sage, and chives.

Lawns and ground cover

Many herbs make excellent and decorative ground cover and some of these also make fragrant lawns. All tend to suppress weeds because they cover the ground densely enough to cut out light from the soil surface and stop seedlings growing, although there are some weeds, such as the perennial thistles, docks, and bindweed, which they will not prevent from pushing through. Another great benefit of ground-cover herbs is that they keep the soil covered in winter, insulating it against frost and protecting it from erosion during heavy rains. In summer, they help the soil's moisture retention and protect it from the baking sun. Not all ground-cover plants are low-growing – some, such as lemon balm and marjoram, form a mat of low-growing foliage during the winter but grow up to 24 ins (60 cm) in the summer. Other plants that are relatively tall but can be used in this way are the dwarf species of comfrey (*Symphytum grandiflorum*), which spreads vigorously and has attractive drooping flowers coloured cream and red, and lady's bedstraw. For shady areas and under large trees, try sweet violet, wood-

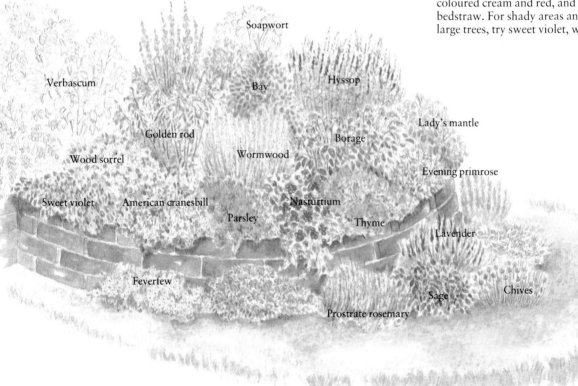

Soapwort
Verbascum
Bay
Hyssop
Lady's mantle
Golden rod
Borage
Wood sorrel
Wormwood
Evening primrose
Sweet violet
American cranesbill
Nasturtium
Parsley
Thyme
Lavender
Feverfew
Sage
Chives
Prostrate rosemary

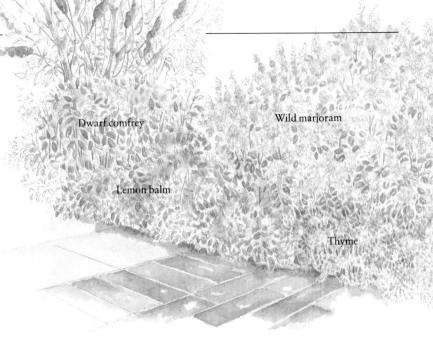

Dwarf comfrey

Wild marjoram

Lemon balm

Thyme

ruff, ground ivy, wild strawberry and lungwort. Before planting these, you should eliminate weeds so that the ground cover plants will have the chance to spread and become established before the weeds start to develop. Make sure that you remove all the roots, particularly of deep-rooting and creeping weeds (see pp. 266–7).

For well drained areas in full sun you can choose from a number of herbs for lawn cover. Most are fragrant and colourful. There are several varieties of carpeting thyme (many strongly scented and edible), which make a fragrant lawn. Another suitable plant is chamomile (*Anthemis nobilis*), which you should keep cut short. The non-flowering variety (*Anthemis nobilis* treneague) requires no cutting and, like the flowering variety, has leaves with the fragrance of apples. Pennyroyal makes a bright green ground cover, and wild white clover attracts bees in early summer. Yarrow is also suitable for lawn growing if you keep it cut short.

Building a raised bed
Construct a raised bed 12 ins (30 cm) above ground level. You can make the walls from stone, old bricks, or even logs, leaving gaps to accommodate trailing plants. Put in a 6 ins (8 cm) bottom layer of stones or rubble to allow good drainage. Fill up the bed with the same soil mix as for a rock garden (see opposite page).

Container gardening

You can grow a wide range of herbs in containers. There is no limit to the types of containers you can use, although those made of natural materials – terracotta pots, wooden troughs and half barrels, and stone troughs and sinks – usually look best with herbs. Every container should have drainage holes in the bottom. Start by putting in a layer of stones or broken pot to aid drainage. If you are using a large container, follow this with a layer of upturned turf or some other bulky organic material. Finally fill up with a soil-based potting compost. (Peat-based composts dry out too rapidly.)

Because a plant container is isolated from the rest of the garden it requires certain special treatment. Be careful not to over-water. Wait until the compost surface is quite dry before watering. If you are growing in a small pot, add water to the saucer beneath; the plant will take up the moisture within a few minutes if needed. You should also give special attention to feeding. When the container garden is a few months old, you should start to feed the plants regularly with an organic fertilizer (see pp. 264–5).

You should grow certain herbs, such as mints, fennel, French tarra-gon, angelica, lovage, sorrel, bergamot, and wormwood, in separate containers, as they tend to be invasive. Shrubs such as rosemary, sage, lavender, lemon verbena, sweet bay, and santolina are also best grown in their own separate containers. Keep annuals to a container of their own, and have another tub or trough of mixed herbs.

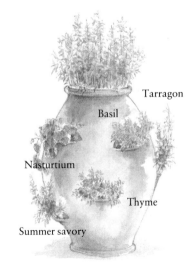

Tarragon

Basil

Nasturtium

Thyme

Summer savory

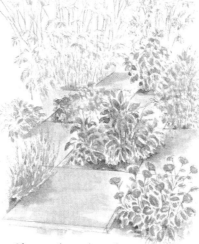

Formal herb gardens

The formal approach to herb gardening, though less natural than the other methods in this section, has several advantages. The convenience of small beds with paths close by means that maintenance and harvesting are straightforward. The resulting patterns of beds, paving, and small hedges are attractive. And the formal design need not prevent you from creating ecological niches appropriate to each plant – areas that are shady and sunny, sheltered and more exposed.

Some of the most effective formal garden designs are very simple. One traditional arrangement groups the beds symmetrically around a central feature such as a bird bath or a clipped bay tree. This type of design can be based on a square divided into four, or a circle with the divisions between the beds like the spokes of a wheel. Within the formal layout, planting can be quite informal, mixing heights, textures, and colours, and making use of companion plants (see pp. 268–9). You can achieve a different decorative effect by planting each of the beds with a particular type of herb, so that one contains carpeting thymes, another grey-leaved plants, and so on.

A chequerboard pattern attractive-

Chequerboard garden
Most paving slabs are between 1 and 2 ft (30–60 cm) square, although many different shapes are available. You can make the garden more sheltered by planting the larger herbs as a screen against the wind.

ly alternates paving slabs with beds of either one species or several smaller plants. This makes each type of plant easily accessible. Whichever system of planting you choose, leave some of the beds free for sowing annual herbs, such as borage, marigold, dill, and basil.

Symmetrical garden
Make the beds large enough to accommodate all the plants you want to grow – but not so large that you cannot reach them easily from paths. If you want a neat border for the beds, use santolina – avoid invasive hedging species such as privet. Gravel makes paths that are easy to install and many herbs will root and seed in them. They need attention to keep them free of weeds.

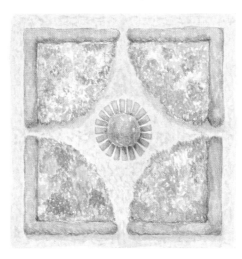

Choosing herbs

Use these lists when planning your garden. They show how you can use herbs for their decorative effects (opposite), for their scent, and to attract bees (below).

Butterfly and bee herbs
Anise (*Pimpinella anisum*)*
Basil (*Ocimum basilicum*)*
Bergamot (*Monarda didyma*)
Betony (*Stachys officinalis*)
Borage (*Borago officinalis*)
Broom (*Cytisus scoparius*)
Burdock (*Arctium lappa*)
Catnip (*Nepeta cataria*)
Chicory (*Cichorium intybus*)
Chives (*Allium schoenoprasum*)*
Clover (*Trifolium pratense*)
Comfrey (*Symphytum officinale*)
Coltsfoot (*Tussilago farfara*)
Dandelion (*Taraxacum officinale*)
Evening primrose (*Oenothera sp.*)
Fennel (*Foeniculum vulgare*)
Heal-all (*Prunella vulgaris*)
Horehound (*Marrubium vulgare*)
Hyssop (*Hyssopus officinalis*)
Lemon balm (*Melissa officinalis*)*
Lavender (*Lavandula officinalis*)*
Marjoram (*Origanum spp*)
Marsh mallow (*Althaea officinalis*)
Mints (*Mentha spp*)*
Meadowsweet (*Filipendula ulmaria*)
Peppermint (*Mentha piperita*)*
Rosemary (*Rosmarinus officinalis*)*
Sage (*Salvia officinalis*)*
Thyme (*Thymus vulgaris*)*
Valerian (*Valeriana officinalis*)*
Yarrow (*Achillea millefolium*)*

Perfumed herbs
Chamomile (*Anthemis nobilis*)
Chervil (*Anthriscus cerefolium*)
Dill (*Anethum graveolens*)
Fennel (*Foeniculum vulgare*)
Lemon verbena (*Aloysia triphylla*)
Parsley (*Petroselinum crispum*)
Pineapple sage (*Salvia sp*)
Rose (*Rosa centifolia*)
Savory (*Satureia spp*)
Sweet violet (*Viola odorata*)
Tansy (*Tanacetum vulgare*)
Tarragon (French) (*Artemisia dracunculus*)
Wormwood (*Artemisia absinthium*)
Plus herbs above marked *

Grey foliage

Catnip (*Nepeta cataria*)
Clary sage (*Salvia sclarea*)
Costmary (*Chrysanthemum balsamita*)
Eucalyptus (*Eucalyptus spp*)
Globe artichoke (*Cynara scolymus*)
Horehound (*Marrubium vulgare*)
Lavender (*Lavandula spp*)
Marsh mallow (*Althaea officinalis*)
Mugwort (*Artemisia vulgaris*)
Opium poppy (*Papaver somniferum*)
Sage (*Salvia officinalis*)
Thyme (*Thymus vulgaris*)
Wormwood (*Artemisia absinthium*)

Evergreen foliage

Chervil (*Anthriscus cerefolium*)
Juniper (*Juniperus communis*)
Horehound (*Marrubium vulgare*)
Lavender (*Lavandula officinalis*)
Lemon balm (*Melissa officinalis*)
Parsley (*Petroselinum crispum*)
Pennyroyal (*Mentha pulegium*)
Rosemary (*Rosmarinus officinalis*)
Rue (*Ruta graveolens*)
Sage (*Salvia officinalis*)
Sweet bay (*Laurus nobilis*)
Thyme (*Thymus spp*)
Winter savory (*Satureja montana*)
Wormwood (*Artemisia absinthium*)

Variegated foliage

Applemint (*variegated*)
Comfrey (*variegated*)
Lemon balm (*gold*)
Lungwort (*variegated*)
Pelargonium (*variegated, scented*)
Thyme (*silver and golden*)
Sage (*golden and tricolor*)

Other colours

Red Sage (*Salvia officinalis*)
Blue/grey Rue (*Ruta graveolens*)
Silver Sea holly (*Eryngium*)
Silver-edged leaves Alpine lady's mantle (*Alchemilla alpina*)

White flowers

Anise (*Pimpinella anisum*)
Blood root (*Sanguinaria canadensis*)
Caraway (*Carum carvi*)
Chamomile (*Anthemis nobilis*)
Chervil (*Anthriscus cerefolium*)
Feverfew (*Chrysanthemum parthenium*)
Garlic mustard (*Alliaria petiolata*)
Hyssop (*Hyssopus officinalis*)
Lavender alba (*Lavandula sp*)
Lily of the valley (*Convallaria majalis*)

Queen Anne's lace (*Daucus carota*)
Solomon's seal (*Polygonatum multiflorum*)
Sweet basil (*Ocimum basilicum*)
Sweet cicely (*Myrrhis odorata*)
Sweet marjoram (*Origanum marjorana*)
White clover (*Trifolium repens*)
Winter savory (*Satureja montana*)
Woodruff (*Asperula odorata*)
Wood sorrel (*Oxalis acetosella*)
Yarrow (*Achillea millefolium*)

Pink flowers

Centaury (*Erythraea centaurium*)
Coriander (*Coriandrum sativum*)
Cumin (*Cuminum cyminum*)
Foxglove (*Digitalis purpurea*)
Gravel root (*Eupatorium purpurea*)
Hollyhock (*Althaea rosea*)
Lavender (pink) (*Lavandula sp*)
Marsh mallow (*Althaea officinalis*)
Motherwort (*Leonorus cardiaca*)
Mountain mint (*Calamintha officinalis*)
Oregano (*Origanum vulgare*)
Pink hyssop (*Hyssopus officinalis*)
Pot marjoram (*Origanum onites*)
Red clover (*Trifolium pratense*)
Rose (dog, sweet briar) (*Rosa spp*)
Soapwort (*Saponaria officinalis*)
Thyme (*Thymus vulgaris*)
Valerian (*Valeriana officinalis*)

Yellow flowers

Agrimony (*Agrimonia eupatoria*)
Arnica (*Arnica montana*)
Avens (*Geum urbanum*)
Blessed thistle (*Cnicus benedictus*)
Broom (*Cytisus scoparius*)
Celandine (*Chelidonium majus / Ranunculus ficaria*)
Coltsfoot (*Tussilago farfara*)
Cowslip (*Primula veris*)
Dandelion (*Taraxacum officinale*)
Dill (*Anethum graveolens*)
Elecampane (*Inula helenium*)

Evening primrose (*Oenothera biennis*)
Fennel (*Foeniculum vulgare*)
Five-finger grass (*Potentilla tormentilla*)
Marigold (orange) (*Calendula officinalis*)
Mullein (*Verbascum thapsus*)
Primrose (*Primula vulgaris*)
Safflower (*Carthamus tinctorius*)
Sunflower (*Helianthus annuus*)
Yellow flag (*Iris pseudacorus*)

Blue flowers

Borage (*Borago officinalis*)
Chicory (*Cichorium intybus*)
Columbine (*Aquilegia vulgaris*)
Flax (*Linum usitatissimum*)
Hyssop (*Hyssopus officinalis*)
Larkspur (*Delphinium consolida*)
Lavender lanata (*Lavandula sp*)
Rosemary (*Rosmarinus officinalis*)
Sea holly (*Eryngium maritimum*)

Purple or mauve flowers

Betony (*Stachys officinalis*)
Black horehound (*Ballota nigra*)
Chives (*Allium schoenoprasum*)
Clary sage (*Salvia sclarea*)
Comfrey (*Symphytum officinale*)
Echinacea (*Echinacea angustifolia*)
Greater burdock (*Arctium lappa*)
Heal-all (*Prunella vulgaris*)
Hedge woundwort (*Stachys sylvatica*)
Hyssop (*Hyssopus officinalis*)
Lavender (*Lavandula spp*)

Lobelia (*Lobelia inflata*)
Mint (*Mentha spp*)
Opium poppy (*Papaver somniferum*)
Pasque flower (*Anemone pulsatilla*)
Pennyroyal (*Mentha pulegium*)
Sage (*Salvia officinalis*)
Scullcap (*Scutellaria laterifolia*)
Sweet violet (*Viola odorata*)
Vervain (*Verbena officinalis*)
Wild bergamot (*Monarda didyma*)
Wild pansy (*Viola tricolor*)

Red flowers

Crimson clover (*Trifolium pratense*)
Field poppy (*Papaver rhoeados*)
Red bergamot (*Monarda sp*)
Red valerian (*Valeriana*)
Pleurisy root (*Asclepias tuberosa*)

See Glossary for cautions on use of particular herbs.

Herbs as a commercial crop

Herbs have been cultivated commercially for centuries in the warm climate of mediterranean Europe. With the release of surplus land in the north from over-production of wheat and beef, and the reaction against intensive agriculture's wastefulness and addiction to chemicals, has come a resurgence in organic farming and the planting of herbs as an alternative crop. Evening primrose, feverfew, and linseed are among the first to take over on land vacated by cereals.

Elsewhere, the value of jojoba oil for engines and cosmetics led to the establishment of the plant as an important plantation crop in the early 1980s. As well as replacing traditional crops in California, it thrives in arid lands where few other plants can survive (see opposite). The sago palm of Malaysia and Indonesia, which takes 15 years to mature, is harvested just before flowering. One tree yields 600–800 lb (270–360 kg) of starch for export as sago, or bread and cakes locally, and the residuary pith is either roasted or fed to the pigs. And sunflower, another oil producer, is grown widely in Europe.

In addition there has been a huge increase in the number of commercial herb farms selling plants and seeds – not just direct to the public for home planting, but to local authorities, for instance, who wish to make herb gardens in public parks. This idea of "community gardens" is not entirely new. There is an ancient custom in the Madrid Botanical Gardens that anyone requesting medicinal herbs before 11 am must be given them free. In London, the Chelsea Physic Garden was started in 1673 specifically for providing a place where apprentice herbalists could grow and learn about their stock in trade. More recently, a community garden at Ashram Acres in the English midlands, where a variety of herbs and vegetables are raised organically by the local people, has proved such a success that another similar project nearby for the training of long-term unemployed people in the growing of Asian and Caribbean vegetables and herbs is being established.

More urgent and on a wider scale is the development of herb gardens in poorer regions of the world. Vietnamese families are encouraged to grow a dozen or so of the 58 recognized "family medicine" plants for local use and for sale to the government, thus providing health care close at hand and extra income. Plant medicines are produced locally in a similar way in Bangladesh, Madagascar, Rwanda, and Thailand.

One consequence of the commercialization of herb-growing is the tendency, seen so clearly in crop development, to modify the wild plants. The cultivated sunflower is bigger-flowered, bigger-leaved and thicker-stemmed than its wild relation. The ancestral forms from which cultivated plums are derived are small-fruited and spiney – two undesirable characteristics for commerce. Another tendency, the use of chemical fertilizers, should also be avoided for fear of polluting the plants. At this point the dividing line between organic vegetable farming and growing herbs as a commercial crop is almost indistinguishable.

Jojoba
*Jojoba (*Simmondsia chinensis*) is a valuable dual-purpose crop. It can be planted to halt desertification of arid grasslands, and its seeds yield a high-quality oil used in shampoos, in engines and as a substitute for sperm whale oil. It now covers 40,000 acres (16,000 ha) of semi-arid land in the U.S.A. There is a danger, however, that its exploitation will lead to loss of desert ecosystems.*

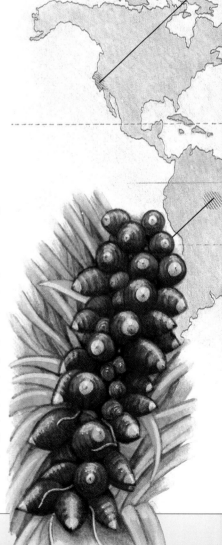

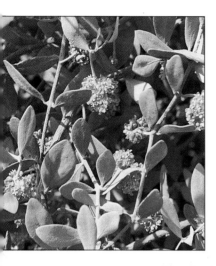

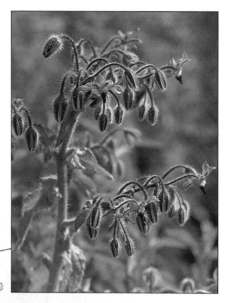

Borage

The bright hopes for the future of borage (Borago officinalis) as a commercial crop have recently dimmed. In the early 1980s borage was found to contain more gamma linoleic acid (GLA) – a valuable medicinal substance – than evening primrose oil. But cultivation problems recently coincided with a dramatic slump in prices as waste blackcurrant pulp proved a cheaper and richer source of GLA.

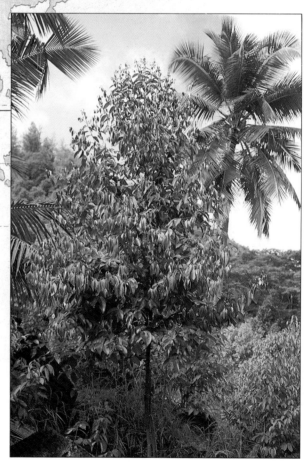

Babassu palm

This palm (Orbignya speciosa) is a commercial success in its native Brazil, where it replaces coconut oil in soaps, cosmetics and food products. In the future, it could help to enrich depleted grasslands. From a yield of 200 lb of nuts per year from each tree, farmers can extract oil, methyl alcohol, charcoal, cattle cake, and pig food.

Cinnamon

One of the oldest spices known to man, cinnamon (Cinnamomum zeylanicum) is native to Sri Lanka and S. India, where wild, self-seeded plants still yield more dried bark each year than cultivated shrubs. Several thousand tons are produced annually, mainly from Sri Lanka. Cinnamomum cassia, a member of the same genus and a native of S.E. China is also a source of the spice.

Seeds

Every seed, no matter how small, contains a tremendous life-force. Unlocking this force and growing plants from seed is one of the most rewarding experiences for any gardener. Once the flower is fertilized, the seeds start to develop and the flower petals, which have now done their job of attracting insects, fall off to reveal the seeds or their swelling containers. As the seeds develop further, they lose their high moisture content until they are usually brown and dry to the touch. At this ripening stage, you can see the enormous range of shapes and sizes of seeds from different plants (see pp. 260–1). This is when the seed is ready to be dispersed – or to be harvested.

Starting with seeds has several advantages over stocking your garden with bought-in plants. They are cheaper, and a much wider variety of species is available from herb seed specialists. Most herbs grow well from seed, although decorative varieties of certain herbs, such as the silver variegated thymes and purple and golden sages, are not suitable for sowing – either they produce no seed or the seedlings do not grow true. French tarragon is another popular herb that does not produce seed. Mints are best grown from cuttings (see pp. 262–3) since most are hybrids and their seedlings do not grow true.

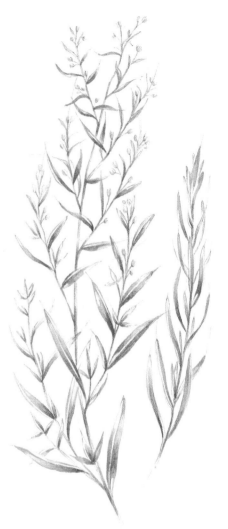

Tarragon
French tarragon (Artemisia dracunculus) *does not produce seeds, but has a superior flavour, more delicate than its close relative Russian tarragon* (A. dracunculoides), *which seeds prolifically. French tarragon should be propagated either by cuttings or root division (see pp. 262–3).*

Successful germination

Most seeds require four things to germinate successfully: the right levels of moisture, air, light, and temperature. In addition, certain wild seeds have a long dormancy period, and special techniques are required to break this (see opposite).

Moisture This is provided via the soil or compost so it is critical, especially with tiny seeds, to make sure that the compost surface does not dry out. A piece of glass or clear plastic over the seed tray will help keep moisture in, provided that you keep the tray away from direct sunlight. Remove the glass as soon as the seeds start to germinate.

Air A well cultivated soil or good, open compost should provide the right aerobic conditions for seeds. An organic, peat-based compost is ideal. Avoid sowing seed in compacted or waterlogged soil, which will eliminate the air that the plant's young roots need. If you are sowing outdoors and your soil is clay or poorly drained, break it up as much as possible.

Light This is vital for most herb seeds – do not sow them too deep. Light will penetrate a thin soil covering but you should sow very fine seeds on the surface. Otherwise, the general rule is the larger the seed, the less light it is likely to need, so you should plant the seed to a depth that is about three times its diameter and sow tiny seed on the surface.

Temperature Many seeds native to northern Europe and North America germinate well at temperatures a few degrees above freezing point. An exception to this is parsley, which requires a much higher temperature. Some seeds from the Mediterranean and from hotter climates, especially rosemary, require temperatures of 60–80 °F (15–21 ° C) though lavender germinates best at low temperatures.

Dormancy

The germination times of many seeds depend on whether the seed lies dormant before germination. Dormancy is a mechanism that enables seeds to germinate at the best time (usually spring) over a long period, to ensure the plant's survival in the wild. Some seeds, such as members of the Umbelliferae or carrot family, will germinate only after a period at a cold temperature. A solution to this problem is to subject seeds to a pregermination period of chilling (a process called "vernalization").

Other species, such as bay and lily of the valley, will germinate when they are very fresh and go into dormancy once they have dried. One technique that can speed up germination of hard-covered seeds such as legumes is scarification – rubbing the seeds with sandpaper to break up the outer coating.

Sowing outside

Although it is best to sow the smaller herb seeds indoors in trays, you can sow larger seeds outside. Ideal times for outdoor sowing vary according to species (see pp. 274–9), but spring is generally the best time to sow annuals and perennials. This gives them the advantage of rising temperatures and longer daylight hours to trigger germination. Chervil and coriander are two annuals that you can sow in the autumn. They will overwinter satisfactorily and this gives them an early start to the growing season. It is best to sow biennial plants in late summer and leave them to overwinter. Autumn sowing is generally best for seeds from temperate climates, since they may need frost to break down the seed coat and break dormancy. This is beneficial for angelica and vital for sweet cicely, which needs all the frost it can get.

When you are sowing outdoors always be careful to mark the place precisely. Include on the label both the name of the plant and the date on which the seeds were sown.

Birds can be a problem with outdoor seeds. You can protect the seedbed by putting a network of thread, attached to sticks at the edge of the bed, across the area.

Special treatment

Some seeds need special treatment. Bulbous plants, such as lily of the valley, do not like their roots to be disturbed until the plants are two or three years old. Sow the seeds around the edge of a 5 ins (13 cm) pot so that they have room to develop without pricking out. They will die down after each season and build up a large bulb.

Self seeding

This is one of the most natural processes in the garden – most plants will produce seedlings themselves if you do not collect the seed or cut off seed heads. Some species, such as elecampane, pot marigold, caraway, motherwort, and lady's mantle, self-seed prolifically. If allowed the seed will germinate when the conditions are right and the resulting plants will be more vigorous and healthy than those grown in seed trays and planted out. The seedlings do not always appear where you want them, but you can move the plants later, or adopt a more flexible, less formal style of gardening, in which chance combinations of plants and colours can occur. An advantage of letting plants self-seed is that you may find an interesting hybrid. Most decorative lavenders (and many other garden plants) are descended from chance seedlings spotted by observant gardeners.

Requirements for germination

Conditions	Plants
Temperature 60–70 °F (15–21 °C)	Most plants from southern latitudes (see also Dormancy, below)
55 °F (13 °C) or less	Most plants from N Europe and N America
40–50 °F (4–10 °C)	Lavender
70 °F (21 °C)	Parsley
80–90 °F (27–32 °C)	Rosemary
Inhibited by high temperature	Juniper, lettuce, lavender, soapwort
Dormancy Period of up to several months before germination	Dried seeds of bay and lily of the valley; see also below
Vernalization Necessary	Arnica, angelica (old seed), woodruff, sweet violet, juniper, pasque flower, rose, hawthorn
Helpful	Agrimony, yellow iris, blood root
Double chilling Two periods of chilling with a warm period between	Tree and shrub seeds, especially hawthorn, that do not germinate easily
Light Germination in the light	Berberis, birch, capsicum, chamomile, foxglove, heather, lobelia, peony, poppy, primula, thyme, winter savory, witch hazel, yarrow

Seed types

Herbs, which come from many different habitats all over the world, have evolved many different mechanisms for survival. Nowhere is this clearer than in their seeds. Place a selection of herb seeds on a sheet of white paper and you will see a whole world of marvellously sculpted forms all beautifully designed for success and survival in their particular environment. Some have very tough coats (often smooth and hard, sometimes ribbed) which can remain in the soil for years without germinating or decomposing. Others are soft and oily and germinate more quickly. They also vary widely in their dispersal mechanisms: some with hooks and spines that will attach themselves to passing animals, others with parachutes that can travel for long distances blown by the wind. One type of seed that is especially good at travelling is the fruit which is eaten by humans or animals – a process that also aids germination.

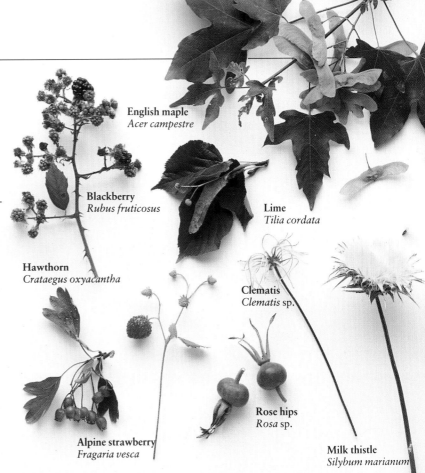

English maple
Acer campestre

Blackberry
Rubus fruticosus

Lime
Tilia cordata

Hawthorn
Crataegus oxyacantha

Clematis
Clematis sp.

Rose hips
Rosa sp.

Alpine strawberry
Fragaria vesca

Milk thistle
Silybum marianum

Windborne seeds

Many herbs have seeds that are distributed by the wind. The dandelion, with its familiar "clock" made up of seeds with tiny parachutes, is typical of this type. It is a member of the Compositae or daisy family, and many other members of this family have similar seeds that travel on the wind. Most of the thistles also have light, windborne seeds – their success in distribution is one reason why these plants are so difficult to eradicate from the garden. There are also a number of trees with seeds that are specially adapted to travel in this way. The familiar maple, sycamore, and ash have winged seeds, while black poplar has a cotton-wool-like substance attached to its seeds, which sometimes travel for miles on the wind. Some plants, such as horsetail, have tiny dust-like seeds that also lend themselves well to distribution by the wind.

Waterborne seeds

Many seeds growing on the seashore or by rivers can survive in the water. The aquatic plant seeds germinate in the water itself and don't require any contact with soil. They are often carried long distances by the tides or currents, eventually coming to rest on a muddy riverbank or a beach, where the seeds will grow. Most fresh-water plants root easily, so their seeds are not as vital for survival as those of other plants.

Ejected seeds

Some plants have a catapult mechanism that throws seeds in all directions. Certain members of the geranium and cabbage families use this method. Some plants of the pea family, such as the vetches, have large seed pods which hold on to the seeds when the pods are damp and violently eject them once the pods dry out.

Gravity

The greatest number of seeds simply fall out of their pods by the force of gravity. This doesn't mean that they all fall in a heap beside the plant. Many of these species are tall like the foxglove, figwort, and purple loosestrife. These tall plants move from side to side in the wind and so their seeds can be scattered over a large patch of ground. Members of the poppy family such as the opium poppy have a hard seed capsule containing hundreds of tiny hard seeds. These tip out when the plant dies down and the dead stems are blown over. If the seeds all came up at once this would be a waste of the plant's resources. But the seeds, with their hard coats, have a time-lapse mechanism. They can remain dormant in the soil for years waiting for the perfect conditions to germinate. Many seeds of the borage family can stay in the soil for a spring germination.

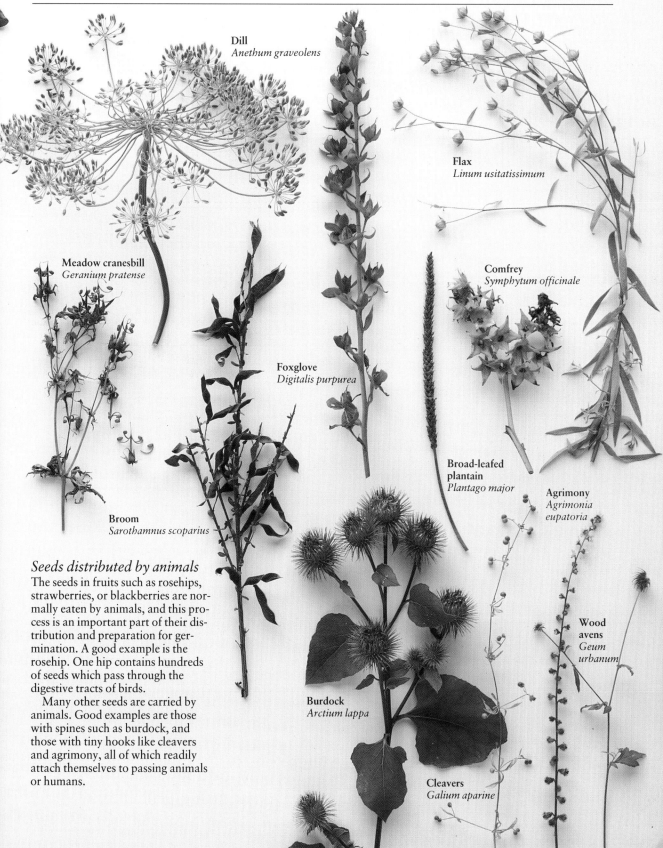

Dill
Anethum graveolens

Flax
Linum usitatissimum

Meadow cranesbill
Geranium pratense

Comfrey
Symphytum officinale

Foxglove
Digitalis purpurea

**Broad-leafed
plantain**
Plantago major

Agrimony
*Agrimonia
eupatoria*

Broom
Sarothamnus scoparius

**Wood
avens**
*Geum
urbanum*

Seeds distributed by animals

The seeds in fruits such as rosehips,
strawberries, or blackberries are normally eaten by animals, and this process is an important part of their distribution and preparation for germination. A good example is the
rosehip. One hip contains hundreds
of seeds which pass through the
digestive tracts of birds.

Many other seeds are carried by
animals. Good examples are those
with spines such as burdock, and
those with tiny hooks like cleavers
and agrimony, all of which readily
attach themselves to passing animals
or humans.

Burdock
Arctium lappa

Cleavers
Galium aparine

Sowing inside

Using a seed tray, sow in late summer or early autumn – most seeds will germinate in the late summer warmth. Half-size seed trays are useful – they take as many seedlings as you are likely to need. Use a peat-based organic compost and cover the seed to about three times its diameter, sowing the tiniest on the surface. After sowing, cover the tray with glass or clear plastic and keep it out of direct sunlight. Once the seedlings emerge, remove the covering and expose them to brighter light (but not direct sun). Plant annuals and biennials into small pots or multi-cell trays. Prick out perennials into 3 ins (7.5 cm) pots to grow on before planting out.

How to sow

1 Fill the tray with seed compost to within ½ in (1.25 cm) of the top, level the surface and firm it gently with a block of wood. Give the compost a thorough soaking using a watering can with a fine head.

2 Sow the seed thinly. If it is fine, tip it into the palm of one hand, pick up a pinch with the thumb and first finger of the other hand, and sprinkle it evenly.

3 Sprinkle compost over the seeds to the required depth. Use a sieve to keep the compost fine.

4 Label the tray clearly with name, date, and source of seed. Give a further light watering to dampen the top layer of compost. Place a sheet of glass over the tray, and keep the tray in a shady, sheltered place until the seeds start to germinate.

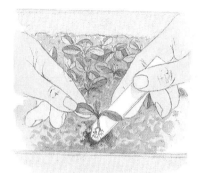

Pricking out

Do this when the first true leaves have developed. Ease them out gently with a knife, holding the leaves carefully between the thumb and finger.

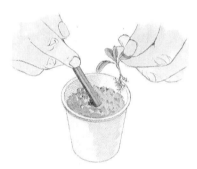

Potting the seedlings

Transplant the seedlings into a small pot containing soil-based compost. Leave them in the pots until the root system grows and starts to emerge from the bottom. Before leaving the plants outside permanently, make sure that they are properly accustomed to outside conditions. For the first 2 to 3 weeks, keep them under cover at night and in bad weather. A cold frame with a lid that can be opened by day is an ideal place to put the seedlings during this period.

Other methods

If you cannot grow a plant from seed, you may be able to propagate it by taking cuttings or by dividing the roots.

Taking cuttings is simple. You cut a short length of stem with leaves attached below a leaf joint, insert this into a suitable soil (often known as a "cutting medium"), and keep the leaves of the cutting humid. Most shrubby herbs (such as thymes, sages, hyssop, marjorams, rosemary, lavender, and winter savory) propagate easily from softwood cuttings taken in late spring or early summer. Rosemary and lavender also do well from semi-ripe cuttings. Some herbs, such as water-loving plants like mints, will root very quickly in a glass of water.

For mature plants that are a few years old, you can use root division as a means of propagation. Plants with thick, fleshy roots, such as comfrey, horseradish, elecampane, and valerian respond well to root division, as do plants that run, such as mints, woodruff, and bedstraw.

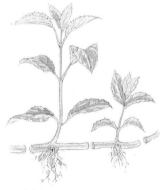

Taking root cuttings

Mint is easy to propagate by cutting sections of its spreading, horizontal roots to create new plants. A section of the stem of mint will also root very easily in a glass of water.

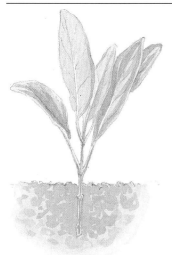

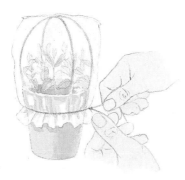

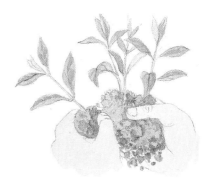

Softwood cuttings
Use a cutting medium that is low in nutrients, well drained, and aerated, such as sharp sand mixed with peat or potting compost. Take softwood cuttings in late spring or summer when the new shoots are soft and full of sap, but not spindly. Cut the shoot just below a leaf node, producing a cutting 2–4 ins (5–10 cm) long. Cut off the lower leaves and insert the stem about 1 in (2.5 cm) into the medium.

Covering cuttings
Keep the cuttings sprayed with water until you cover the pot. For this you can use a plastic bag with a thin wire hoop to prevent the plastic touching the leaves, or an upturned glass jar. Keep the cuttings out of direct sunlight; in hot weather quite heavy shade is desirable for the first week. The cutting medium is low in nutrients, so give regular foliar feeds when the cuttings start to root.

Potting cuttings
When the cuttings are well rooted, pot in small individual pots in a seed or multi-purpose compost. Allow to grow on before planting out. Take semi-ripe cuttings towards the end of the growing season. Dipping the cut end in a hormone rooting powder is often beneficial. Use the same method as for softwood cuttings, but leave them in a cold greenhouse or conservatory over the winter and they will be ready to prick out in spring.

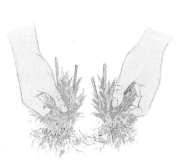

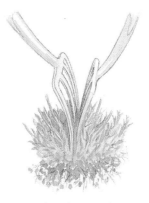

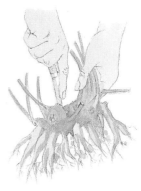

Dividing perennials
You can divide the roots of many perennials that have been established for two years or more. Divide them in spring or autumn using your fingers or a knife.

Dividing larger clumps
Old, vigorously rooting plants require a different technique of root division. The best way is to gain extra leverage by prising the roots apart with two forks.

Dividing fleshy roots
Fleshy-rooted plants such as horseradish can be propagated by root division. Cut the roots carefully into short lengths. Use a sharp knife to give a clean cut through the root.

Organic cultivation

The basic principle of organic cultivation is to feed the soil and build up its structure, so encouraging the teeming mass of micro-organisms that convert plant foods in the soil into a soluble form that the plant can use (see pp. 244–5). Most garden soils contain more than adequate nutrients for herbs, and for most other plants except green vegetables, which require extra nitrogen each season. The essential elements in soil nutrition are well known to gardeners as nitrogen (chemical symbol N), phosphorous (P_2O_5), and potassium (K_2O), or NPK for short. In addition the soil also needs traces of many other elements (boron, calcium, chlorine, copper, fluorine, magnesium, manganese, nickel, silica, and zinc). But adding a chemical fertilizer containing these elements bypasses the natural process of feeding the plant; it can prevent the plant taking up the nutrients it requires, making it over-reliant on artificial feeding. To avoid this you need to give the soil organisms the right conditions to live and multiply. Chemical fertilizers can have the opposite effect. They can kill off beneficial fungi that live on the plant roots and feed the plant. The best way to encourage soil micro-organisms is to build up the humus layer and to use good compost or organic fertilizer. Spread compost on the soil in autumn or work it into the topsoil layer during spring. The plants and soil bacteria will then feed each other, the plants releasing protein and carbohydrates that can be used by the bacteria, which in turn convert the insoluble nutrients into a soluble form which the roots can take up. An organic soil will also encourage root fungi. If plants are under particular stress (when conditions are unusually hot or dry, or when you are growing them in containers) you can feed them through the leaves with a seaweed feed. This has a quicker effect and is a useful supplement to, but not a substitute for, feeding the soil with organic material.

If you build up and cherish your soil in this way, the top few inches of soil in your garden will be dark, crumbly, and fertile. Keep this topsoil on the top, where it will be most beneficial, do not turn it under by repeated digging. Even if you have a heavy clay soil that does not drain well, resist the temptation to dig and bring the clay to the top. Plant roots are very good at penetrating into clay and breaking it up given a little encouragement. The best and simplest method is to plunge a fork into the soil at regular intervals, working it backwards and forwards. This will let in the oxygen needed by the soil organisms. It will also enable water to drain away more easily. In these drier, more aerobic conditions both roots and earthworms will penetrate deeper into the subsoil. If you are starting a new garden, it is worthwhile preventing waterlogged soil by laying drains. Alternatively, creating a well drained rock garden or raised bed (see pp. 252–3) will allow you to introduce better soil into a small area of your garden and ensure that it does not get waterlogged.

Composting

As well as feeding the soil and improving its structure and water retention, compost enables you to make good use of many materials that would otherwise go to waste. You can use any plant material that is not woody, together with organic kitchen wastes (except for meat products, which attract vermin), the contents of the vacuum cleaner, grass mowings, and most weeds (provided that they do not have too much soil attached to their roots). A perfect compost heap heats up to as much as 190°F (90°C). This will kill off plant disease and weed seeds, but many heaps fail to reach this temperature, so it is best to avoid seeding plants, particularly vigorous species, such as docks and thistles.

Compost containers can come in many shapes and sizes, from compact bins and baskets ideal for the small garden, to large wooden boxes built side-by-side. But they are all variations on the traditional compost heap and the method for making the compost is similar for each. Build the heap directly on the soil. Build up the base layer with thick stems and coarse material, which will remain open, allowing air to enter the heap. Add material in layers of about 8 ins (20 cm) thick. Alternate with a sprinkling of activator and dolomite lime. The activator can consist of chicken, rabbit, or guinea pig droppings, seaweed meal, or blood, fish and bone meal. Build up the heap well over the top of the container – it will sink rapidly as it breaks down. Top the heap with a piece of old carpet or a sheet of plastic to keep in the heat and moisture.

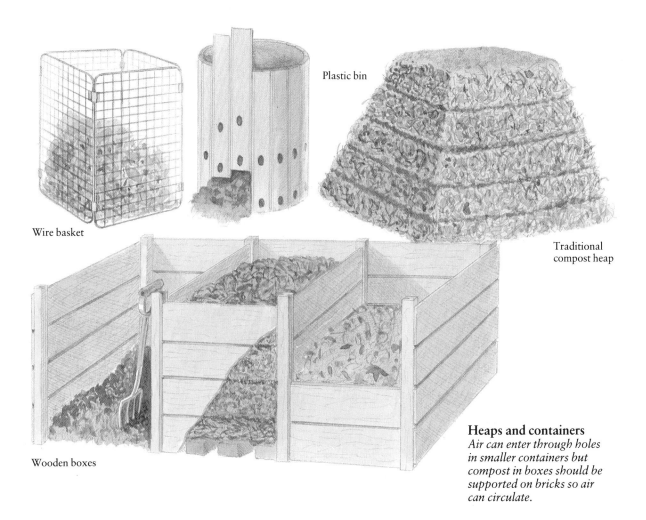

Plastic bin

Wire basket

Traditional
compost heap

Wooden boxes

Heaps and containers
*Air can enter through holes
in smaller containers but
compost in boxes should be
supported on bricks so air
can circulate.*

Other organic fertilizers

If you cannot make compost, or if
you do not have enough to go round,
you can use one of the many organic
fertilizers that are available. You can
buy these from garden centres, high
street shops or specialist suppliers
and they are highly beneficial to
plants during the main growing season. The table shows their principal
nutrient constituents, although most
also contain numerous additional
trace elements.

Fertilizer	Main nutrients
Dried blood	Nitrogen
Hoof and horn	Slow-release nitrogen and some phosphate
Bonemeal	Phosphorous
Blood, fish and bone	Combination of dried blood, fish meal, and bonemeal containing: nitrogen, phosphorous, and small amount of potash
Rock phosphate	Phosphate
Seaweed meal	Nitrogen, phosphorous, and potassium
Calcified seaweed	Calcium (50%), magnesium, sodium, numerous trace elements
Liquid seaweed leaf and soil feed	Small amounts of nitrogen, phosphorous, and potassium; rich in trace elements

Creative weeding

If you mulch your garden (see opposite) you should keep weeds to a minimum. But if apparent weeds do occur in your herb beds, do not pull them up without first examining them closely. They may prove to be seedlings of hardy annuals and biennials which appear in the autumn and often make strong plants for the following season. If they do appear in the wrong place, transplant them while the weather is still mild and the soil warm, so that they can settle in before winter. More seedlings will appear in spring and you can choose to move these while they are still small, or leave them and thin them out later. Look out for any unusual seedlings. Some plants, such as pansies, cross with each other to produce a variety of different flower colours. Let them self-seed and they will produce ground cover and colour throughout the season. If you are not sure of the identity of a weed, consult a field guide or the Glossary (see pp. 26–128) – it may be a useful plant that you want to grow. But there are a few weeds that are particularly invasive, and you should eradicate these as soon as you see them. Bindweed, creeping buttercup, and creeping thistle are three of the most common examples. Pull these out, root and shoot, and burn them: they do nothing to improve the compost heap either.

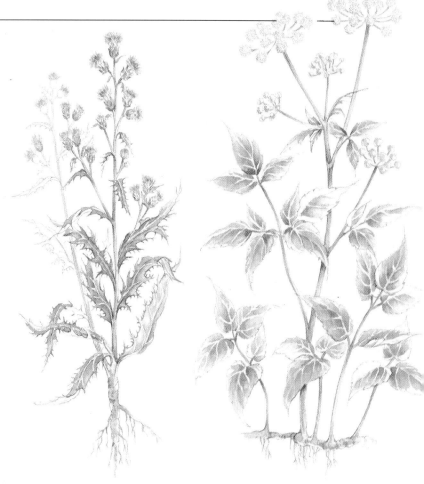

Creeping thistle
The vigorous roots send up shoots away from the parent. Remove each plant carefully with a fork.

Ground elder
Spreading by creeping roots, ground elder smothers neighbouring plants if you do not keep it in check.

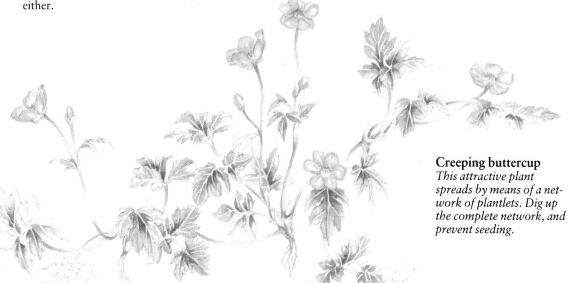

Creeping buttercup
This attractive plant spreads by means of a network of plantlets. Dig up the complete network, and prevent seeding.

Couch grass
The creeping roots of couch grass grow near to the surface and are easy to remove if you use a fork. Do not use a spade.

Lesser celandine
A useful plant if kept under control, this celandine spreads rapidly, particularly in damp, shady places.

Bindweed
Long, trailing stems help this very persistent plant to take hold. Pull up the plants as soon as they appear.

Manures and mulches

One of the essentials of caring for your soil is to keep it covered. This will protect the soil from erosion and deter weeds. Compost or pulverized bark make excellent mulches, but even a simple covering of black plastic or newspaper will keep down the weeds, stop nutrients being washed away in wet weather, and help prevent baking and drying out when it is hot. A better-looking solution, which is also more beneficial, is to use a green manure crop. This is a fast-growing crop that can be useful in one of two ways. Either it produces masses of leaves that hold nutrients over the winter and that you can turn into the soil in spring; or it has extensive roots that break up the soil and hold nutrients over the winter. Both types add valuable organic material to the soil, although they have the drawback of taking up valuable growing space in the garden. Three of the best are mustard, which is a good suppressor of weeds and produces plenty of leaves to work into the soil; buckwheat, which has a vigorous root system and also attracts bees; and grazing rye, which has the most penetrating root system of all and can be sown as late as October. Other legumes that are useful, particularly in vegetable gardens, are clover, lupins, and tares.

Pest and disease control

Grow your plants organically and you will keep pests and diseases down to a minimum (see p. 264). There are natural solutions to most of the problems that do occur.

Treat aphids with a commercially available insect-repellant powder. Choose one which is harmless to bees. Other natural preparations for aphids are pyrethrum (see p. 160), quassia (wood chippings from which you make a liquid spray), and soft soap (a cleansing mixture of vegetable oils and potash). An elder leaf infusion (1 lb/450 g of leaves to 6 pt/ 3.4 l of water) makes an effective spray.

Remove slugs by hand as they emerge in the evening. Thyme bushes will attract slugs away from other species, and a jar of beer sunk into the ground is also a slug attractant.

Mints are sometimes subject to rust. This is difficult to eradicate without removing all the contaminated foliage down to the soil level and burning it. Applying a flame gun to the crown of the plant and surrounding soil is also effective. Another method is to soak the root in water at about 105–115 °F (41–46 °C) for 10 minutes. Replant in clean soil.

Leaf scale is a frequent problem on bay trees. Wipe regularly or spray with derris when the bugs emerge.

Mildew can be a problem on bergamot, hyssop, the thymes, and the sages. Avoid hot dry conditions and keep the atmosphere humid with overhead spraying if you are growing these plants under cover.

Companion planting

"No plant is an island" and neighbouring species affect each other in many different ways. Large, leafy plants can offer shade or wind protection to less robust species. Many flowering plants attract beneficial insects that act as predators for pests or as valuable pollinators – borage, hyssop, marjoram, and thyme are among the most popular for bees. Other herbs act as insect repellants (see below). Other plants produce strong root secretions which affect the surrounding soil and may be taken up by neighbouring plant roots. Plants with deep root systems survive when the topsoil dries out and so produce a microclimate for neighbouring shallow-rooted plants. They also bring up minerals from the subsoil when the plant decays. Alfalfa is a good example of such a plant. Buckwheat is another plant with a useful extensive root system. It collects calcium and will enrich poor soils when you dig it well in. Its vigorous roots also help to break up heavy soils such as clay.

Traditional companions

There are several traditional plant combinations: garlic, with its strong odour is thought to be beneficial to roses; chives have a folk reputation for preventing black spot on roses; tarragon is reputed to be generally beneficial in the garden; and sage and rosemary are thought to be mutually beneficial. Certain fragrant herbs are useful when planted amongst vegetables. For example, pests like carrot fly locate their victims by scent, which can be masked by aromatic herbs planted nearby. Many herbs act as insect repellants when grown near other plants or when you make an infusion and use it as a spray. These are some of the most effective: tansy, pennyroyal, nasturtium, stinging nettle, garlic,

chives, thyme, hyssop, sage, wormwood, lavender, and southernwood (see also pp. 160–1 for further information on insect repellents).

As a general rule, fragrant herbs – hyssop, thyme, sage, marjoram, chives, and parsley – are beneficial in maintaining the health of the vegetable garden. Their benefits have not been analysed scientifically but a number of gardeners have reported

improvements in the general health of their vegetables when interplanting with these herbs.

Some plants affect their neighbours adversely. Members of the buttercup family (Ranunculaceae) are vigorous and heavy feeders, and other plants do not grow well with them. Fennel and wormwood are poor companions, while dandelion's emissions of ethylene gas hinder growth.

Nasturtium
This herb has an excellent reputation as a companion plant. It keeps pests away from cabbages and broad beans, attracting some, such as blackfly, away from vegetables. It also gives ground cover.

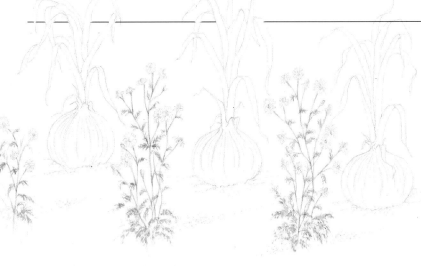

Chamomile
Chamomile (left) repels many insects and is known as "the plants' physician".

Yarrow
The uses of yarrow (below) are less well documented; it is thought to be generally good for the garden.

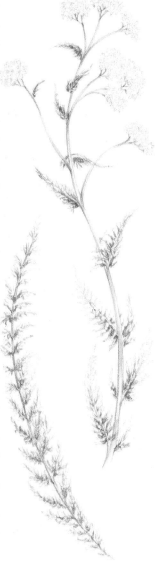

Herb	Plant with	Effect
Pennyroyal	General	Repels ants
Nasturtium	Brassicas	Repels aphids
	Apple trees	Repels aphids
	Tomatoes	Attracts blackfly to itself
	Broad beans	
	General	Repels ants; keeps garden healthy
French marigold	Tomatoes	Repels aphids
Chives	Apple trees	Prevent scab
	Roses	Prevent black spot
Garlic	Roses	Generally beneficial
Sage	Cabbages	Repels cabbage moth
	Vines	Generally beneficial
	Rosemary	Generally beneficial
	General	Repels a number of harmful flying insects
Summer savory	Beans	Generally beneficial; attracts bees
Nettle	General	Controls blackfly
	Angelica	Improves oil content
Caraway, buckwheat, flax	General	Improve heavy soil
Basil	Tomatoes	Repels flying insects
Borage	Strawberries	Improves crop yield; attracts bees
Chamomile	General	Repels flying insects
	Onions	Improves crop yield
Coriander	General	Attracts bees
	Anise	Improves flavour
Hyssop	Grape vines	Improves crop yield
Mint	General	Repels flies
	Cabbage	Repels cabbage grubs
Rosemary	Carrot	Repels carrot fly
	Sage	Generally beneficial
Dill, fennel	General	Attract beneficial insects

Harvesting and storage

The climax of your herb growing comes when you collect the parts of each plant that you want to use, and gather the seeds that you can sow to produce next season's plants. If you harvest correctly, you will preserve the plant's useful properties. This means gathering your herbs at the right moment during the day and the right point in the growing season. (For information on drying and preserving herbs after harvesting, see p. 272).

Harvesting leaves

For culinary flavouring, you can pick a sprig of leaves at any point during the season when a herb plant is green and healthy. But the timing of the harvest is much more critical if you need to retain all the medicinal properties of your herbs. It is best to gather the leaves when the flowers are in bud and before any have opened. This is true whether you are cutting the whole plant or a single stem, and whether you are going to use the herb fresh or dried. When you are cutting leaves for drying, you should do so early in the day, as soon as the dew has evaporated from the plant.

Harvesting flowers

Take flowers at the same time of day as leaves and as soon as possible after they are fully open. After removing each flower, shake off any tiny insects in the head.

Harvesting roots

Harvest roots at the end of the growing season – this is when the maximum nutrients are stored in the roots for the winter. Try not to damage the roots when you are lifting them, and discard any that have been damaged in any way. Wash the roots in cold water to remove all soil and dirt before drying, but do not soak them for any length of time.

Collecting seeds

To know when seeds are ready to collect, get used to looking at the various seed heads. Each plant has different characteristics, but there are often similarities between members of particular families.

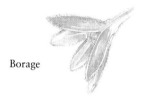

Borage

Boraginaceae (borage family)

The seeds of this family turn black when ripe and fall to the ground immediately. Catch them by tying muslin over the stem, or gather a few seeds every day as they ripen. Alternatively, cut a stem before all the seed has ripened and hang it up in a well ventilated, dry place.

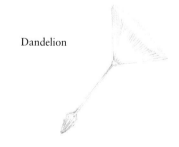

Dandelion

Compositae (daisy family)

The seed is ready when the heads have turned brown and dry-looking and the petals have dropped off. Rub the seeds off the heads and gently blow off the debris from the flower or leave it with the seeds.

Labiatae (mint family)

This family includes the mints and thymes, which retain their seeds until after the stem and sepals have turned brown. The seeds ripen more or less all at once. Thyme seeds are so tiny that it is easy to miss them.

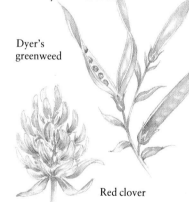

Dyer's greenweed

Red clover

Leguminosae (pea family)

A wide variety of seed types is produced by this family. Clover seeds, for example, are contained in the soft calyx and you should collect this when it looks dry and brown. Do not leave it too long, otherwise the seed will be dispersed. Other members of this family, such as peas, vetches, trefoils, and dyer's greenweed, hold their seeds in pods.

Paperavaceae (poppy family)

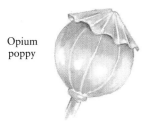

Opium poppy

When ripe, tip the large seed capsules into a container; the tiny seeds will drop out.

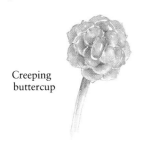

Creeping buttercup

Ranunculaceae (buttercup family)

The exposed seeds are attached to a head. Pick it when it is brown and dry-looking.

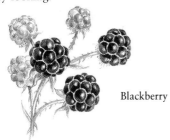

Blackberry

Rosaceae (rose family)

This family contains a wide range of plants. Some have seeds contained in hips, others have seed capsules. Both are easy to collect. The seeds germinate most easily if they have passed through a bird's intestine, so you can feed chickens on rose hips and collect seed from the droppings. Otherwise hips and berries require two winters outside before germination.

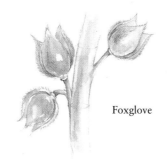

Foxglove

Scrophulariaceae (figwort family)

The small seed capsules of this family are easy to collect when they are brown and ripe. The tiny seeds tip out easily.

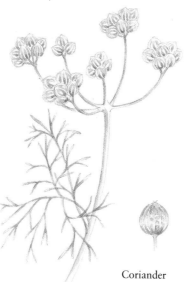

Coriander

Umbelliferae (carrot family)

Plants of this family can bear prodigious quantities of seed. The family includes many useful culinary herbs, including angelica, parsley, and coriander. The dry, usually ridged seeds typical of this family appear exposed on the flat flower heads or umbels where it is easy to see them ripening, usually in August or September. You can rub or shake them off the head when ripe.

Storing herbs

When your home-dried herbs have cooled, you can start the rubbing down process. Choose a well-ventilated place such as a kitchen or shed with the doors and windows left open. Put aside those herbs you prefer to keep whole such as some twigs of thyme, marjoram, and tarragon, for bouquets garnis (see pp. 168–9). Keep bay leaves whole for soups and casseroles. You should also leave chamomile, mullein, and similar small flowers whole, although you can detach marigold petals if you prefer. Strip other leafy herbs by hand, picking the leaves from the stalks. Discard stalks and crush the leaves in a grinder or with a rolling pin, one kind at a time. A fine mesh sieve is useful for feathery herbs such as dill and fennel.

Dried herbs can be adversely affected by light, heat, and air. To keep them at their best, store them immediately after drying and rubbing down. This helps to prevent the herbs from picking up moisture from the air. Dark-glass, airtight jars are ideal since you can see how much herb you have at a glance. Keep them in a cool place. If you only have standard glass, the jars must be stored in a dark closet. Light destroys the essential oils. Plastic is unsuitable since it encourages condensation inside the container. Other suitable vessels are earthenware pots with airtight lids or tight-fitting corks; any other opaque air-tight container; airtight wooden boxes.

Label each container immediately and date it. This way you will not confuse different batches of leafy herbs which, all together, can look very similar.

If you have dried a large amount of material, keep some of it separately in a smaller jar for regular use. Opening and closing a large container will only speed up the deterioration of the contents.

Store seeds in packets in the refrigerator, or in air-tight jars.

Drying herbs

Home-dried herbs are far superior to most packaged, shop-bought varieties. Dried correctly, their colour, flavour, taste, and healing properties will be largely preserved. The three essentials for successful herb drying are shade, ventilation, and some warmth. Herb drying is simple if you live in a warm, dry climate. In cool, damp, conditions an additional source of heat may be necessary.

Places to dry herbs

A warm, shady, airy part of the house such as an attic or shed is ideal for hanging up bunches or paper bags of herbs for drying. For smaller quantities of herbs, a well-ventilated closet, or a very cool oven with the door left ajar, are all suitable. Spread the herbs on trays or sheets of wrapping paper or newspaper and turn them frequently. If you are using the oven, spread the herbs on baking trays.

When drying herbs in an attic or shed, make sure the bunches hang well away from the wall. A line or old-fashioned wooden clothes rack is ideal. If drying large quantities, you can construct your own drying rack. Stretch muslin or net material over wooden frames and stack them in levels on a framework, like a chest of drawers but open at the sides. Or, if you have sufficient space, simply stand the drying frames on legs made from wooden blocks or bricks. If the weather is cool and damp you can use a fan or convector heater to maintain a steady temperature.

How long to dry?

Drying times vary depending on the particular plant and the part you want to use. In general, leaves should be brittle and break between the fingers. If the leaves are dry before the stems, strip them off and store them. Stems and stalks should break when they are dry, and not bend. Flower petals are ready when they rustle, but do not crumble. Bark and roots should be dry enough to snap, or if they are very thick, to chip with a small hammer. A very rough guide is three to seven days for drying; some herbs may be ready at five. Dried herbs should look, smell, and taste very much like the fresh plant, but will be about one eighth the weight.

Preparing herbs for drying

As soon as you have harvested your herbs, take them out of direct sunlight. Bright light will draw out the essential oils and bleach the leaves. Next pick out any weeds or discoloured leaves. Leaves for drying, except for large kinds like borage, are best left on the stalk. Finally, separate the herbs into bunches and tie loosely with string or thread.

Gently cut off flower heads, such as marigold or elder, for drying.

Wipe roots and barks carefully to remove any soil. Then chop them into pieces about 1 in (2.5 cm) thick.

Drying temperatures

Herbs dry best slowly and steadily. Artificial heat speeds up the process but should not exceed 93 °F (34 °C). An ideal temperature is between 90° and 93° F (32° and 34° C). Make sure the drying area has reached this before introducing your herbs. After one or two days, the temperature can be reduced to 77° to 81 °F (25° to 27 °C) to complete the process. Free circulation of air is essential.

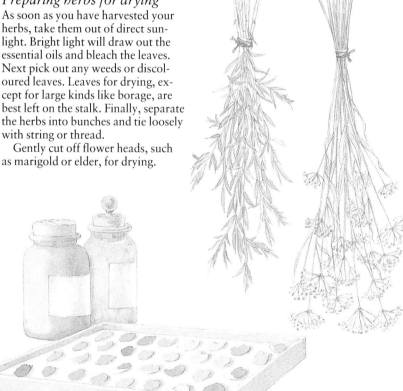

Drying methods
Whether you use frames or hang up your herbs, good air circulation is vital.

Herbs in the garden

The previous pages in this chapter give the basic ground rules for organic herb cultivation. Follow these and you should be able to grow herbs successfully. But particular species vary in the conditions and growing techniques they prefer. The chart on the following pages gives cultivation details for a selection of the most popular herbs which can be grown with success in both northern and southern latitudes. They will provide a range of useful plants for cooking, healing, and other uses in the home.

The chart gives the common and Latin names of each herb, together with its growing type (annual, biennial, or perennial). Further information is included which will help when you are planning your herb garden – the plant's preferred soil and situation; its approximate size (indicating how much space you should allow for it and its position in the bed); and its flower and foliage colours, so that you can assess its decorative potential. When planning a herb garden, you should use this chart in conjunction with the other plant lists throughout the chapter – especially those showing herbs that suit particular soil types (see pp. 248–9), herbs with particular decorative characteristics and plants that attract bees and butterflies to the garden (see p. 254).

Information on sowing and propagation shows the best times and techniques to use for each herb, and any particular requirements for each species – whether you should sow in a tray indoors or in situ; whether the plants require a high temperature for germination; whether seeds germinate poorly or erratically and an alternative method such as taking cuttings or dividing roots is recommended. Many herbs are very tolerant and will grow in a variety of soils and situations, adapting to the prevailing conditions – but the main exceptions to this are covered in the chart.

Some plants self-seed particularly well. This fact is noted in the chart because it can be either a blessing or a curse to the gardener. Self-seeding usually produces strong, healthy plants, but it can also mean that these plants take over the garden if they are not kept in check. Another feature included in the chart is the fact that some plants spread rapidly. This obviously makes their size in the garden difficult to predict and in some cases (such as the mints) makes them invasive. Such plants need to be managed carefully if they are not to overrun the garden – it is often best to grow them in containers.

The chart's final column gives any additional points relevant to cultivation. Details of closely related species or varieties that you can grow in a similar way are shown here. This column also highlights any problems that you are likely to have with low temperatures. Most of the herbs are hardy enough to grow in northern latitudes, but a few (such as sweet bay and lemon verbena) require sheltered or frost-free positions.

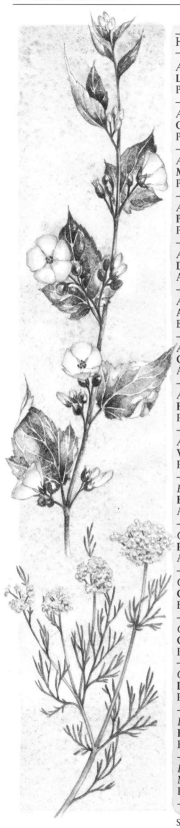

Herb	Soil & situation	Height × spread	Sowing
Alchemilla vulgaris **Lady's mantle** Perennial	Moist loam or gravel over loam	20 × 16 ins 50 × 40 cm	Late summer in tray; self seeds
Allium sativum **Garlic** Perennial bulb	Well drained, rich to medium, light	h 12 ins h 30 cm	
Althea officinalis **Marsh mallow** Perennial	Moist, rich Full sun	40–80 × 36 ins 100–200 × 90 cm	Late spring to summer, seed tray at 21 °C (70 °F)
Anemone pulsatilla **Pasque flower** Perennial	Well drained, chalky Sun	4–12 × 8 ins 10–30 × 20 cm	Spring/early summer, fresh seed; otherwise vernalization
Anethum graveolens **Dill** Annual	Most soils Full sun	h 80 ins h 200 cm	Spring in situ
Angelica archangelica **Angelica** Biennial	Moist, rich Sun	60–100 × 36 ins 150–250 × 90 cm	When ripe summer or early spring; older seed in autumn
Anthriscus cerefolium **Chervil** Annual or biennial	Most moisture-retentive soils Sun or part shade	28 × 12 ins 70 × 30 cm	Summer in situ; or spring
Artemisia drancunculus **French tarragon** Perennial	Well drained, fertile Sun	36 × 24 ins 90 × 60 cm	Produces no seed
Asperula odorata **Woodruff** Perennial	Well drained, rich Semi- or deep shade	h 10 ins h 25 cm (spreading)	Late summer, fresh seed
Borago officinalis **Borage** Annual	Well drained Full sun	24 × 20 ins 60 × 50 cm	Late spring; self seeds
Calendula officinalis **Pot marigold** Annual	Most soils Full sun	20 × 10 ins 50 × 25 cm	Late spring in situ; self seeds
Carum carvi **Caraway** Biennial	Most soils Sun	32 × 8 ins 80 × 20 cm	Summer in situ; self seeds
Chelidonium majus **Greater celandine** Perennial	Well drained Sun or semi-shade	12–36 × 16 ins 30–90 × 40 cm	Spring or late summer
Convallaria majalis **Lily of the valley** Perennial	Moist, calcareous Woodland or semi-shade	h 4–8 ins h 10–20 cm (spreading)	When fresh in situ
Digitalis purpurea **Foxglove** Biennial	Well drained, acid Sun or semi-shade	h 80 ins h 200 cm	Spring in situ, or seed tray; on surface of soil
Filipendula ulmaria **Meadowsweet** Perennial	Moist, rich Sun or semi-shade	24–36 × 12 ins 60–90 × 30 cm	Autumn or spring in situ

See Glossary for cautions on use of particular herbs.

Propagation	Flowers	Foliage	Harvest	Further notes
Divide roots early spring or autumn	Greenish-yellow panicles; early summer	Decorative, clear green, rounded, many-lobed	Leaves, summer	*A. alpina* is decorative dwarf sp. *A. mollis* is garden form
Bulbs split into cloves after harvest; plant autumn or early spring	White; late summer	Long, flat, pointed leaves	Leaves, early summer; bulbs, late summer	Many named varieties available with pink and purple skins
Divide roots spring or autumn	Large, delicate, pink; late summer	Large, soft, green/grey	Flowers, leaves, root autumn	Decorative
Divide rhizomes after flowering	Dark, violet; at Easter	Rosette of leaves after flowering	Flowers, leaves	Distinctive and decorative seed heads; poisonous
	Yellow umbels; mid summer	Feathery blue/green; very aromatic	Flowers, leaves	Named varieties for leaf or seed production
	Greenish white in large, spherical umbels; early summer	Large, light green, few leaves	Young leaves, seeds, rhizome, green stems	Stately, decorative plant
	Delicate, white umbels; spring to summer	Delicate, deeply cut and sweetly scented	Young leaves	Runs rapidly to seed in summer
Divide roots spring; cuttings spring	Insignificant, white; summer	Small, thin, shiny, green	Leaves, spring to summer	Divide and re-plant every few years to retain flavour
Divide roots, spring or autumn	White, star-like; late spring	Decorative, whorled leaves, divided into 6	Flowers, leaves	Dried leaves smell of new-mown hay
	Intense blue; from early summer	Large, rough, hairy	Flowers, leaves, root, summer	Good bee plant
	Bright orange, yellow, single or double; summer	Grey/green	Flowers when open and dry	
	White umbels; from early summer	Feathery leaves in first year	Ripe seed, late summer or autumn	Decorative plant; grows vigorously
Divide roots, spring	Bright yellow, 4 petals; summer	Light green/grey	Flowering stems	Juice poisonous in large doses
Divide roots, autumn	White bells, fragrant; spring	Wide, pointed, flat, mid-green	Flowers	Poisonous
	Tall spire of purple (or white) thimbles; mid summer	Large, downy, grey/green	Leaves	Many garden varieties available; poisonous
Divide roots, spring	Cream, giving a frothy appearance, scented; late summer	Decorative, dark green	Flower heads and roots, autumn	A good plant to grow by water

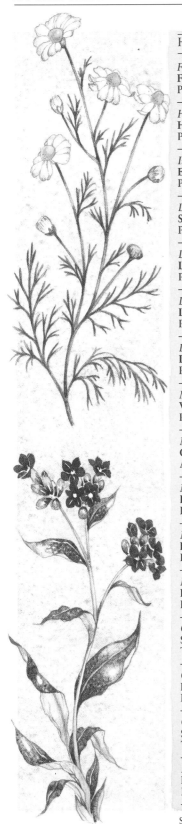

Herb	Soil & situation	Height × spread	Sowing
Foeniculum vulgare **Fennel** Perennial	Very well drained, light	80 × 36 ins 200 × 90 cm	Late summer in situ
Hyssopus officinalis **Hyssop** Perennial sub-shrub	Dry, rocky, calcareous Full sun	20 × 16 ins 50 × 40 cm	Spring
Inula helenium **Elecampane** Perennial	Moist, rich Sun or semi-shade	120 × 40 ins 300 × 100 cm	Spring; self seeds
Laurus nobilis **Sweet bay** Perennial shrub; evergreen	Rich Full sun Sheltered from wind	26 × 13 ft 800 × 400 cm	Fresh seed in pots
Lavandula officinalis **Lavender** Perennial shrub; evergreen	Well drained, poor, calcareous Full sun	32 × 24 ins 80 × 60 cm	Autumn without heat or early spring
Levisticum officinale **Lovage** Perennial	Most soils Sun	80 × 40 ins 200 × 100 cm	Spring in situ or late summer
Lippia citriodora **Lemon verbena** Perennial shrub	Well drained Very sheltered (half-hardy)	80 × 40 ins 200 × 100 cm	Seed not available
Marrubium vulgare **White horehound** Perennial	Well drained to dry Sun	24 × 20 ins 60 × 50 cm	Late spring; slow, erratic germination
Matricaria chamomilla **German chamomile** Annual	Most soils, especially light	24 × 4 ins 60 × 10 cm	Late summer to autumn
Melissa officinalis **Lemon balm** Perennial	Moist, rich Sun or semi-shade	32 × 24 ins 80 × 60 cm	Late spring; slow germination
Mentha piperata **Peppermint** Perennial	Moist, rich Sun or semi-shade	h 12–20 ins h 30–50 cm (spreading)	Does not come true from seed
Monarda didyma **Bergamot** Perennial	Moist, rich, medium to light Some shade preferred	20–40 × 12 ins 50–100 × 30 cm	Spring
Ocimum basilicum **Sweet basil** Tender annual	Fertile loam Sun	10–24 × 12 ins 25–60 × 30 cm	Spring inside with heat; outside mid-summer full sun, shelter
Oenothera biennis **Evening primrose** Biennial	Dry, stony Full sun	60 × 24 ins 150 × 60 cm	Late summer in situ
Origanum majorana **Sweet marjoram** Tender perennial	Well drained, rich Full sun	10–20 × 10 ins 25–50 × 25 cm	Inside with heat; outside in June
Petroselinum crispum **Parsley** Biennial	Moisture-retaining rich Sun or semi-shade	24 × 16 ins 60 × 40 cm	Early summer or August in situ

See Glossary for cautions on use of particular herbs.

Propagation	Flowers	Foliage	Harvest	Further notes
	Large yellow umbels; summer	Soft, feathery, blue/green, very aromatic	Young leaves green stems, ripe seed	Bronze, wild, and bulbous fennels also available
Cuttings, late spring, early summer	Rich blue, sometimes pink, white, or purple; summer	Thin, dark green, aromatic	Leaves, before flowers open	Superb bee plant
Divide roots, autumn	Large, bright yellow; summer	Basal leaves very large, light green	Roots, autumn	Very dramatic plant; self-seeds profusely
Cuttings late July, early August; best with mist and bottom heat	Yellow/cream; late spring	Dark green, shiny aromatic	Leaves	Grows well in containers; if cut down by frost will shoot from base
Softwood cuttings, spring; hardwood cuttings, autumn	Pale mauve; mid summer	Narrow, grey/green	Flowers, mid to late summer	Good hedging plant; cut back after flowering
Divide roots, spring or autumn	Greenish/yellow umbels; summer	Very large, mid-green, aromatic	Seed, leaves, root, autumn	
Cuttings, early, summer	Small, pale lavender; late summer	Light green aromatic	Leaves	Will only survive outside in very sheltered southern sites
Divide roots, spring; cuttings, summer	White; from mid summer	Grey/green, hairy, wrinkled, aromatic, decorative	Leaves or flowering stem, when in bud	Decorative plant with unusual grey foliage
	Small, daisy-like; from early summer	Feathery, bright green	Flowers when fully open	
Divide roots, spring or autumn	Small, white to pink; summer	Nettle-like, with lemon fragrance	Leaves, in growing season	Good bee plant; gold variegated form available
Divide root runners in growing season; cuttings root in water	Mauve on terminal spike; late summer	Shiny dark green/purple, very aromatic	Leaves and flowering stems	Can be invasive; white form is less aromatic than black
Divide roots, spring; cuttings, summer (root in water)	Scarlet, summer	Dark green tinged with red, highly aromatic	Leaves and flowering stems; roots in autumn	Garden forms available with variety of flower colours
Cuttings	White or purplish; mid to late summer	Delicate, clear green, very aromatic	Leaves as required; stems before flowering	Many varieties, including decorative purple form
	Large, bright, yellow on spikes, very fragrant; mid–late summer	Long, pointed, shiny	Flowers, seeds, root	Many other species some with large flowers
	White or pinkish spikes in knot formation; late summer	Greyish, with spicy scent	Leaves, flowering stems	Will overwinter if kept frost-free
	Small, greenish yellow; summer	Dark green, curled	Leaves, seed, root	Allow to self-seed; flat-leaved French and giant Italian varieties available

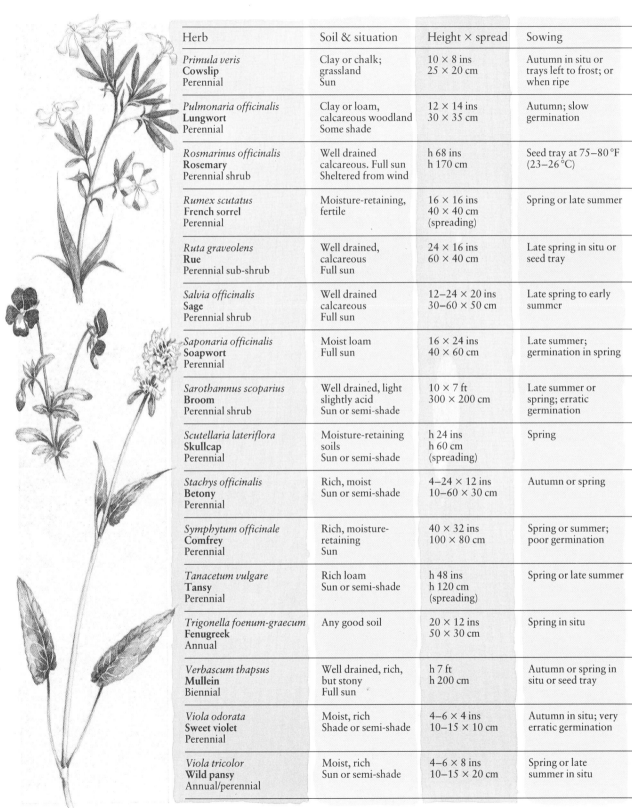

Herb	Soil & situation	Height × spread	Sowing
Primula veris **Cowslip** Perennial	Clay or chalk; grassland Sun	10 × 8 ins 25 × 20 cm	Autumn in situ or trays left to frost; or when ripe
Pulmonaria officinalis **Lungwort** Perennial	Clay or loam, calcareous woodland Some shade	12 × 14 ins 30 × 35 cm	Autumn; slow germination
Rosmarinus officinalis **Rosemary** Perennial shrub	Well drained calcareous. Full sun Sheltered from wind	h 68 ins h 170 cm	Seed tray at 75–80 °F (23–26 °C)
Rumex scutatus **French sorrel** Perennial	Moisture-retaining, fertile	16 × 16 ins 40 × 40 cm (spreading)	Spring or late summer
Ruta graveolens **Rue** Perennial sub-shrub	Well drained, calcareous Full sun	24 × 16 ins 60 × 40 cm	Late spring in situ or seed tray
Salvia officinalis **Sage** Perennial shrub	Well drained calcareous Full sun	12–24 × 20 ins 30–60 × 50 cm	Late spring to early summer
Saponaria officinalis **Soapwort** Perennial	Moist loam Full sun	16 × 24 ins 40 × 60 cm	Late summer; germination in spring
Sarothamnus scoparius **Broom** Perennial shrub	Well drained, light slightly acid Sun or semi-shade	10 × 7 ft 300 × 200 cm	Late summer or spring; erratic germination
Scutellaria lateriflora **Skullcap** Perennial	Moisture-retaining soils Sun or semi-shade	h 24 ins h 60 cm (spreading)	Spring
Stachys officinalis **Betony** Perennial	Rich, moist Sun or semi-shade	4–24 × 12 ins 10–60 × 30 cm	Autumn or spring
Symphytum officinale **Comfrey** Perennial	Rich, moisture- retaining Sun	40 × 32 ins 100 × 80 cm	Spring or summer; poor germination
Tanacetum vulgare **Tansy** Perennial	Rich loam Sun or semi-shade	h 48 ins h 120 cm (spreading)	Spring or late summer
Trigonella foenum-graecum **Fenugreek** Annual	Any good soil	20 × 12 ins 50 × 30 cm	Spring in situ
Verbascum thapsus **Mullein** Biennial	Well drained, rich, but stony Full sun	h 7 ft h 200 cm	Autumn or spring in situ or seed tray
Viola odorata **Sweet violet** Perennial	Moist, rich Shade or semi-shade	4–6 × 4 ins 10–15 × 10 cm	Autumn in situ; very erratic germination
Viola tricolor **Wild pansy** Annual/perennial	Moist, rich Sun or semi-shade	4–6 × 8 ins 10–15 × 20 cm	Spring or late summer in situ

See Glossary for cautions on use of particular herbs.

Propagation	Flowers	Foliage	Harvest	Further notes
Divide roots, autumn	Yellow trumpet; spring	Wrinkled	Flowers, leaves, roots	
Divide roots after flowering	Red, purple; spring	Oval, pointed, with white blotches	Whole plant, when flowers open	
Cuttings of non-flowering shoots, from early summer	Pale to deep blue; late spring	Thin, leathery, grey/green, oily, very aromatic	Leaves	Many decorative sub-species and varieties
Divide roots, spring or autumn	Reddish; mid–late summer	Green/grey, rounded, fleshy	Leaves, before flowering	*R. acetosa* is large-leaved species
Cuttings, spring to early summer	Small, yellow; summer	Green/blue, deeply divided strong scent	Leaves	Jackman's rue is a decorative garden variety
Cuttings, spring to early summer	Violet/blue, sometimes white or pink; from early summer	Soft, grey/green, aromatic	Leaves	Decorative red and golden leaved forms available
Divide root, spring	Soft pink, single or double; mid to late summer	Smooth, light green	Leaves, summer; root, autumn	Spreading rootstock
Cuttings, summer	Bright yellow, pea-like; spring	Dark green, short, thin, hard, pointed	Flowering tops	
Divide roots, early spring	Small blue; summer	Small, yellow/green	Whole herb, before flowering	
Divide plant, autumn or spring	Purple/red; dense terminal spikes; mid–late summer	Dark green, tooth-edged	Flower spikes, leaves	
Divide roots in growing season	Cream to pink, bell-shaped; from early summer	Light green, long, soft, hairy	Leaf, summer; roots, autumn	Bee plant; valuable compost and animal feed
Divide roots, spring or autumn	Heads of scented yellow buttons; mid summer–early autumn	Feathery, very aromatic	Leaves, before flowers open	
	Whitish; mid summer	Trifoliate	Seeds and leaves	Good agricultural hay crop
	Tall spire of yellow flowers; late summer	Grey/green, large, soft, downy	Leaves and flowers	Many other very decorative species
Propagate from offsets, winter or early spring	Violet, pink, or white, highly scented; spring	Dark green oval	Flowers, leaves, roots	Spreads rapidly in suitable situations
Cuttings, spring or summer	Single, violet and yellow; spring to summer	Sparse, straggly	Flowers, leaves	Readily self-seeds and hybridizes

Resources

Herb suppliers

Suppliers marked * offer a mail-order service

Aphrodisia*
282 Bleeker Street, New York,
NY 10014
212–989–6440

Bio-Botanica
75 Commerce Drive, Hauppauge,
NY 11788
516–231–5522

The Herb Shop*
278 South Main, Springville,
UT 84663
801–489–8787

House of Quality Herbs
PB Box 14, Woodland Iills,
CA 91365

Meer Corporation
9500 Railroad Avenue,
North Bergen, NJ 07047
201–861–9500

Nature's Herb Company*
281 Ellis Street, San Francisco,
CA 94102
415–474–2756

Angelica Herb and Spice*
137 1st Avenue, New York,
NY 10003
212–677–1549

Glie Farms*
1600 Bathgate Avenue, Bronx,
NY 10457
212–731–2130

Meadowsweet Herbal Apothecary
77 East 4th Street, New York,
NY 10003
212–254–2870

Canadian suppliers

For Your Health
Box 307, 1136 Eglinton Avenue West,
Willowdale, Ontario, Canada

Organisations

American Herb Society
300 Massachusetts Avenue
Boston, MA 02115

Chemical glossary

Alcohols A large group of compounds often found in volatile oils. Waxes are combinations of alcohols and fatty acids.

Alkaloids Compounds containing a nitrogen atom, alkaloids are usually present in plants as groups of chemicals. Their physical effects include killing pain, poisoning, and causing hallucinations.

Anthraquinones Glycoside compounds that produce dyes and purgatives.

Bitters Herbs containing a range of chemicals that have a bitter taste. Some are useful as appetite stimulants, others as anti-inflammatories, still others as relaxants.

Carbohydrates The most common plant carbohydrates are the nutritionally important sugars and starches, and cellulose. Polysaccharides are sugars that join with other chemicals to produce compounds such as pectin and mucilage which soothe, protect, and relax the alimentary canal.

Coumarins Glycoside compounds that are responsible for the "new mown hay" smell of many grasses.

Flavonoid glycosides Common group of plant chemicals named from their yellow colour (the Latin *flavus* means yellow). They have a wide variety of actions and include diuretics, circulatory stimulants, and anti-spasmodics.

Glycosides These common plant chemicals consist of molecules made up of two sections, one of which is a sugar. Some have a strong effect on the heart and are known a cardio-active glycosides (e g foxglove/digitalis). Some are purgative (e g the anthraquinones in cascara, senna, rhubarb, buckthorn).

Mucilages Gel-like substances with molecules made up of long chains of sugar units. Mucilages have a soothing effect when applied to inflamed tissues, and their gel is useful in some cosmetic preparations.

Phenol A basic building-block of many plant constituents: many different phenolic compounds exist that are based on it. One such compound is salicylic acid, which is often combined with a sugar to form a glycoside that is antiseptic (e g in meadowsweet).

Saponins These glycosides form a soap-like lather when shaken in water. There are two broad groups: the steroidal saponins, which seem to mimic the precursors of female sex hormones, and the tri-terpenoid saponins, which mimic the adrenal hormone ACTH.

Tannins These are compounds that react with protein to produce a leather-like coating on animal tissue (as in the process of tanning). They promote healing and numbing (to reduce irritation), reduce inflammation, and halt infection.

Volatile oils These complex compounds are chemical mixtures of hydrocarbons and alcohols. In the plant they often enhance the moisture-retaining properties of the leaves. They lend many herbs their characteristic taste and flavour. They can be antiseptic, antifungal, or aromatic, and some are thought to help the body fight infection.

References

ARALIACEAE

Oriental ginseng 1. See accounts in P. Dixon, *Ginseng*, Duckworth, 1976 and S. Fulder, *The Root of Being*, Hutchinson, 1980. **2.** W. Court, *Pulse*, October 20 1984. **3.** I. I. Brekhman, *Zhen-shen*, State Publishing House for Medical Literature, Leningrad, 1957. See also W. Petkov, *Panax ginseng, a Response Regulator*, Faculty of Pharmacology, Sofia, *Pharmazeutische Zeitung*, 31, 1 August 1968. **4.** Fulder, op. cit., p. 122. **5.** R. K. Siegal, *Ginseng Abuse Syndrome; Problems with the Panacea*, *J. Amer. Med. Assoc.*, 241, 1614–15, 1979. **6.** M. McIntyre, *Herbal Medicines*, B.H. M.A. report to BMA working party on Alternative Therapy, July 1986. **7.** D. Bensky and A. Gamble, *Chinese Herbal Medicine*, Eastland Press, p. 360, 1980.

BERBERIDACEAE

Barberry 1. Martindale, *Extra Pharmacopeia*, 26th edn, p. 324. **2.** See *Chem. Abstr.*, 77, 135606n, 1972. **3.** See *Chem. Abstr.*, 81, 100062n. **4.** Bensky, Gamble, op. cit., p. 111. **5.** See *Chem. Abstr.*, 86, 1149746, 1977. **6.** V. Preininger, *The Alkaloids*, vol. 15, RHF Manske, ed. Academic Press, New York, p. 207, 1975. **7.** *Ind. Med. J.*, 65, 683, 1930. **8.** Martindale, op. cit. **9.** Lascarato, 1899 La. *Grece Medicale* No. 2.

BETULACEAE

Silver birch 1. H. Leclerc, *Rev. Phytotherap*, 2, 65, 1938. **2.** A. Ellianowska and F. Kaczmarck, *Herba pol*, 11, 47, 1966. **3.** M. Tissut and P. Rowanel, *Phytochemistry*, 19, 2077, 1980. **4.** R. R. Paris and H. Moyse, *Matière Medicale*, Masson ed, Paris 1981.

BORAGINACEAE

Comfrey 1. S. Times Colour Suppl., April 1981. **2.** I. F. Stanford and I. A. Tavares *J. Pharm. Pharmacol.*, 35, 1983. **3.** T. Furuya and K. Asaki, *Chem. Pharm. Bull.* 16 (12), 2512–6, 1968. **4.** S. Times Colour Suppl., April 1981. **5.** T. Furuya op. cit., p. 2515. Also A. Taylor and N. C. Taylor, *Proc. Soc. Exper. Biol. Med.*, 114, 772, 774, 1963. **6.** S. Times Colour Suppl., April 1981. **7.** Ibid.

BURSERACEAE

Myrrh 1. BPC (1973) p. 317. **2.** Martindale, 27th edn, p. 252. **3.** Kiangsu – 1167 through A. Leung *Encyclopedia of Natural Ingredients*, Wiley, N. York, 1980.

Balm of Gilead 1. L. S. Goodman and Gilman eds., *The Pharmacological Basis of Therapeutics*, 5th edn, Macmillan, N. York, 1975. **2.** Martindale, 1977.

CAMPANULACEAE

Lobelia 1. L. S. Goodman and Gilman, op. cit.

CANNABIDACEAE

Hops 1. R. Wohlfart, R. Hansel and H. Schmidt, *Planta medica*, 48, 120, 1983. **2.** See *Chem. Abstr.*, 72, 41267x, 1970. **3.** See *Chem. Abstr.*, 86, 70045t, 1977. **4.** L. Bezanger-Beauquesne et. al., *Plantes Medicinales des Régions Temperées*, p. 78, Maloine, ed. Paris 1980. **5.** R. Hansel and H. H. Wagner, *Arneim-Forsch*, 17, 79, 1967. See also, Koch Wand Heim G. *Munch Med. Wschr*, 31/32, 844, 1953.

CAPRIFOLIACEAE

Black haw 1. C. H. Janboe, *J. Med. Chem.*, 10, 488, 1967; see also C. H. Janboe et. al., *Nature*, 212, 837, 1966.

COMPOSITAE

Yarrow 1. See *Chem. Abstr.*, 67, 62837v, 1967. **2.** A. Leung, op. cit., p. 327. **3.** Ibid. **4.** A. S. Goroberg and E. C. Mueller, *J. Pharm. Sci.*, 58, 938, 1969. **5.** G. Verzan-Petri and Banh-Nhu *Scienta Pharm.*, 45, c.24, 1977. **6.** See *Chem. Abstr.*, 73, 102048w, 1970.

Burdock 1. K. E. Schulte et. al., *Arzneim-Forsch*, 17, 829, 1967, see also Delaveau P., *Les Plantes Medicinales*, vol. 1, ed. Paris. **2.** See *Chem. Abstr.*, 66, 1451e, 1967. **3.** J. L. Hartwell, *Lloydia*, 31, 71, 1968.

Arnica 1. See *Chem. Abstr.*, 81, 1309102, 1974.

Chicory 1. *IRCS Medical Science, ab*14, 212, 1986. **2.** Benoit et. al., *Lloydia*, 39, 160, 1976. **3.** Balbaa et. al. *Planta Medica*, 24, 133, 1973. **4.** See *Chem. Abstr.*, 59, 5535c, 1963.

Globe artichoke 1. See *Chem. Abstr.*, 67, 896676, 1967. **2.** W. H. Hammeri et. al., *Wiener Med. Wochensch*, 41, 601, 1973. **3.** P. Preziosi and B. Loscalzo, *Arch. Int. Pharmacodyn*, 117, 1–2, 63, 1958.

Echinacea 1. E. Koch and H. Haaze, *Arzneimittel Forschung*, 2, 464, 1952. **2.** K. H. Busing, *Arzneimittel Forschung*, 2, 467, 1952. **3.** E. Koch and Vebel, op. cit., *1*, 16, 1953; *Quadriput S.A.*, Ther. Ggw., *115*, 1072, 1976. **4.** A. Stoll et. al., *Helvetica Chimica Acta*, 33, 6, 1950. **5.** O. Kuhn, *Arzneimittel Forschung* 2, 467, 1952. **6.** D. Orinda, J. Diederich and A. Wacker, *Arzeneimittel Forschung* 23 (3), 1973. **7.** A. Wacker and W. Hilbig, *Planta Medica*, 33, 89–102, 1978. **8.** H. Wagner and A. Proksch, *Zeitschrift für Agnewande Phytotherapie*, 2(5), 166–8, 171, 1981. **9.** F. J. Reith, *Ger. Offen*, 2, 721,014, November 1978. **10.** D. J. Voaden and M. Jacobsen, *Journal of Medicinal Chemistry* 15 (6), p. 619–23 (1952).

Boneset 1. Benoit et. al., *Lloydia*, 39, 160, 1976. **2.** E. P. Claus, *Pharmacognosy*, 4th Edition, Lea and Febiger, 1961. **3.** M. D. Midge and A. V. Rao, *Indian J. Chem.*, 13, 541, 1975. **4.** K. H. Lee et. al., *Phytochemistry*, 16, 1068, 1977. **5.** E. O. Arene et. al., *Lloydia*, 41, 186, 1978. **6.** Z. Rodrigue et. al., *Phytochemistry*, 15, 1573, 1976, through A. Leung, op. cit.

Elecampane 1. See *Chem. Abstr.*, 87, 162117, 1977. **2.** A. Leung, op. cit. **3.** R. Kiesewette and M. Muller, *Pharmazie*, 13, 777, 1958.

German chamomile 1. Martindale, op. cit. **2.** S. Times Colour Suppl., April 1981. **3.** Martindale. **4.** List P. H. and Norhammer L. Hajer's *Handbuch der Pharmazeutischen Praxis*, Springer-Verlag; through A. Y. Leung, op. cit. **5.** M. Szalontai et. al., *Parfum, Kosmet*, 58, 121, 1977. **6, 8, 9, 10.** S. Times Colour Suppl., April 1981. **7.** Martindale.

Dandelion 1. Martindale. **2.** E. Chabrole et. al., *C.R. Soc. Biol.*, 108, 1100, 1931. **3.** R. Benigni et. al., *Plante medicinali Invernie Della Betta*, 11, 1593, 1964. **4.** E. Popowska et. al., *Acta pol Pharm*, 32, 491, 1975. **5.** See research at university of Tigu-Mures in Romania and that carried out at North East London Polytechnic, 1978 – through Sunday Times Colour Suppl. **6.** Racz-Kotilla et. al., *Planta Medica*, 26, 212, 1974. **7.** F. Fletcher-Hyde, *Mims 2*, 127–136, 1978.

Coltsfoot 1. C. C. J. Culvenor et. al., *Aust. J. Chem.*, 29, 229–30, 1976. **2.** A. Flock et. al., Dept, Pharmacog, Univ. Uppsala, 1978.

CRUCIFERAE

Black mustard 1. K. K. Abdullin, *Zap Dazansk,*

Vet. Inst., 84, 75, 1962; through *Chem. Abstr.*, 60, 11843b, 1964. **2.** I. Slavenas, *Chem. Abstr.*, 58, 8244c, 1963.

CUPRESSACEAE

Thuja 1. S. Mills, *Dictionary of Modern Herbalism*, Thorsons, 1985.

EQUISETACEAE

Horsetail 1. K. Schwatz and D. Milne, *Nature*, 1972, 239, 334. **2.** E. M. Carlisle, *Fed. Proc.*, 1974, 6, 33, 1958. **3.** J. Loeper et. al., *La Presse Medicale*, 74, 17,865, 1966. **4.** J. Loeper et. al., *Atherosclerosis*, 33, 397, 1979. **5.** E. L. Franck Bakke and B. Hillestad, *Medd Nursk Farm. Selsk*, 42, 9, 1980.

ERICACEAE

Bearberry 1. Martindale. **2.** D. Fiohne, *Planta Med.*, 18, 1, 1970.

FUCACEAE

Bladderwrack 1. L. Bezamger-Beauquesne et. al., *Plantes Medicinales des Régions Temperées*, p. 13, Maloine ed. 1980.

FUMARIACEAE

Fumitory 1. Symposium de phytotherapie Lourmarin, June 1981. Proceedings of the college of Phyto-Aromatherapie et de Medicine de Terraine de Langue Francaise. **2.** R. Cahen et. al., *Therapie*, 19, 357, 1964.

GENTIANACEAE

Centaury 1. See *Chem. Abstr.*, 82, 7590u, 1975. **2.** *The Merck Index, An Encyclopedia of Chemicals and Drugs* 9 edn., 1976, Merck, Rahway, N. Jersey. **3.** See *Chem. Abstr.*, 78, 79634b, 1973. **4.** A. Leung, op. cit.

GRAMINEAE

Couch grass 1. Paris and Moyse, op. cit., *11*, p. 13. **2.** P. H. List and L. Horhammer, *Hagers Handbuch der Pharmazeutischen Praxis*, vols 2–5. Springer-Verlag, Berlin, through A. Leung, op. cit.
Corn 1. Bensky, Gamble, op. cit.

HIPPOCASTANACEAE

Horse chestnut 1. P. Delaveau, *Les Plantes Medicinales*, ed. Paris.

HYPERICACEAE

St John's wort 1. O. Gessner, *Diegilt und Arnsnei Planzen von Mittel Europe*, 1974. **2.** Martindale, 26th edn.

LABIATAE

Hyssop 1. A. Leung, op. cit. **2.** E. C. Harrmann and L. S. Kucera, *Proc. Soc. Exp. Biol. Med.*, 124, 874, 1967.

Lavender 1. See *Chem. Abstr.*, 77, 84292x, 1972. **2.** See *Chem. Abstr.*, 81, 58356, 1974.

Motherwort 1. P. Schauenberg and F. Paris, *Guide to Medicinal Plants*, Lutterworth, 1977. **2.** Bensky, Gamble, op. cit.

White horehound 1. List and Norhammer, through A. Leung, op. cit. **2.** See *Chem. Abstr.*, 86, 2355u, 1977. **3.** List and Norhammer through A. Leung, op. cit. **4.** As for 1 and 3.

Lemon balm 1. A. M. Debelmas and J. Rochat, *Pl. med et Phytoth*, 1, 23, 1967. **2.** Howagner et. al., *Planta Medica*, 37, 9, 1979. **3.** H. B. Forster et. al., *Planta Medica*, 40, 4, 309, 1980. **4.** A. M.

Debelmas and J. Rochat, *Plant. Med. Phytother., 1,* 23, 1967. 5. H. Wagner and Sprinkmeyer, *Dtsch, Apoth.-Ztg, 113,* 11159, 1973. 6. L. S. Kucera and E. C. Herrmann, *Proc. Soc. Exp. Biol. Med., 124,* 865, 1967. 7. Herrmann and Kucera, ibid., 869.

Peppermint 1. A. Sanyal and K. C. Varma, *Indian J. Microbiol, 9,* 23, 1969. **2.** Herrmann and Kucera, op. cit., 874. **3.** Martindale, op. cit., 1024. **4.** See *Chem. Abstr., 80,* 19365w, 1974. **5.** See *Chem. Abstr., 62,* 3285c, 1965.

Rosemary 1. A. Boido et al., *Studi Sarsan, Sez. 2, 53,* 383, 1975; through *Chem. Abstr., 88,* 69046d, 1978. **2.** B. G. Rao and S. S. Nigam, *Indian J. Med. Res., 58,* 627, 1970. **3.** As for note 1, above. **4.** A. Leung, op. cit.

Sage 1. See *Chem. Abstr., 86,* 117603r, 1977. **2.** See *Chem. Abstr., 82,* 167491r, 1975. **3.** H. Leclerc, *Précis de Phytotherapie,* p. 90, ed. Masson, Paris. **4.** J. C. Bourret, *Les Nouveaux Succes de la Medicine par les Plantes,* p. 281, ed. Hachette, Paris, 1981.

Thyme 1. See *Chem. Abstr., 86,* 84201c, 1977. **2.** See *Chem. Abstr., 71,* 58264w, 1969.

LAURACEAE
Bay 1. See *Chem. Abstr., 69,* 944k, 1968.

LEGUMINOSAE
Astragalus 1. See also *Medical Tribune Report,* G. Mavglit et al., University of Texas, M. D. Anderson Hospital and Tumour Institute.

Licorice 1. Martindale, op. cit., 26th edn., p. 714. **2.** R. J. Calvert, *Lancet,* i/805, 1954, see also E. J. Ross, *Br. Med. J., ii,* 733, 1970. **3.** A. G. G. Turpie et al., *Gut, 10,* 299, 1969. See also E. Schulze et al., *J. Am. Med. Ass., 155,* 1448, 1954. **4.** M. R. Gibson, *Lloydia, 41,* 4, 348 et. seq., 1978. **5.** C. Van Hulle, *Pharmazie, 25,* 620, 1970.

LILIACEAE
Garlic 1. See E. Block, *The Chemistry of Garlic and Onions, Scientific American,* 1985. **2.** R. C. Jain, *Lancet, 1,* 1240, 1975. See also A. Bordia et al., *Atherosclerosis, 21,* 15, 1975. **3.** Martindale, op. cit., 26th edn.

False unicorn root 1. C. L. Butler and C. H. Costello, *J. Am. Pharm. Assoc., 33,* 177, 1944.

Lily of the valley 1. F. Fletcher Hyde, *Mims, 2,* 127–136, 1978.

Sarsaparilla 1. A. Leung, op. cit. See also Bensky and Gamble, op. cit.

Squill 1. A. Leung, op. cit.

LORANTHACEAE
Mistletoe 1. S. Rosell and G. Samuelsson, *G. Toxicon, 4,* 107, 1966. **2.** P. N. Nguyen-Luong et. al., *Plantes Med et Phyt, 13,* 1, 66, 1979. **3.** *BMJ, 282,* 187, 1981. **4.** F. F. Hyot, *Proceedings of First International Conference on Herbal Medicine JAM.* See also *JAM,* January 1984. **5.** F. Vester et al., *Hoppe-Seyleris Z. Physiol. Chem., 349,* 125, 495, 1968.

MALVACEAE
Marsh mallow 1. P. Delaveau et. al., *Planta Medica, 40,* 49, 1980.

MONIMIACEAE
Boldo 1. J. Levy et. al., *J. Pharm. Belg., 32,* 1, 13, 1977. **2.** H. Schindler, *Arzneim-Forsch, 7,* 747, 1957.

MYRICACEAE
Bayberry 1. B. D. Paul et. al., *J. Pharm. Sci., 63,* 958, 1974.

ONAGRACEAE
Evening primrose 1. M. Brush, *Understanding Premenstrual Tension,* Pan, 1984. **2.** S. Wright and J. Burton, *Lancet,* 20 November 1982. **3.** Judy Graham, *Evening Primrose Oil,* Thorsons, 1984. **4.** E. Glen et. al., Highland Psychiatric Research Group, Craig Dunain Hospital, Inverness. **5.** J. Rotrosen et. al., *Life Science, 26,* 1867–76, 1980. **6.** A. C. Campbell and G. C. MacEwan, *British Journal of Dermatology,* 1984. **7.** A. K. Sim and A. P. McCraw, *Thrombosis Research, 10,* 385–397, 1977.

PAPAVERACEAE
Blood root 1. A. Leung, op. cit.

PAPILIONACEAE
Broom 1. Martindale, 26th edn.

Fenugreek 1. A. Leung, op. cit.

PARMELIACEAE
Iceland moss 1. A. Leung, op. cit.

PASSIFLORACEAE
Passion flower 1. J. Lutomski et. al., *Planta Med., 27,* 112, 1975.

PEDALIACEAE
Devil's claw 1. B. Zom, *Zeitschrift für Rheumaforschung,* 1958. **2.** O. Eichler and E. Koch, *Arzheim, Forsch, 20,* 107, 1970. **3.** Erdos et. al., *Planta Medica, 34,* 97, 1978. **4.** W. Zimmermann, *Deutsch. Apoth. Ztg., 116,* 937, 1976. **5.** P. Belaiche, *Phytotherapy, 21,* 22, 1982. **6.** G. Sens-Olive, *Phytotherapy, 1.*

PLANTAGINACEAE
Plantain 1. L. Bezanger-Beauquesne et. al., *Plantes Medicinales des Régions Temperées,* p. 347, ed. Paris, 1980.

RANUNCULACEAE
Black cohosh 1. E. Genazzi and L. Sorrentino, *Nature, 194,* 544, 1962. **2.** N. R. Farnsworth and A. B. Segelman, *Tile Till, 57,* 52, 1971.

Golden seal 1. K. Genest and D. W. Hughes, *Can. J. Pharm. Sci., 4,* 41, 1969. **2.** V. Preininger, *The Alkaloids,* vol. 15, Academic Press, N.Y., 1975.

ROSACEAE
Agrimony 1. Bensky, Gamble, op. cit.

Hawthorn 1. H. P. T. Ammon and M. Handel, *Planta Medica, 3,* 3,209, 1981. **2.** T. Beisin et. al., *Arzneim Forsch, 5,* 490, 1955. **3.** R. R. Paris and H. Moyse, op. cit., *11,* p. 4111.

Meadowsweet 1. F. Decaux *F. Rev. Phyto therap, 6,* 125, 1942.

RUTACEAE
Rue 1. D. L. J. Opdyke, *Food Cosmet. Toxicol., 13,* 455, 1976.

Prickly ash 1. J. Phillipson and L. Anderson, *Pharmaceutical Journal,* July 28 1984. **2.** J. L. Hartwell, *Lloydia, 34,* 103, 1971.

SOLANACEAE
Chillies 1. See *Chem. Abstr., 78,* 80226b, 1973.

Thornapple 1. Martindale, 26th edn.

TILIACEAE
Lime 1. R. Cahen and S. C. R. Aubron, *Soc. Biol., 155,* 1218, 1961. **2.** I. S. Beaulaton and J. Tanbouriech, *J. Soc. Pharm. Montpellier, 20,* 3, 197, 1960.

TROPAEOLACEAE
Nasturtium 1. P. Schauenberg and F. Paris, *Guide to Medicinal Plants,* Lutterworth, 1977.

TURNERACEAE
Damiana 1. E. F. Steinmetz, *Acta Phytother., 7,* 1, 1960.

UMBELLIFERAE
Angelica 1. R. F. Weiss, *Lehbuch der Phytotherapie,* 62, Hippocrates verlag Ed. Stuttgart, 1980. **2.** D. L. J. Opdyke, *Food Cosmet. Toxicol, 13 (suppl.),* 713, 1975. **3.** H. Wagner et. al., *Planta Medica, 37,* 9, 1979.

Wild carrot 1. A. Leung, op. cit.

Fennel 1. H. Wagner et. al., op. cit., 37, 9, 1979. **2.** F. M. Ramadan et. al., *Chem. Microbiol. Technol. Lebensm., 2,* 51, 1972. **3.** R. R. Paris and H. Moyse, op. cit., *II,* 474.

Lovage 1. List and Norhammer, through A. Y. Leung, op. cit.

Parsley 1. A. Y. Leung, op. cit.

Anise 1. A. Y. Leung, op. cit.

URTICACEAE
Nettle 1. R. F. Weiss, op. cit., 296. **2.** R. K. Alier and I. A. Damirov, *Chem. Zentialbl.,* 4437, 1961.

VALERIANACEAE
Valerian 1. H. Hendriks et. al., *Planta Medica, 45,* 150, 1982. **2.** K. W. Von Eickstedt and S. Rahman. **3.** E. Cionga, *Pharmazie, 16,* 43, 1961. **4.** A. Y. Leung, op. cit. **5.** R. R. Paris and H. Moyse, op. cit., *III,* 386, 1971. **6.** E. Skramlik, *Pharmazie, 14,* 435, 1959.

VERBENACEAE
Vervain 1. Otto Gessner, *Diegilt und Planzen von Mitteleuropa,* 1974.

Chaste tree 1. H. W. Kayser and S. Istanbulluoglu, *Hippokrates, 25,* 717, 1954. **2.** V. Probst and D. A. Roth, *Deutsch Med. Wschr,* 1943, 204. **3.** H. Mohr, *Deutsch Med. Wschr, 79,* 1513, 1954. **4.** H. Attelmann et. al., *Geriatrie, 2,* 239, 1972. **5.** W. Amann, *Selecta, XIX,* 3688, 1977.

VIOLACEAE
Wild pansy 1. A. Y. Leung, op. cit.

ZINGIBERACEAE
Ginger 1. H. Walker, Vermont University, reported in *Yorkshire Ev. Press,* 27 May 1985.

Index

Acknowledgments

Text

Introduction and feature spreads	Richard Mabey
Glossary of Herbs	Michael McIntyre (additional entries Gaia)
Herbs for Natural Living	Pamela Michael (additional material Gaia)
Herbs for Nutrition	Gail Duff (addtional recipes Sara Mathews)
Herbs for Healing	Michael McIntyre
Herb Gardening	John Stevens

Gaia would like to extend particular thanks to the following:

Olive Ashmore, for the germ of an idea; Rosanne Hooper, Libby Hoseason, and Susan McKeever, for additional editorial work; Margaret Sadler for design assistance; Juliet Bailey for botanical advice and checking; Helen Banbury for editorial assistance; Lesley Gilbert for copy preparation; Cathy Gill for compiling the index; Caroline Stevens for tirelessly answering queries, providing live plants for photography, and giving advice on herb cultivation; David Philipson for pharmacological advice; Dr John Allfree for his patient reading of the glossary and healing sections; Sara Mathews for providing recipes and advice on culinary matters; Elizabeth Fenwick for advice on medical and physiological matters; Harry Dagnall of Baldwins for cheerfully and efficiently supplying dried herbs for photography; Caroline Ungode Thomas, Duncan Donald of Chelsea Physic Garden, and the University Botanic Gardens Cambridge, for supplying live plants; Steve Davis and Professor Heywood of the IUCN Conservation Monitoring Centre, Kew, for advice; the staff of the library, Kew; John Hancock of the British Herb Trade Association and Farmers' Weekly magazine, for information on herb farming; the Soil Association and the Biodynamic Agricultural Association, for advice on organic growing; the Lancet, New Scientist, and Efamol Ltd., for articles and statistics; the Nature Conservancy Council, UK, and the Garden Club of America for conservation information; and Odyssey Books for research resources.

Additional illustrations by Andrew MacDonald (pp. 18–19, 136–7, 174–5, 190–1, 256–7) and Anne Savage (pp. 134–5, 246–7, 262–3, 272).

The authors would like to give special thanks to Keith Loudoun-Shand and Arthur Shwartz for providing spices from Malawi; to Frances Mount, Cees and Hedy Stapel-Valk, Mr King of the University Botanic Garden, Cambridge, Patrick Hughes, Mrs Minns, Mrs Rowling, Susan Cutmore, and Duncan Ross of Poyntzfield Herb Nursery for giving or loaning plant material for photography; to Caroline Stevens for her research and co-ordination of the plant material used for photography and for the long hours she spent proof-reading. All the photographic spreads except one were taken in a special studio set-up at Sawyers Farm. Special thanks and admiration are due to Kate Poole and Philip Dowell for long hours in cramped conditions coaxing often uncooperative plant material into glorious colour spreads.

Photographic credits

Planet Earth Pictures: pp. 10–11 and 186–7 (Georgette Douwma), pp. 136–7 (Peter Stevenson), pp. 138–9 (Geoff du Feu). Heather Angel: pp. 18–19, 26–7, 190–1, 256–7. South American Pictures: pp. 136–7 (Tony Morrison, Bill Leimbach), 256–7. Bruce Coleman: pp. 6–7 (Peter Davey), 130–1 (John Shaw), 154–5 (N. French, L. Lee Rue). Ardea London: pp. 154–5 (A. P. Paterson, John Mason), pp. 162–3 (Bob Gibbons). A-Z Botanical Collection: pp. 242–3. Tropix Photographic Library: pp. 190–1 (John Schmid). Tony Stone Worldwide: p. 15 (Hans P. Merten)